The Physiology of Physical Stress

A Selective Bibliography, 1500-1964

The Physiology of Physical Stress

A Selective Bibliography, 1500-1964

Carleton B. Chapman and Elinor C. Reinmiller

Harvard University Press, Cambridge, Massachusetts, 1975

Preface

Thousands of physiological studies involving physical exercise have been carried out in the last several hundred years and, at present, the number and complexity of such studies that appear annually is increasing prodigiously. The reason is not far to seek. In the mammalian organism, physical activity may be viewed as the means by which the organism recovers from previous inactivity and prepares for the next episode of physical stress. Physiological data obtained during the resting state are in themselves incomplete and serve mainly as control information with which data obtained during and after physical stress can be compared. The value of physical conditioning, and the damage wrought by prolonged inactivity, are finally beginning to be understood in objective physiological terms.

Because of these and other considerations, and as technological barriers to studies on human subjects (especially during physical stress) are in the process of being overcome, the literature on physical stress has become so vast that detailed access to it has become increasingly difficult.

In the course of working on the physiology of physical stress over some two decades, one of us (C.B.C.) began a card file of pertinent references which, by the early sixties, had become fairly extensive. When the MEDLARS plan of the National Library of Medicine was constructed, it was realized that this system would not, for a long time to come, provide references published before 1962 or thereabouts. For this reason, the decision was made to expand the collection of references with special emphasis on basic nineteenth and early twentieth century literature and to make them available as an organized bibliography. During 1963 and 1964, a methodical search was made in libraries in the United States, Britain, and Sweden in order to identify and verify references to basic physiologic work on physical stress. Books, review articles, original articles, standard indexes, and (in some instances) long runs of scientific journals were searched. The emphasis throughout was on basic articles in their original locus and format. But (especially in the nineteen forties and fifties) extensions were made into clinical areas that had basic implications. The intent was to find sources of concepts and basic techniques, plus later articles that expanded concepts or resulted in significant modifications of techniques. We excluded, however, most items that had to do solely with the techniques of sports. Also, there is a vast and largely inconsequential literature on the effects of exercise on the electrocardiogram. Of these, we included only a few key entries.

It is hardly surprising that a great deal of classical physiology of the eighteenth, nineteenth, and early twentieth centuries is included, since most of it bears directly or tangentially on physical stress in man

v

or animal. For example, Lavoisier's work in the late eighteenth century focused on mammalian respiration but used physical stress as an investigative tool. So did Regnault and Reiset (1849). So also did E. A. Scharling in 1843; all of which preceded the very elegant and largely unsung work of the English physiologist Edward Smith, done in the 1850's. It was in some measure on these foundations that most of the great late nineteenth and early twentieth century physiologists built their work on circulatory and respiratory function.

It is hoped, therefore, that the bibliography may be of use to those interested in the emergence of physiology as a basic medical science, as well as to stress physiologists. But very few who have worked at construction of special bibliographies are rash enough to claim that their final effort includes all relevant references. We have been at considerable pains to make our listing as complete as possible within the framework of the original intent; but we dare make no more sweeping claim.

In Part One, the Author Index, individual references are listed alphabetically by author, and the individual entries are as complete as we were able to make them. Abbreviations of titles of journals have been modified (and usually extended) for purposes of clarity.

Titles of articles have, for the most part, been left in the original language but English translations are supplied in instances where the original language is one not usually known to Western investigators. Thus, titles in the Romance languages and German are untranslated; those in Slavic, Scandinavian, and Oriental languages are. In some instances, the only title available to us was the English translation, and in such cases, titles appear in brackets.

Where possible, we have consulted the original article in order to verify the author's name and location, titles, pagination, and content.

In Part Two, the Subject Index, we have tried as much as possible to use headings that are familiar to those working in the field. Usage is often inconsistent and unsystematic, a fact that is reflected in the structure of the Subject Index. Rigid adherance to a system of headings, which was tried at first, appeared to impair the usefulness of the bibliography. The final result is a compromise, far more pragmatic than systematic.

Librarians in five countries have uncomplainingly lent a hand in locating and verifying individual references, and are too numerous to be listed. The National Library of Medicine supplied the services of MEDLARS which, in turn, printed out several hundred references for 1963 and 1964 (heading: Exertion). About one-fourth were unsuitable, and a few relevant titles were missing. Even so, the potential for automated retrieval was amply demonstrated, and the services of the staff at the National Library of Medicine are gratefully acknowledged.

The initial Subject Index was prepared by Mrs. Doreen Blake of Addlestone near Weybridge, England. Suggestions for revision came from bibliographers and colleagues in many parts of the United States and Britain, especially from Dr. Jere Mitchell and staff, Dr. Arthur Grollman, and Dr. Ivan Danhoff.

The enormous chore of checking references, and the labor of putting the work in its present form, were done by Brigitta Payne and Patricia Wells, and the library staff at the University of Texas Health Science Center, Dallas.

Finally, some of the work (1964) was carried out during the tenure of a Guggenheim fellowship (C.B.C.) and final preparation of the alphabetical listing and subject index was made possible by a small grant-in-aid from the Commonwealth Fund (1972).

Carleton B. Chapman
Elinor C. Reinmiller

Contents

Part One   Author Index

Abarquez, Ramon F., Jr.; Kintar, Quintin, L.; Valdez, Ernesto V.; and Dayrit, Conrado: Evaluation of some criteria for the dynamic and postexercise electrocardiogram in diagnosing coronary insufficiency. Amer. J. Cardiol. 13:310-319, Mar., 1954. (Manila)

Abbott, B. C.; and Bigland, Brenda: The effects of force and speed changes on the rate of oxygen consumption during negative work. J. Physiol. 120:319-325, May 28, 1953. (London)

----, ----, and Ritchie, J. M.: The physiological cost of negative work. J. Physiol. 117:380-390, July 29, 1952. (London)

----, and Lowy, J.: Contraction in molluscan smooth muscle. J. Physiol. 141:385-397, May 28, 1958. (Plymouth and London)

Abelin, T.; and Scherrer, M.: Ventilation und Säurebasen haushalt des Gesunden bei schwerer Arbeit. Untersuchungen am Metabographen von Fleisch mit fortlaufender arterieller Blutgasanalyse. Schweiz. med. Wschr. 90:369-374, Mar. 26, 1960. (Bern)

Abramova, N. D.; Goldberg, A. F.; Gurevich, T. Z.; et al: Iskhod infarkta miokarda i trudosposobnost' posie nego u lits umstvennogo truda srednego i pozhilogo vozrasta. (The outcome of myocardial infarct and work capacity thereafter in middle-aged and elderly persons engaged in metal work) (Russ). Sovet. Med. 26:22-26, May, 1963.

Abramson, David, I.; and Fierst, Sidney, M.: Peripheral vascular response in hyperthyroid state. J. Clin. Invest. 20:517-519, Sept., 1941. (Cincinnati)

----, ----, and Flacks, K.: Effect of muscular exercise upon peripheral circulation in patients with valvular heart disease. J. Clin. Invest. 21:747-750, Nov., 1942.

----, Tuck, Samuel, Jr.; Bell, Yvonne; Burnett, Carolyn; and Rejal, Habib: Relationship between a range of tissue temperature and local oxygen uptake in the human forearm. III. Changes observed after anaerobic work, in the postexercise period. J. Clin. Invest. 38: 1126-1133, July, 1959. (Chicago)

Abramson, Ernst: Energieumsatz bei Muskelarbeit. Arbeitsphysiol. 1:480-502, 1929. (Stockholm)

----: Der Energieumsatz bei Muskelarbeit. IV. Die Wirkungsgrad. Arbeitsphysiol. 2:85-96, 1930. (Stockholm)

Acker, J. E., Jr.: Work and the heart. J. Tenn. Med. Ass. 56:46-48, Feb., 1963. (Knoxville, Tenn.)

Adam, A.: Über den Einfluss des Fiebers auf den Phosphorsaurehaushalt des Muskels. Hoppe-Seyler Zeits. physiol. Chem. 113:281-300, Apr. 5, 1921. (Frankfurt)

Adams, Thomas; Funkhouser, Gordon E.; and Kendall, Warren W.: Measurement of evaporative water loss by a thermal conductivity cell. J. Appl. Physiol. 18:1291-1293, Nov., 1963. (Oklahoma City and Norman)

Adler, E. L.: Relation between blood pressure and physical exertion. Med. Press 205: 181-183, Feb. 26, 1941. (London)

Adler, Erich: Einfluss der Aussentemperatur auf den Lactacidogengehalt des Frosches. Hoppe-Seyler Zeits. physiol. Chem. 113:174-186, Mar. 30, 1921. (Frankfurt)

----: Über den Einfluss der Jahreszeit auf den Lactacidogengehalt des Froschmuskels (Rana esculenta und Rana temporaxia). Hoppe-Seyler Zeits. physiol. Chem. 113:193-200, Apr. 5, 1921. (Frankfurt)

----, and Günzburg, L.: Einfluss der Aussentemperatur auf den Lactacidogengehalt des Froschmuskels. II. Hoppe-Seyler Zeits. physiol. Chem. 113:187-192, Apr. 5, 1921. (Frankfurt)

----, and Isaac, S.: Über den Einfluss der Phosphorvergiftung auf den Lactacidogengehalt des Froschmuskels. Hoppe-Seyler Zeits. physiol. Chem. 113:271-280, Apr. 5, 1921. (Frankfurt)

Adrower, Giulio: Tromboflebite della vena ascellare da sforzo. Minerva Med. 54:2243-2245, Aug. 4, 1963.

Afar, J. M.; and Rogozkin, V. A.: Influence of ingested casein hydrolyzate on the high energy nucleotide content of working muscle. Canad. J. Biochem. Physiol. 41: 1531-1536, July, 1963. (Sofia and Leningrad)

Agadzhanian, N. A.; Bizin, U. P.; Doronin, G. P.; et al: Izmenenie vysshei nervanoi deiatel'nosti i nekotorykh vegetativnykh reaktsii pri dlitel'nom prebyvanii v usloniiakh otnositel'noi adinamii i izoliatsil. (Changes in higher nervous activity and some autonomic reactions in a long stay in conditions of relative adynamia and isolation) (Russ). Zh. Vyssh. Nerv. Deiat. Pavlov 13:953-962, Nov.-Dec., 1963.

Aghemo, P.; Gsell, D.; and Mangili, F.: The relation of work performance to heart rate in aged men. Gerontologia 9:91-97, 1964.

Agostini, E.; Taglietta, A.; and Agostini, A. Ferrario: Composizione dell'aria alveolare a spazio morto respiratorio a diversi livelli metabolia. Boll. Soc. Ital. Biol. Sper. 34: 674-676, July 15, 1958.

Ahlman, K.; and Karvonen, M. J.; Stimulation of sweating by exercise after heat induced "fatigue" of the sweating mechanism. Acta Physiol. Scand. 53:381-386, Nov.-Dec., 1961. (Helsinki)

Äikäs, E.; Karvonen, M. J.; Piironen, P.; and Ruosteenoja, R.: Intramuscular, rectal and oesophageal temperature during exercise. Acta Physiol. Scand. 54:366-370, Mar.-Apr., 1962. (Helsinki)

Akerblom, H.; and Maijala, L.: Acetone bodies in the blood of diabetic children after exercise. Preliminary report. Ann. Paediat. Fenn. 10:36-41, 1964.

Akzhigton, G. N.: Vliianie fizicheskoi nagruzki na kronoobrashchenie. (Effect of physical exercise on blood circulation) (Russ). Ter. Arkh. 36:90-97, Mar., 1964.

Albanes, Alfonso R.: Acute thrombosis of the anterior tibial artery. Angiology 9:172-175, June, 1958. (Buenos Aires)

Albeaux-Fernet, M.; and Romani, J. D.: Les pertubations endocrino-métaboliques observées
au cours d'efforts importants. Agressologie 1:155-162, Apr., 1960. (Paris)

----, ----: Les perturbations endocrino-métaboliques observéees au cours d'efforts importants
chez l'homme. Bull. Acad. Nat. Med. 144:96-102, Feb. 2, 1960. (Paris)

Albrecht, H.; Valentin, H.; and Venrath, H.: Über die Atmung und das Herzminutenvolumen
bei Arbeit und Sport, sowie die Herzleistung. Zeits. ges. exp. Med. 122:356-368, Dec.
17, 1953. (Köln)

Aleksandrow, D.; Klopstowski, T.; and Smietańsk, Z.: Effect of physical activity upon
cholesterol synthesis in the rat liver. J. Atheroscler. Res. 4:351-355, July-Aug.,
1964. (Warsaw)

Alexander, James K.: Obesity and cardiac performance. Amer. J. Cardiol. 14:860-865,
Dec., 1964. (Houston)

Allbutt, Sir Thomas Clifford: The effect of exercise on the bodily temperature. J. Anat.
Physiol. 7:106-119, Nov., 1873. (London)

Allébé, G. A. N.: Over beweging en rust. Schat d. Gezondh. (Haarlem) 3:225;257, 1860.

Allen, Nathan: Physical culture, and its influence on the body. J. Psych. Med. (London),
new series 2:156-160, 1876.

Allen, Scott; and Conn, Harold O.: Observations on the effect of exercise on blood ammonia
concentration in man. Yale J. Biol. Med. 33:133-144, Oct., 1960. (New Haven)

Allen, T. H.; Krzywicki, H. J.; and Isaac, G. H.: Energy requirements and physical
achievements according to body composition of young soldiers offered food to satiety.
U.S. Army Med. Res. Nutr. Lab. Rep. 243:1-30, Feb. 18, 1960.

Allen, William; and Pepys, William Hasledine: On respiration. Phil. Trans. Roy. Soc.
99:404-429, 1809.

Alov, I. A.; and Abramson, E. N.: Mitotic activity during muscular exertion. Biull.
Eksp. Biol. Med. 51:710-714, Nov., 1961.

Altilla, F.; Borgatti, E.; Pascucci, E.; et al: Sui rapporti tra portata ematica e sforzo
fisico nell'avambraccio. Boll. Soc. Ital. Cardiol. 8:490-493, 1963.

Altland, Paul D.; and Highman, Benjamin: Effects of exercise on serum enzyme values
and tissues of rats. Amer. J. Physiol. 201:393-395, Aug., 1961. (Bethesda)

----- ----, and Garbus, Joel: Exercise training and altitude tolerance in rats: blood,
tissue, enzyme and isoenzyme changes. Aerospace Med. 35:1034-1039, Nov.,
1964. (Bethesda)

Altman, Joseph: Differences in the utilization of tritiated leucine by single neurones in
normal and exercised rats: an autoradiographic investigation with microdensitometry.
Nature 199:777-780, Aug. 24, 1963. (Cambridge, Mass.)

Alwall, Nils: Studien über die Einwirkung von Benzedin und Pervitin auf die physische und psychische Leistungs-fähigkeit hochgradig ermüdeter Menschen. Acta Med. Scand. 114:33-58, Apr. 29, 1943. (Lund)

Alyea, Edwin P.; and Boone, Alex W.: Urinary findings resulting from nontraumatic exercise. Southern Med. J. 50:905-910, July, 1957. (Durham)

Amels, E.: Geschichtlicher Ueberblick über die Physiologie der Atmung bis zum Anfange des 19. Jahrhunderts. Leipzig, 1903.

Anastasi, Gaspar W.; Wertheimer, Haskell M.; and Brown, James R.: Popliteal aneurysm with osteochondroma of the femur. Arch. Surg. 87:636-639, Oct., 1963. (St. Albans, New York)

Anders, M.; Nieschke, W.; Dahm, H., and Taugner, R.: Vergleichende pharmakologische Untersuchungen am ermüdeten bzw, anoxämischen und normalen Skeletmuskel. Naunyn Schmiedberg Arch. exp. Path. 217:406-412, Mar. 23, 1953. (Heidelberg)

Andersen, K. Lange: (Aerobic working capacity) (Nor.). T. Norsk. Laegeforen. 80: 1087-1091, Nov. 15, 1960.

----: Kondisjonsundersøkelser av idrettsmenn. Nord. Med. 54:1246-1248, Aug. 11, 1955.

----: Leucocyte response to brief, severe exercise. J. Appl. Physiol. 7:671-674, May, 1955. (Urbana)

----: Measurement of work capacity. J. Sport Med. 4:236-240, Dec., 1964.

----: Respiratory recovery from muscular exercise of short duration: a functional study of healthy adults in relation to age, sex, and physical activity. Oslo, Oslo University Press, 1959. (Oslo)

----; Bolstad, Atle;and Sand, S.: The blood lactate during recovery from sprint runs. Acta Physiol. Scand. 48:231-237, Mar. 18, 1960. (Oslo)

----; and Bugge-Asperheim, B.: Reduction of CO_2 stores of man due to muscular exercise. Acta Physiol. Scand. 47:91-96, Sept. 30, 1959.

----; and Hart, J. S.: Aerobic working capacity of Eskimos. J. Appl. Physiol. 18:764-768, July, 1963. (Oslo and Ottowa)

Anderson, Albert D.: The use of the heart rate as a monitoring device in an ambulation program: a progress report. Arch. Phys. Med. 45:140-146, Mar., 1964. (New York)

Anderson, R. J.; and Lusk, G.: The interrelation between diet and body condition and the energy production during mechanical work in the dog. Proc. Nat. Acad. Sci. 3:386-389, 1917.

Anderson, W. G.: Studies in the effects of physical training. Amer. Phys. Educat. Rev. 4:265-278, 1899.

Andrieu: Ventilation et échange gazeux pulmonaires au cours de l'exercice musculaire prolongé. Montpellier, Mari-Lavit, 1937.

Angelino, P. F.; Dulbecco, A.; and Gallo, C.: Attivita fisica à fibrinolisi. Minerva Med. 55: 2111-2113, July 4, 1964.

Anstie, Francis E.: Note on the relations of muscular exercise to urea and food. Practitioner 5:353-357, Dec., 1870. (London)

Apthorp, G. H.; Chamberlain, D. A.; and Hayward, G. W.: The effects of sympathectomy on the electrocardiogram and effort tolerance in angina pectoris. Brit. Heart J. 26: 218-226, Mar., 1964.

Aramendía, P.; Fermoso, J. D.; Barrios, A.; and Taquini, A. C.: Response of the pulmonary circulation to infusion of norepinephrine and isoproterenol. Acta Physiol. Lat. Amer. 13:20-25, 1963. (Buenos Aires)

Arborelius, M.; and Liljestrand, G.: Muskelarbeit und Blutreaktion. Skand. Arch. Physiol. 44:215, 1923.

Arenander, Eric; and Carlsten, Arne: Physical work capacity in patients with varicose veins. Acta. Chir. Scand. 122:520-525, Dec., 1961. (Göteborg)

Areno, W.: Os exercicios fisicos no periodo catamenial. Hospital 25:289-293, Feb., 1944.

Aresu, G.: I mutamenti del tratto finale dell'elettrocardiogramma durante e dopo il lavoro muscolare nell'uomo. Rapporti fra entità del consumo di ossigeno e detti mutamenti elettrocardiografici. Rass. Med. Sarda 63:125-146, Mar.-Apr., 1961.

Arienzo, F.; and Russo, E.: (Influence of digoxin on the changes in guinea pigs caused by the effort of swimming) (It). Gior. Med. Milit. 110:575-587, Nov.-Dec., 1960.

Armstrong, Bruce W.; Hurt, Holcombe, H.; Blide, Richard W.; and Workman, John M.: The humoral regulation of breathing. A concept based on the physicochemical composition of mixed venous and arterial blood. Science 133:1897-1906, June 16, 1961.

Arnett, John H.; and Gardner, Kenneth D., Jr.: Urinary abnormalities from over-use of muscles. Amer. J. Med. Sci. 241:55-58, Jan., 1961. (Philadelphia)

Aronson, Elliot: Effort, attractiveness, and the anticipation of reward: a reply to Lott's critique. J. Abnorm. Soc. Psychol. 67:522-526, Nov., 1963. (Minneapolis)

Arturson, G.; and Kjellmer, Ingemar: Capillary permeability in skeletal muscle during rest and activity. Acta Physiol. Scand. 62:41-45, Sept.-Oct., 1964. (Uppsala and Göteborg)

Asahina, Kazuo; Itahara, Fujiko; Yamanara, Miyoko; and Akiba, Toshiko: Influence of excessive exercise on the structure and function of rat organs. Jap. J. Physiol. 9: 322-326, Sept. 15, 1959. (Tokyo)

Asdell, S. A.; Doornenbal, H.; and Sperling, G.A.: Sex steroid hormones and voluntary exercise in rats. J. Reprod. Fertil. 3:26-32, February, 1962. (Ithaca)

----; and Sperling, G. A.: Sex steroid hormones and voluntary exercise in rats. A correction. J. Reprod. Fertil. 5:123-124, Feb., 1963. (Ithaca)

Asher, L.: Beträge zur Physiologie der Drüsen. XVII. Die innere Sekretion der Nebenniere und deren Innervation. Zeits. Biol. 58:274-304, 1912.

Asher, L.: Einfluss der Bewegung auf Nervensystem. Trans. XV Internat. Congr. Hyg. and
   Demog. Washington, 1912. 2:640-646, 1913.

Ashkar, Edmundo; and Hamilton, William F.: Cardiovascular response to graded exercise in
   the sympathectomized-vagotomized dog. Amer. J. Physiol. 204:291-296, Feb., 1963.
   (Augusta)

Ashmarin, B. A.: Do stsinky rezal'tativ doslidshennia na kinematometri Zhukovs'kogo.
   (On evaluation of the results of examination on a Zhukovs'kil cinematometer) (Uk).
   Fiziol. Zh. 9:479-484, Aug.-Sept., 1963.

Asmussen, Erling: Aerobic recovery after anaerobiosis in rest and work. Acta Physiol. Scand.
   11:197-210, Apr. 27, 1946. (Copenhagen)

----: Observations on experimental muscular soreness. Acta Rheumat. Scand. 2:109-116,
   1956. (Copenhagen)

----, and Bøje, Ove: Body temperature and capacity for work. Acta Physiol. Scand. 10:1-22,
   Aug. 2, 1945. (Copenhagen)

----, and Christensen, E. Hohwü: Einfluss der Blutverurteilung auf den Kreislauf bei körperlicher
   Arbeit. Scand. Arch. Physiol. 82:185-192, 1939. (Copenhagen)

----, ----, and Nielsen, Marius: Humoral or nervous control of respiration during muscular work?
   Acta Physiol. Scand. 6:160-167, 1943.

----, ----, and ----: Die O_2-Aufnahme der ruhenden und der arbeitenden Skelettmuskeln. Scand.
   Arch. Physiol. 82:212-220, 1939.

----, ----, and ----: Pulsfrequenz und Körperstellung. Scand. Arch. Physiol. 81:190-203, 1939.
   (Copenhagen)

----, and Consolazio, Frank C.: The circulation in rest and work on Mount Evans (4,300 m.).
   Amer. J. Physiol. 132:555-563, Mar., 1941. (Boston)

----, Hemmingsen, I.: Determination of maximum working capacity at different ages in work
   with the legs or with the arms. Scand. J. Clin. Lab. Invest. 10:67-71, 1958. (Copenhagen)

----, and Nielsen, Marius: Cardiac output during muscular work and its regulation. Physiol. Rev.
   35:778-800, Oct., 1955. (Copenhagen)

----, and ----: The cardiac output in exercise. Ann. Vol. Physiol. Exp. Med. Sci. India 2:21-26,
   1958-1959. (Copenhagen)

----, and ----: The cardiac output in rest and work determined simultaneously by the acetylene
   and the dye injection methods. Acta Physiol. Scand. 27:217-230, Jan. 25, 1953. (Copenhagen)

----, and ----: The effect of auto-transfusion of "work-blood" on the pulmonary ventilation. Acta
   Physiol. Scand. 20:79-87, Feb. 20, 1950. (Copenhagen)

----, and ----: Experiments on nervous factors controlling respiration and circulation during exercise
   employing blocking of the blood flow. Acta Physiol. Scand. 60:103-111, Jan.-Feb., 1964.
   (Copenhagen)

Asmussen, Erling; and Nielsen, Marius: Measurement of arterial pO_2 in light and heavy exercise. Acta Physiol. Scand. 42 (suppl. 145):17, 1957. (Copenhagen)

----, and ----: Studies on the initial changes in respiration at the transition from rest to work and from work to rest. Acta Physiol. Scand. 16:270-285, Dec. 29, 1948.

----, and ----: Studies on the regulation of respiration in heavy work. Acta Physiol. Scand. 12: 171-188, Nov. 26, 1946. (Copenhagen)

----, and ----: Physiological dead space and alveolar gas pressures at rest and during muscular exercise. Acta Physiol. Scand. 38:1-21, Dec. 29, 1956. (Copenhagen)

----, and ----: Pulmonary ventilation and effect of oxygen breathing in heavy exercise. Acta Physiol. Scand. 43:365-378, Oct. 8, 1958. (Copenhagen)

----, and ----: Ventilatory response to CO_2 during work at normal and at low oxygen tensions. Acta Physiol. Scand. 39:27-35, Apr. 10, 1957. (Copenhagen)

----, ----, and Wieth-Pedersen, G.: Cortical or reflex control of respiration during muscular work. Acta Physiol. Scand. 6:168-175, 1943.

Åstrand, Irma: Aerobic work capacity in men and women with special reference to age. Acta Physiol. Scand. 49 (Suppl. 169):1-92, 1960. (Stockholm)

----: Clinical and physiological studies of manual workers 50-64 years old at rest and during work. Acta Med. Scand. 162:155-164, 1958. (Stockholm)

----: Exercise electrocardiograms in a 5-year follow-up study. Acta Med. Scand. 173:257-268, Mar., 1963. (Stockholm)

----: Lactate content in sweat. Acta Physiol. Scand. 58:359-367, Aug., 1963. (Stockholm)

----: The physical work capacity of workers 50-64 years old. Acta Physiol. Scand. 42:73-87, Feb. 10, 1958. (Stockholm)

----, Åstrand, Per-Olof; Christensen, Erik Höhwu; and Hedman, Rune: Circulatory and respiratory adaptation to serve muscular work. Acta Physiol. Scand. 50:254-258, Dec. 30, 1960. (Stockholm)

----, ----, ----, and ----: Intermittent muscular work. Acta Physiol. Scand. 48:448-453, Apr. 25, 1960. (Stockholm)

----, ----, ----, and ----: Myohemoglobin as an oxygen store in man. Acta Physiol. Scand. 48:454-460, Apr. 25, 1960. (Stockholm)

----, ----, and Stunkard, Albert: Oxygen intake of obese individuals during work on a bicycle ergometer. Acta Physiol. Scand. 50:294-299, Dec. 30, 1960. (Stockholm)

----, Cuddy, T. Edward; Landgren, Johan; Malmborg, Robert O.; and Saltin, Bengt: Hemodynamic response to exercise during atrial flutter and sinus rhythm. Acta Med. Scand. 173:121-127, Jan., 1963. (Stockholm)

Åstrand, Irma, and Hedman, Rune: Muscular strength and aerobic capacity in men 50-64 years old. Int. Zeits. angew. Physiol. 19:425-429, Feb. 7, 1963. (Stockholm)

Åstrand, Per-Olof: Breath holding during and after muscular exercise. J. Appl. Physiol. 15: 220-224, Mar., 1960. (Stockholm)

----: Experimental studies of physical working capacity in relation to sex and age. Copenhagen, Ejnar Munksgaard, 1952. (Stockholm)

----: Human physical fitness with special reference to sex and age. Physiol. Rev. 36:307-335, July, 1956. (Stockholm)

----: New records in human power. Nature 176:922-923, Nov. 12, 1955. (Stockholm)

----: The respiratory activity in man exposed to prolonged hypoxia. Acta Physiol. Scand. 30: 343-368, May 13, 1954. (Stockholm)

----, Cuddy, T. Edward; Saltin, Bengt; and Sternberg, Jesper: Cardiac output during submaximal and maximal work. J. Appl. Physiol. 19:268-274, Mar., 1964. (Stockholm)

----, and Ryhming, Irma: A nomogram for calculation of aerobic capacity (physical fitness) from pulse rate during submaximal work. J. Appl. Physiol. 7:218-221, Sept., 1954. (Stockholm)

----, and Saltin, Bengt: Maximal oxygen uptake and heart rate in various types of muscular activity. J. Appl. Physiol. 16:977-981, Nov., 1961. (Stockholm)

----, and ----: Oxygen uptake during the first minutes of heavy muscular exercise. J. Appl. Physiol. 16:971-976, 1961. (Stockholm)

----, and ----: Plasma and red cell volume after prolonged severe exercise. J. Appl. Physiol. 19:829-832, Sept., 1964. (Stockholm)

Astrup, Christian; and Gantt, W. Horsley: Effects of muscular exertion and verbal stimuli on heart rate and blood pressure in the human. Recent Advances Biol. Psychiat. 4:39-42, 1961. (Baltimore)

Atkins, A. R.; and Nicholson, J. D.: An acute constant-workrate ergometer. J. Appl. Physiol. 18:205-208, Jan., 1963. (Johannesburg)

Atwater, W. O.; and Benedict, F. G.: Experiments on the metabolism of matter and energy in the human body. U. S. Dept. Agriculture, Bull. no. 136, 1903.

Atzler, E. and Meyer, Fritz: Schwerarbeit des Alkoholgewohnten unter dem Einfluss des Alkohols. Arbeitsphysiol. 4:410-432, 1931. (Dortmund-Münster)

Aubert, X.: Expériences sur le mécanisme de l'effort. Lyon Med. 5:383-391, July 17, 1890.

----: L' intervention musculaire dans les phénomènes de fatigue. Acta Belg. Arte Med. Pharm. Milit. 110 (part 2):513-520, Dec., 1957.

Auchincloss, J. Howland, Jr.; Sipple, John; and Gilbert, Robert: Effect of obesity on ventilatory adjustment to exercise. J. Appl. Physiol. 18:19-24, Jan., 1963. (Syracuse)

Aull, J. C.; and McCord, William M.: Effects of posture and activity on the major fractions of serum protein as determined by the phosphate turbidity method. Amer. J. Clin. Path. 27:52-55, Jan., 1957. (Charleston)

Aulo, T. A.: Weiteres über die Ursache der Herzbeschleunigung bei der Muskelarbeit. Skand. Arch. Physiol. 25:347-360, 1911. (Helsingfors)

Austin, W. T. S.; and Harris, E. A.: Measurement of heart rate in exercise. Quart. J. Exp. Physiol. 42:126-129, Jan., 1957. (Edinburgh)

Auvergnat, R.: Effets immédiats du travail musculaire sur le nombre des hématies, le taux de l'hémoglobine et la valeur de l'hématocrite. Comptes Rend. Soc. Biol. 152:176-181, Aug. 25, 1958. (Montpellier)

----: Variations de pH et de la pression osmotique du plasma sanguin au cours du travail musculaire. J. Physiologie 42:531, 1950. (Montpellier)

----: Variations du taux sérique des protéines et des électrolytes au cours du travail musculaire. J. Physiologie 49:30-33, Jan.-Mar., 1957. (Toulouse)

Aykut, Resit; Terzioglu, Meliha; and Bilge, Muamma: Energy exchange under basal conditions at rest and during exercise at 1850 m. altitude. Arch. Int. Physiol. 68:285-298, Mar., 1960. (Istambul)

Azuma, R.: Thermodynamic phenomena exhibited in a shortening or lengthening muscle. Proc. Roy. Soc. 96B:338, 1924.

Babarin, P. M.; Romanova, L. S.; and Chibich'ian, D. A.: Izmenenie soderzhaniia kholesterina v krovi lits srednego i pozhilogo vozrasta pod vliianiem fizicheskikh uprazhnenii. (Changes in the blood cholesterol content of the middle-aged and aged under the influence of physical exercise). (Russ). Sovet. Med. 26:109-111, May, 1963.

Babbitt, J. A.: Blood corpuscle count, haemoglobin, ... as influenced by athletic and gymnastic exercise. Amer. Phys. Educat. Rev. 6:240-245, 1901.

Babinet, J. P.; and Heraud, G.: (Muscular activity and glucides) (Fr). Bull. Soc. Sci. Hyg. Aliment. 48:3-10, 1960.

----, and ----: (Muscular work and glucose consumption) (Fr). Diàbete 10:15-17, Jan., 1962.

Backman, P.; Pirilä, V.; Raekallio, T.; and Väänänen, I.: Die Schwankungen im Kreatin, und Kreatiningehalt des Blutes bei fortgesetztem starken Training. Scand. Arch. Physiol. 78: 304-312, 1938.

Baer, Adrian D.; Gersten, Jerome W.; Robertson, Barbara M.; and Dinken, Harold: Effect of various exercise programs on isometric tension, endurance and reaction time in the human. Arch. Phys. Med. 36:495-502, Aug., 1955. (Denver)

Baglioni, S.: L'educazione fisica e la fisiologia. Gior. Med. Milit. 68:425-440, 1920.

Bahnson, E. R.; Horvath, S. M.; and Comroe, Julius H.: Effects of active and passive limb movements upon respiration and O_2 consumption in man. J. Appl. Physiol. 2:169-173, Sept., 1949. (Philadelphia)

Bailie, Michael D.; Robinson, Sid; Rostorfer, Howard H.; and Newton, Jerry L.: Effects of exercise on heart output of the dog. J. Appl. Physiol. 16:107-111, Jan., 1961. (Bloomington)

Bainbridge, Francis Arthur: The influence of venous filling upon the rate of the heart. J. Physiol. 50:65-84, Dec. 24, 1915. (London)

----: On some cardiac reflexes. J. Physiol. 48:332-340, July 14, 1914. (Durham)

----: Physiology of muscular exercise. London, Longmans Green, 1919.

----: Physiology of muscular exercise. Second edition. Revised by G. V. Anrep. London, Longmans Green, 1923.

----: The physiology of muscular exercise. Third edition. Rewritten by A. V. Bock and D. B. Dill. London, Longmans Green, 1931.

----, and Hilton, R.: The relation between respiration and the pulse rate. J. Physiol. 52:lxv-lxvi, Jan. 25, 1919. (London)

----, and Trevan, J. W.: Some actions of adrenalin upon the liver. J. Physiol. 51:460-468, Dec. 6, 1917. (London)

Bajusz, E.; Jasmin, G.; and Mongeau, A.: Dissociation by forced muscular exercise of the cardiotoxic from the myotoxic actions of plasmocid. Rev. Canad. Biol. 23:29-36, Mar., 1964.

Baker, Mary Ann; and Horvath, Steven M.: Influence of water temperature on heart rate and rectal temperature of swimming rats. Amer. J. Physiol. 207:1073-1076, Nov., 1964. (Santa Barbara)

Bakst, Hyman; and Rinzler, Seymour H.: Effect of intravenous cytochrome C on capacity for effort without pain in angina of effort. Proc. Soc. Exp. Biol. Med. 67:531-533, Apr., 1948. (New York)

Baldes; Heichelheim; and Metzger: Untersuchungen über den Einfluss grosser Körperanstrengungen auf Zirkulations apparat, Nieren und Nervensystem. München med. Wschr. 53:1865-1866, Sept. 18, 1906. (Frankfurt)

Balgairies, E.; Quinot, E.; and Claeys, C.: La dynamique respiratoire an cours d'efforts importants. Arch. Mal. Prof. 17:508-512, Sept.-Oct., 1956.

Baliuk, I. G.; O trudosposobnosti lits, perenesshikh rezektsiiu legkogo po povodu tuberkuleza. (On the work capacity of persons having undergone lung resection for tuberculosis) (Russ). Probl. Tuberk. 41:40-43, 1963.

Balke, Bruno: Cardiac performance in relation to altitude. Amer. J. Cardiol. 14:796-810, Dec., 1964. (Oklahoma City)

----: Experimental evaluation of work capacity as related to chronological and physiological aging. Report 63-18. U. S. Civil Aeromed. Res. Institute 1-6, Sept., 1963.

----: Optimale körperliche Leistungsfähigkeit, ihre Messung und Veränderung infolge Arbeitsermüdung. Arbeitsphysiol. 15:311-323, 1954.

----, Grillo, G. P.; Konecci, E. B.; and Luft, U. C.: Work capacity after blood donation. J. Appl. Physiol. 7:231-238, Nov., 1954. (Randolph Air Force Base)

----, and Ware, Ray W.: An experimental study of "physical fitness" of air force personnel. U. S. Armed Forces Med. J. 10:675-688, June, 1959. (Randolph Air Force Base)

Ball, A. Brayton: Physical exercise. In Cyclopedia of the practice of medicine, vol. 18, H. von Ziemssen (editor). New York, William Wood, 1879.

Ball, Jerry R.: Effect of eating at various times on subsequent performances in swimming. New York J. Med. 63:600-603, Feb. 15, 1963. (Iowa City)

Bande, J.; and Van de Woestijne, K. P.: (The significance of the end-expiratory PCO_2 during the effort test) (Dut). Acta Tuberc. Belg. 52:99-113, Mar.-Apr., 1961.

Banerjee, Sachchedananda; Acharya, K. N.; and Chattopadhyay, D. P.: Studies on energy expenditure of rickshaw pullers. Indian J. Physiol. Pharmacol. 3:147-160, July, 1959. (Bikaner)

----, and Mahindra, Santosh Kumari: Energy intake and expenditure of medical college women. J. Appl. Physiol. 17:971-973, Nov., 1962. (Bikaner)

Bang, Ole: The lactate content of the blood during and after muscular exercise in man. Scand. Arch. Physiol. 74(Suppl. 10):49-82, 1936.

Bang, Ole: Lactic acid in the blood during muscular work. Bibliot.Laeger 128:106-110, May, 1936.

----: Undersøgelser over Maelkesyren i Blodet ved Muskelarbejde. (Studies on lactic acid in blood during muscular work) (Dan). Levin and Munksgaard, 1935.

Bannister, Roger G.: Muscular effort. Brit. Med. Bull. 12:222-225, Sept., 1956. (London)

----, and Cunningham, Daniel John Chapman: The effects on the respiration and performance during exercise of adding oxygen to the inspired air. J. Physiol. 125:118-137, July 28, 1954. (Oxford)

Bansi, H. W.; and Groscurth, G.: Funktionsprufung des Kreislaufs durch Messung der Herzarbeit. Klin. Wschr. 41:1902-1907, Oct. 11, 1930. (Berlin)

Bara, B.: Wydalanie magnezu i wapnia w pocie termicznym. (Excretion of magnesium and calcium with thermal sweat) (Pol). Pol. Arch. Med. Wewnet. 33:1125-1132, 1963.

Barach, Joseph H.: Physiological and pathological effects of severe exertion (the marathon race) on the circulatory and renal systems. Arch. Intern. Med. 5:382-405, Apr., 1910. (Pittsburgh)

Barclay, J. A.; Cooke, W. T.; Kenney, R. A.; and Nutt, M. E.: The effects of water diuresis and exercise on volume and composition of urine. Amer. J. Physiol. 148:327-337, Feb., 1947. (Birmingham, Eng.)

Barcroft, Henry: Circulatory changes accompanying the contraction of voluntary muscle. Aust. J. Exp. Biol. Med. Sci. 42:1-16, Feb., 1964.

----, Basnayake, V.; Celander, O.; Cobbold, A. F.; Cunningham, D. J. C.; Jukes, M. G. M.; and Young, I. Maureen: The effect of carbon dioxide on the respiratory response to noradrenaline in man. J. Physiol. 137:365-373, Aug. 6, 1957. (London and Oxford)

----, Bock, K. D.; Hensel, H.; and Kitchin, A. H.: Die Muskeldurchblutung des Menschen bei indirekter Erwärmung und Abkühlung. Pflüger Arch. ges. Physiol. 261:199-210, July 12, 1955. (London and Heidelberg)

Barcroft, Henry; Greenwood, B.; and Rutt, D. L.: pH, standard bicarbonate and pCO_2 of the blood in the deep veins of the forearm before, during and after strong sustained contraction of the forearm muscles. J. Physiol. 169:34P-35P, July, 1963. (London)

----, ----, and Whelan, R. F.: Blood flow and venous oxygen saturation during sustained contraction of the forearm muscles. J. Physiol. 168:848-856, Oct., 1963. (London)

----, and Millen, J. L. E.: The blood flow through muscle during sustained contraction. J. Physiol. 97:17-31, Nov. 14, 1939. (Belfast)

Barcroft, Joseph: Features in the architecture of physiological function. Cambridge, University Press, 1934.

----; Binger, C. A.; Bock, A. V.; Doggart, J. H.; Forbes, H. S.; Harrop, G.; Meakins, J. C.; and Redfield, A. C.: Observations upon the effect of high altitude upon the physiological processes of the human body, carried out in the Peruvian Andes, chiefly at Sierro de Pasco. Philos. Trans. Roy. Soc. 211:351-480, Jan., 1923.

Barcroft, Joseph; and Florey, Howard: The effects of exercise on the vascular conditions in the spleen and the colon. J. Physiol. 68:181-189, Oct. 23, 1929. (Cambridge, Eng.)

----, and Kato, Toyojiro: The effect of functional activity upon the metabolism, blood-flow, and exudation in organs. Proc. Roy. Soc. 88B:541-543, 1915. (Cambridge, Eng.)

----, and Roberts, F.: The dissociation curve of haemoglobin. J. Physiol. 39:143-148, Aug. 26, 1909. (Cambridge, Eng.)

Bard, Gregory: Energy expenditure of hemiplegic subjects during walking. Arch. Phys. Med. 44:268-270, July, 1963. (San Francisco)

Bardino, M.; and Quatrini, U.: Influenza degli ormoni sui processi di proteosintesi e di proteolisi durante il lavora. I. Influenza dell'adrenalina. Boll. Soc. Ital. Biol. Sper. 35:453-456, Apr. 30, 1959.

Bardswell, N. D.; and Chapman, J. E.: Some observations upon the deep temperature of the human body at rest and after muscular exertion. Brit. Med. J. 1:1106-1110, May 13, 1911. (Midhurst)

Barger, A. C.; Metcalfe, J.; Richards, V.; and Günther, B. Circulation during exercise in normal dogs and dogs with cardiac valvular lesions. Amer. J. Physiol. 201:480-484, Sept., 1961. (Boston)

----; Richards, V.; Metcalfe, J.; and Günther, B.: Regulation of the circulation during exercise; cardiac output (direct Fick) and metabolic adjustments in the normal dog. Amer. J. Physiol. 184:613-623, Mar., 1956. (Boston)

----; Roe, B. B.; and Richardson, G. S.: Relation of valvular lesions and of exercise to auricular pressure, work tolerance, and to development of chronic, congestive failure in dogs. Amer. J. Physiol. 169:384-399, May, 1952. (Boston)

Bariocco, A.: Modificazioni dei diametri cardiaci, del polso e della pressione; esercizio muscolare. Cron. Clin. Med. Genova 26:75; 123; 155, 1920.

Barman, Julio M.; Consolazio, Frank; and Moreira, Manoel F.: Relation between pulmonary ventilation and oxygen consumption after exercise. Amer. J. Physiol. 138:16-19, Dec., 1942. (Boston)

----, Moreira, Manoel F.; and Consolazio, F.: The effective stimulus for increased pulmonary ventilation during muscular exertion. J. Clin. Invest. 22:53-56, Jan., 1943. (Boston)

Barnes, LeRoy L.: The deposition of calcium in the hearts and kidneys of rats in relation to age, source of calcium, exercise and diet. Amer. J. Path. 18:41-47, Jan., 1942. (Ithaca)

Barnes, Richard H.; Labadan, Beatriz Alcazar; Siyamoglu, Bahriye; and Bradfield, Robert B.: Effects of exercise and administration of aspartic acid on blood ammonia in the rat. Amer. J. Physiol. 207:1242-1246, Dec., 1946. (Ithaca)

Baron, J. B.; Kahn, J.; Rey, P.; Thieffry, P.; and Dubois: Les variations de la fréquence critique de fusion an cours d'un travail intellectuel et physique. Arch. Mal. Prof. 24:429-433, Apr.-May, 1963. (Geneva)

Barr, David P.: Studies in the physiology of muscular exercise. IV. Blood reaction and breathing. J. Biol. Chem. 56:171-182, May, 1923. (New York)

----, and Himwich, Harold E.: Studies in the physiology of muscular exercise. II. Comparison of arterial and venous blood following vigorous exercise. J. Biol. Chem. 55:525-537, Mar., 1923. (New York)

----, and ----: Studies in the physiology of muscular exercise. III. Development and duration of changes in acid-base equilibrium. J. Biol. Chem. 55:539-555, Mar., 1923.

----, ----, and Green, Robert P.: Studies in the physiology of muscular exercise. I. Changes in acid-base equilibrium following short periods of vigorous muscular exercise. J. Biol. Chem. 55:495-523, Mar., 1923. (New York)

Barr, P. O.; Beckman, M.; Bjurstedt, H.; Brismar, J.; Hesser, C. M.; and Matell, G.: Time courses of blood gas changes provoked by light and moderate exercise in man. Acta Physiol. Scand. 60:1-17, Jan.-Feb., 1964. (Stockholm)

Barratt-Boyes, Brian G.; and Wood, Earl H.: Hemodynamic response of healthy subjects to exercise in the supine position while breathing oxygen. J. Appl. Physiol. 11:129-135, July, 1957. (Rochester, Minn.)

Barrion, Georges: De l'entrainement. Paris, Thèse Numero 494, 1877.

Bartelheimer, H.: Über Empfindlichkeitsreaktionen durch körperliche Anstrengung. Deutsch. med. Wschr. 70:175, Mar. 31, 1944.

Bartels, H.; Beer, R.; Koepchen, H.-P.; Wenner, J.; and Witt, I.: Messung der alveolär-arteriellen O_2-Druckdifferenz mit verschiedenen Methoden am Menschen bei Ruhe und Arbeit. Pfluger Arch. ges. Physiol. 261:133-151, June 7, 1955. (Göttingen)

Bartlett, Frederic: Psychological criteria of fatigue. In Symposium on fatigue, edited by W. F. Floyd and A. T. Welford. London, H. K. Lewis and Co., 1953. (Cambridge, Eng.)

Bartlett, R. G., Jr.: Physiologic responses during coitus. J. Appl. Physiol. 9:469-472, Nov., 1956. (Rockville, Md.)

Baschieri, L.; Ricci, P. D.; Mazzuoli, G. F.; and Lotti, P.: Les variations on débit sanguin hépatique au cours de l'activité physique. Cardiologia 29:229-237, 1956. (Rome)

Basevi, A.; and Dagnini, G.: L'emodinamica renale e l'diminazione di cloruro di sodio in condizioni basali e durante il moto nei portatori di lesioni croniche diffuse polmonari. Folia Cardiol. 14:25-35, Feb. 28, 1955.

----, ----, and de Castro, B.: I gas del sangue nella cardiopatie compensate in condizioni basali e dopo l'esencizio muscolare. Folia Cardiol. 16:323-330, Aug. 31, 1957.

----, ----, and ----: La pressione venosa, la velocità di circolo e la massa sanguigna circolante nei cardiopatici compensati in condizioni basali e dopo l'esercizio muscolare. Folia Cardiol. 14:37-51, Feb. 28, 1955.

Bashenina, N. V.: K voprosu o deistvii letal' noi nizkoĭ temperaturg na melkikh polevok preimashchestvenno Microtus arvalis Pall pri estestvennom Zamerzanii. (On the problem of the effect of lethal low temperature on small voles (particularly microtus arvalis pall) during natural freezing) (Russ). Zh. Obshch. Biol. 24:366-373, Sept.-Oct., 1963.

Basler, Adolf: Die Physiologie der Leibesüngen. Med. Klin. 32:1356-1359, Oct. 2, 1936.

----: Ueber die gewöhnliche Schrittlänge und Geschwindigkeit bei einigen Formen des Gehens. Arbeitsphysiol. 1:271-277, Jan. 9, 1929. (Canton, China)

Bass, David E.; Buskirk, E, R.; Iampietro, P. F.; and Mager, Milton: Comparison of blood volume during physical conditioning, heat acclimatization and sedentary living. J. Appl. Physiol. 12:186-188, Mar., 1958. (Natick)

Basu, Archona; Passmore, R.; and Strong, J. A.: The effects of exercise on the level of non-esterified fatty acids in the blood. Quart. J. Exp. Physiol. 45:312-317, July, 1960. (Edinburgh)

Baum, William S.; Malmo, Robert B.; and Sievers, Rudolph F.: A comparative study of the effects of exercise and anoxia upon the human electrocardiogram. J. Aviation Med. 16:422-428, Dec., 1945. (Bethesda)

Baumann, Hans; and Grollman, Arthur: Über die theoretischen und praktischen Grundlagen und die klinische Zuverlässigkeit der Acetylenmethode zur Bestimmung des Minuten-volumens. Zeits. klin. Med. 115:41-53, 1930. (Düsseldorf)

Baumann, P.; Escher, J.; and Richterich, R.: (The behavior of serum enzymes in muscular work) (Ger). Schweiz. Zeits. Sportmed. 10:33-51, 1962.

Bayley, T. J.; Segel, N.; and Bishop, J. M.: The circulatory changes in patients with cirrhosis of the liver at rest and during exercise. Clin. Sci. 26:227-235, Apr., 1964. (Birmingham, Eng.)

Bayliss, William Maddox: The action of carbon dioxide on blood vessels. J. Physiol. 26:xxxii-xxxiii, Mar. 16, 1901. (London)

Bazett, H. C.: Theory of reflex controls to explain regulation of body temperature at rest and during exercise. J. Appl. Physiol. 4:245-262, Oct., 1951. (Philadelphia)

Beauvallet, M.; Fugazza, J.; and Solier, M.: Étude comparée du faux de la noradrénaline des surrénales et du cerveau avant et après travail musculaire. Comptes Rend. Soc. Biol. 155:2252-2254, Dec. 9, 1961. (Paris)

----, ----, and ----: Variations de la teneur en adrénaline et noradrénaline des surrénales et du cerveau avant et après travail musculaire. Action de l'amphétamine. Comptes Rend. Soc. Biol. 156:1258-1260, July 7, 1962. (Paris)

----, and Solier, Madeleine: Effet d'un exercice forcé sur la toxicité de l'amphétamine et la teneur en noradrénaline du cerveau. Comptes Rend. Soc. Biol. 158:2306-2309, 1964. (Paris)

Becklake, Margaret R.; Varvis, C. J.; Pengelly, L. D.; Kenning, S.; McGregor, M.; and Bates, D. V.: Measurement of pulmonary blood flow during exercise using nitrous oxide. J. Appl. Physiol. 17:579-586, July, 1962. (Montreal)

Beckner, George L.; and Winsor, Travis: Cardiovascular adaptations to prolonged physical effort. Circulation 9:835-846, June, 1954. (Los Angeles)

Béclard, Jules Auguste: De la contraction musculaire dans ses rapports avec la température animale. Paris, P. Asselin, 1861. (Also in Arch. Gen. Med. 17:24-40; 157-180; 257-279, 1861)

Bedell, George N.; and Adams, Richard W.: Pulmonary diffusing capacity during rest and exercise. A study of normal persons and persons with atrial septal defect, pregnancy, and pulmonary disease. J. Clin. Invest. 41:1908-1914, Oct., 1962. (Iowa City)

Bedrak, E.; Beer, G.; and Furman, K. I.: Fibrinolytic activity and muscular exercise in heat. J. Appl. Physiol. 19:469-471, May, 1964. (Beersheba)

Beevor, Charles E.: Muscular movements and their representation in the central nervous system. Croonian Lecture. London, Adlard and Son, 1904.

Beickert, A.: Zur Entstehung und Bewertung der Arbeitshypertrophie des Herzens, der Nebenniere und Hypophyse (tierexperimentelle Untersuchungen). Arch. Kreislaufforsch. 21:115-126, July, 1954.

----, Mannstadt, C.; and Klupsch, E.: Tierexperimentelle Untersuchungen über die Beeinflussung des Grundumsatzes durch körperliches Training. Zeits. ges. exp. Med. 129:60-68, July 8, 1957. (Jena)

Bekeny, Georg; and Kraft, Franciska: Ischämische Muskel-Nerven-Schädigung des Beines nach muskulärer Überanstrengung. Wien. Zeits. Nervenheilk. 20:336-348, Mar., 1963.

Belagyi, J.; and Felker, J. S.: Muscle fatigue and the crystallization of myosin. Acta Physiol. Acad. Sci. Hung. 22:327-330, 1962.

Beliaeva, R. A.: Kotsenke sostoianie sistemy krouoobrashcheniia u bol'nykh mitral'nym stenozom po dannym gazoobmena. (On assessment of the state of the circulatory system in patients with mitral stenosis based on gas exchange data) (Russ). Ter. Arkh. 35:60-65, May, 1963.

Bell, A. M.: March haemoglobinuria. Canad. Med. Ass. J. 57:43-46, July, 1947. (Alvinston)

Bell, G. H.; and Knox, J. A. C.: Recording of pulse rate during exercise. J. Physiol. 93:36P-37P, June 4, 1938. (Glasgow)

Bellet, Samuel; Deliyiannis, Stavros; and Eliakim, Marcel: The electrocardiogram during exercise as recorded by radioelectrocardiography. Comparison with the postexercise electrocardiogram (Master two-step test). Amer. J. Cardiol. 8:385-400, Sept., 1961. (Philadelphia)

----, Eliakim, Marcel; Deliyiannis, Stavros; and Figallo, Eduardo M.: Radioelectrocardiographic changes during strenuous exercise in normal subjects. Circulation 25:686-694, Apr., 1962. (Philadelphia)

----, Muller, Otto F.; Herring, Allen B.; and LaVan, Donald W.: Effect of erythrityl tetranitrate on the electrocardiogram as recorded during exercise by radioelectrocardiography. Amer. J. Cardiol. 11:600-608, May, 1963. (Philadelphia)

Bellet, Samuel; Muller, Otto F.; LaVan, Donald W.; Nichols, George J.; and Herring, Allen B. Radioelectrocardiography during exercise in patients with the anginal syndrome: use of multiple leads. Circulation 29:366-375, Mar., 1964. (Philadelphia)

Benchimol, Alberto; Li, Yeou-Bing; Dimond, E. Grey; Voth, Robert B.; and Roland, Arnold S.: Effect of heart rate, exercise, and nitroglycerin on the cardiac dynamics in complete heart block. Circulation 28:510-519, Oct., 1963. (La Jolla)

Bender, Jay A.; Kaplan, Harold M.; and Pierson, Joe K.: Relation between measured muscular force and success in selected tasks in physically handicapped patients. Arch. Phys. Med. 45:30-40, Jan., 1964. (Carbondale)

Benedict, Francis Gano; and Cathcart, Edward P.: Muscular work. A metabolic study with special reference to the efficiency of the human body as a machine. Publication no. 187. Washington, Carnegie Institution, 1913.

Benedict, Francis Gano; and Smith, H. Monmouth: The metabolism of athletes as compared with normal individuals of similar height and weight. J. Biol. Chem. 20:243-252, 1915. (Washington and Syracuse)

Bengtsson, Elias: The exercise electrocardiogram in healthy children and in comparison with adults. Acta Med. Scand. 154:225-244, May 3, 1956. (Stockholm)

Benjamin, F. B.; and Peyser, L.: Physiological effects of active and passive exercise. J. Appl. Physiol. 19:1212-1214, Nov., 1964. (Farmingdale, Long Island)

Berdan, C.; Gavrilescu, N.; and Vaida, I.: A study of oxygen consumption during effort at various temperatures and air current velocities. Rumanian Med. Rev. 5:95-96, 1961.

Berg, William E.: Individual differences in respiratory gas exchange during recovery from moderate exercise. Amer. J. Physiol. 149:597-610, June, 1947. (Berkeley)

----: Individual differences in respiratory gas exchange during recovery from moderate exercise. Mem. Rep. Aero Med. Lab. (MCREXD-696-114), 103-131, Mar. 3, 1948.

----: Metabolic recovery rates from exercise after alteration of alkaline reserve. Amer. J. Physiol. 152:465-469, Feb., 1948.

Bergamaschi, P.; Capodaglio, E.; and Fre, B.: Aspetti cardiorespiratori e metabolici del lavoro muscolare in granidanza. Minerva Ginec. 16:831-838, Oct., 1964.

Berggren, G.; and Christensen, E. H.: Heart rate and body temperature as indices of metabolic rate during work. Arbeitsphysiol. 14:255-260, 1950.

Berglund, Erik; Borst, Hans G.; Duff, Frank; and Schreiner, Günther L.: Effect of heart rate on cardiac work, myocardial oxygen consumption and coronary blood flow in the dog. Acta Physiol. Scand. 42:185-198, Apr. 2, 1958. (Boston)

Bergman, A.: Variaciones de la presión arterial, pulso, y fórmula leucocitaria, durante el ejercicio en sujetos de corazón clínicamente normal; en algunas afecciones pulmonares y en las insuficiencias cardiacas. Rev. Asoc. Méd. Argent., Sect. Soc. Biol. 35:289-296, 1922.

Bergström, J.: Muscle electrolytes in man: determined by neutron activation analysis on needle biopsy specimens; a study on normal subjects, kidney patients, and patients with chronic diarrhoea. Scand. J. Clin. Lab. Invest. 14(Suppl. 68):1-110, 1962.

Bergström, R. M.: The kinetic energy produced by voluntarily controlled muscle action and the frequency of the motor discharge. Acta Physiol. Scand. 47:179-190, Nov. 15, 1959. (Helsinki)

----: The mechanical work produced by voluntarily controlled muscle action and the frequency of the motor discharge. Acta Physiol. Scand. 47:191-198, Nov. 15, 1959. (Helsinki)

Berloco, N.; Caspani, F.; and Grassi, F.: (The energy yield of pulmonary ventilation during muscular work in the study of the efficiency of the respiratory tract) (It). Gior. Ital. Tuberc. 15:141-145, May-June, 1961.

----, ----, and Masserini, C.: (Relations between muscular activity and respiratory function in healthy subjects of different ages: I. Oxygen absorption) (It). Gior. Ital. Tuberc. 16:101-104, May-June, 1962.

----, ----, and ----: (Relations between muscular activity and respiratory function in healthy subjects of different ages: II. Pulmonary ventilation) (It). Gior. Ital. Tuberc. 16:105-110, May-June, 1962.

----, ----, and ----: (Relations between muscular activity and respiratory function in healthy subjects of different ages: III. The energy yield of ventilation) (It). Gior. Ital. Tuberc. 16:111-113, May-June, 1962.

----, ----, and Stringa, C.: (Respiratory function during inhalations of pure oxygen. I. Energetic consumption in conditions of rest and muscular activity) (It). Gior. Ital. Tuberc. 15:185-188, July-Aug., 1961.

----, ----, and ----: (Respiratory function during inhalations of pure oxygen. II. Pulmonary ventilation during rest and during muscular activity) (It). Gior. Ital. Tuberc. 15:191-195, July-Aug., 1961.

----, ----, and ----: (Respiratory function during inhalations of pure oxygen. III. The energetic efficiency of pulmonary ventilation in conditions of rest and muscular exercise) (It). Gior. Ital. Tuberc. 15:197-199, July-Aug., 1961.

Berner, G. E.; Garrett, C. C.; Jones, D. C.; and Noer, R. J.: The effect of external temperature on second wind. Amer. J. Physiol. 76:586-592, May, 1926. (Philadelphia)

Bernstein, Daniel S.; and Guri, Charles D.: Osteoporosis: etiology and therapy. Postgrad. Med. 34:407-409, Oct., 1963. (Boston)

Bernstein, J.: Zur Thermodynamik des Muskelkontraktion. I. Über die Temperaturkoeffizienten der Muskelenergie. Nebst Versuchen über den Temperaturkoeffizienten der Oberflächenspannung kolloider Lösungen. Pflüger Arch. ges. Physiol. 122:129-195, Apr. 1, 1908.

Bernstein, Nik.; and Popowa, Tatiana: Untersuchung über die Biodynamik des Klavieranschlags. Arbeitsphysiol. 1:396-432, 1929. (Moscow)

Berry, J. Norman; Thompson, Howard K., Jr.; Miller, D. Edmond; and McIntosh, Henry D.: Changes in cardiac output, stroke volume, and central venous pressure induced by atropine in man. Amer. Heart J. 58:204-213, Aug., 1959. (Durham)

Berséus, S.: The influence of heart glucosides, theophylline, and analeptics on the cardiac output in congestive heart failure. Acta Med. Scand. 113(Suppl. 145):1-76, 1943. (Stockholm)

Berven, Hans: The physical working capacity of healthy children. Seasonal variations and effect of ultraviolet irradiation and vitamin-D supply. Acta Paediat. Suppl. 148:1-22, 1963. (Stockholm)

Bessou, P.; Dejours, Pierre; and Laporte, Y.: Effets ventilatoires réflexes de la stimulation de fibres afférentes de grand diamètre, j'origine musculaire, chez le chat. Comptes Rend. Soc. Biol. 153:477-481, June 30, 1959. (Toulouse)

Best, Charles H.; Furusawa, K.; and Ridout, J. H.: The respiratory quotient of the excess metabolism of exercise. Proc. Roy. Soc. 104B:119-151, Jan. 1, 1929. (Toronto and London)

----, and Partridge, Ruth C.: The equation of motion of a runner, exerting a maximal effort. Proc. Roy. Soc. 103B:218-225, Aug. 1, 1928. (Toronto)

----, and ----: Observations on Olympic athletes. Proc. Roy. Soc. 105B:323-332, Sept. 2, 1929. (Toronto)

Best, Lincoln R.: "False positive" post-exercise electrocardiogram in a digitalized patient. J. Nat. Med. Ass. 55:277-279, July, 1963. (Los Angeles)

Beuret, J.: Essai sur l'influence du mouvement et de l'exercice. Strasbourg, 1827.

Bevegård, Sture: The effect of cardioacceleration by methyl scopolamine nitrate on the circulation at rest and during exercise in supine position with special reference to the stroke volume. Acta Physiol. Scand. 57:61-80, Jan.-Feb., 1963. (Stockholm)

----: Observations on the effect of varying ventricular rate on the circulation at rest and during exercise in two patients with an artificial pacemaker. Acta Med. Scand. 172:615-622, Nov., 1962. (Stockholm)

----: Studies on the regulation of the circulation in man. With special reference to the stroke volume and the effect of muscular work, body position, and artificially induced variations of the heart rate. Acta Physiol. Scand. 57(Suppl. 200):1-36, 1962. (Stockholm)

----, Holmgren, A.; and Jonsson, B.: Circulatory studies in well trained athletes at rest and during heavy exercise, with special reference to stroke volume and the influence of body position. Acta Physiol. Scand. 57:26-50, Jan.-Feb., 1963. (Stockholm)

----, ----, and ----: The effect of body position on the circulation at rest and during exercise, with special reference to the influence on the stroke volume. Acta Physiol. Scand. 49:279-298, July 15, 1960. (Stockholm)

Beznák, Margit; Hajdu, István; and Korényi, Zoltán: The role of the increase in the concentration of certain blood constituents in the production of suprarenal hypertrophy caused by muscular exercise. Arch. Int. Pharmacodyn. 67:242-256, Mar. 31, 1942. (Budapest)

Bhatnagar, D. S.; and Chaudhary, N. C.: Effect of exposure to sun and exercise on heat tolerance coefficient in Murrah buffalo calves. Nature 189:844-845, Mar. 11, 1961. (Mhow)

Białeclo, Mieczysław; and Nijakowski, Feliks: Influence of physical effort on the level of thiamine in tissues and blood. Acta Physiol. Pol. 15:192-197, 1964. (Poznán)

Bianucci, G.; and Guarnieri, E.: Effetti dell'attività muscolare intensa sulla lipidemia in soggetti allenati del colesterolo e dei fosfolipidi ematici. Riv. Crit. Clin. Med. 64:120-134, Apr., 1964.

Bickelmann, Albert G.; Lippschutz, Eugene J.; and Weinstein, Leonard: The response of the normal and abnormal heart to exercise: a functional evaluation. Circulation 28:238-250, Aug., 1963. (Buffalo)

Biggs, Rosemary; MacFarlane, R. G.; and Pilling, J.: Observations on fibrinolysis; experimental activity produced by exercise or adrenaline. Lancet 1:402-405, Mar. 29, 1947. (Oxford)

Billewicz-Stankiewicz, J.; and Tyburczyk, W.: Experimentelle Untersuchungen über den Einfluss der physische Arbeit auf die Aktivität der Cholinesterase des Blutes. Int. Zeits. angew. Physiol. 18:361-375, Dec. 27, 1960.

----, and ----: (On changes in adrenalin-oxidases in the blood plasma during physical work) (Ger). Int. Zeits. angew. Physiol. 20:62-74, 1963.

Billimoria, J. D.; Drysdale, Jean; James, D. C. O.; and Maclagan, N. F.: Determination of fibrinolytic activity of whole blood. With special reference to the effects of exercise and fat feeding. Lancet 2:471-475, Oct. 3, 1959. (London)

Billings, Charles E., Jr.; Tomashefski, Joseph F.; Carter, Earl T.; and Ashe, William F.: Measurement of human capacity for aerobic muscular work. J. Appl. Physiol. 15:1001-1006, Nov., 1960. (Columbus)

Binet, Léon: Sur la polyglobulie de l'exercise et sur la polyglobulie adrénalinique chez l'homme. Comptes Rend. Soc. Biol. 100:463-465, Feb. 16, 1929.

----, and Bargeton, Daniel: Etude de la course a vitesse forcée chez le rat. Technique et représentation des résultats. Comptes Rend. Soc. Biol. 139:255-256, Mar. 10, 1945. (Paris)

----, and Bochet, M.: Réactions ventilatoires et circulatoires chez des sujets âgés an cours d'un effort statique exécuté dans l'air normal et sans inhalation d'oxygène. Rev. Franc. Geront. 10:7-19, Feb., 1964.

----, and Contamin, F.: L'action défatigante de l'oxygene chez l'homme. Comptes Rend. Acad. Sci. 227:248-251, July 26, 1948.

Bini, L.; Colonna, L.; and Brindicci, G.: I volumi di sangue del piccolo circolo e dei ventricoli cardiaci a riposo e dopo esercizio fisico nella cirrosi epatica. Cuore Circ. 48:67-81, Apr., 1964.

Bink, B.: Relatie tussen arbeidsbelasting en arbeidscapaciteit. (Relation between work load and work capacity) (Dut). T. Soc. Geneesk. 41:698-701, Nov. 8, 1963.

Binkhorst, R. A.; and Leeuwen, P. van: A rapid method for the determination of aerobic capacity. Int. Zeits. angew. Physiol. 19:459-467, Feb. 7, 1963. (Leiden)

Biörck, Gunnar: On myoglobin and its occurrence in man. Acta Med. Scand. 133(Suppl. 226):1-216, 1949. (Stockholm)

Biörck, Gunnar: Studies on the influence of exercise on the serum iron in man. Acta Physiol.
    Scand. 15:193-197, Apr. 20, 1948. (Stockholm)

Bírčák, J.; and Nikš, M.: Funkčná zdatnosi kardiopulmonálneho systému v období dospievani.
    V. Vplyr pracovného zatazenia na ventiláciu. (Functional efficiency of the cardiopulmonary
    system during the period of adolescence. V. Effect of the work load on ventilation) (Cz).
    Bratisl. Lek. Listy 2:701-709, 1963.

----, ----, Steiner, J.; et al: Funkčná zdatnosi kardiopulmonálneho systému v období dospievania.
    III. Vplyv pracovného zatazenia na niektoré základné ukazovatele vykonnosti krvného obehu.
    (Functional capacity of the cardiopulmonary system in adolescence. III. Effect of work stress
    on some basic indices of blood circulatory efficiency) (Cz). Bratisl. Lek. Listy 2:541-558, 1963.

----, ----, ----, et al: Funkčná zdatnosi kardiopulmonálneho systému v období dospievania. IV.
    Vztah telesného výkonu k niektorým somatickým ukazovatel'om. (Functional efficiency of
    the cardiopulmonary system during the period of adolescence. IV. Relation of physical per-
    formance to some somatic indices) (Cz). Bratisl. Lek. Listy 2:637-648, 1963.

Birkhead, Newton C.; Blizzard, J. J.; Daly, J. W.; et al: Cardiodynamic and metabolic effects
    of prolonged bed rest with daily recumbent or sitting exercise and with sitting inactivity.
    Techn. Docum. Rep. No. AMRL-TDR-64-61. U. S. Air Force 6570 Aerospace Med. Res.
    Lab.:1-28, Aug., 1964.

----, Haupt, George J.; Issekutz, B., Jr.; and Rodahl, K.: Circulatory metabolic effects of different
    types of prolonged inactivity. Amer. J. Med. Sci. 247:243, Feb., 1964. (Philadelphia)

Bishop, J. M.; Donald, Kenneth W.; Taylor, Stanley H.; and Wormald, P. N.: The blood flow in
    the human arm during supine leg exercise. J. Physiol. 137:294-308, July 11, 1957. (Birmingham,
    Eng.)

----, ----, ----, and ----: Changes in arterial-hepatic venous oxygen content difference during
    and after supine leg exercise. J. Physiol. 137:309-317, July 11, 1957. (Birmingham, Eng.)

----, ----, and Wade, Oliver L.: Changes in the oxygen content of hepatic venous blood during
    exercise in patients with rheumatic heart disease. J. Clin. Invest. 34:1114-1125, July
    (Part 1), 1955. (Birmingham, Eng.)

----, ----, and ----: Circulatory dynamics at rest and on exercise in the hyperkinetic states.
    Clin. Sci. 14:329-360, May, 1955. (Birmingham, Eng.)

----, and Wade, O. L.: Relationships between cardiac output and rhythm, pulmonary vascular pressures
    and disability in mitral stenosis. Clin. Sci. 24:391-404, June, 1963. (Birmingham, Eng. and
    Belfast)

----, ----, and Donald, Kenneth W.: Changes in jugular and renal arterio-venous oxygen content
    difference during exercise in heart disease. Clin. Sci. 17:611-619, Nov., 1958. (Birmingham,
    Eng.)

Bisset, Sheenah K.; and Alexander, W. D.: Effect of muscular activity prior to venepuncture on the
    respiration of leucocytes in vitro. Nature 181:909-910, Mar. 29, 1958. (Glasgow)

Black, John E.: Blood flow requirements of the human calf after walking and running. Clin. Sci.
    18:89-93, Feb., 1959. (Belfast)

Black, William A.; and Karpovich, Peter V.: Effect of exercise on erythrocyte sedimentation rate. Amer. J. Physiol. 144:224-226, July, 1945. (San Antonio)

Blackburn, Henry; and Katigbak, Raymundo: What electrocardiographic leads to take after exercise: Amer. Heart J. 67:184-185, Feb., 1964. (Minneapolis)

----, Mitchell, Paul; and Imbimbo, Bruno: The exercise ECG test. At what intervals to record after exercise? Amer. Heart J. 67:186-188, Feb., 1964.

Blair, David A.; Glover, Walter E.; and Roddie, Ian C.: Vasomotor responses in the human arm during leg exercise. Circ. Res. 9:264-274, Mar., 1961. (Belfast)

Blake, William D.: Effect of exercise and emotional stress on renal hemodynamics, water and sodium excretion in the dog. Amer. J. Physiol. 165:149-157, Apr., 1951. (New Haven)

Blandy, John P.; and Fuller, Robert: March gangrene; ischaemic myositis of the leg muscles from exercise. J. Bone Joint Surg. 39B:679-693, Nov., 1957. (Glasgow)

Blasius, W.: Beitrag zur Schlagvolumenbestimmung aus den Blutdruckwerten. Zeits. Kreislaufforsch. 33:201-208, Apr. 1, 1941.

----, Bach, G.; and Sachs, D.: Die Frontal- und Horizontal-projektionen der QRS- und T-Vektoren und ihre Beziehungen zu Schlagvolumen und Herzfrequenz in Ruhe und nach definierter Arbeitsbelastung beim Menschen. Zeits. Kreislaufforsch. 51:105-117, Jan., 1961. (Giessen)

----, ----, and Schafe, M. K.: Der Herzminutenvolumen-Quotient (Qvm) nach dosierter Arbeit und in der Erholungsphase bei Trainierten und Untrainierten. Arch. Kreislaufforsch. 36:58-77, Sept., 1961. (Giessen)

Bliss, Harry A.; and Graettinger, John S.: Caloric expenditure at two types of factory work. Arch. Environ. Health 9:201-215, Aug., 1964. (Chicago)

Blix, Magnus: Die Länge und die Spannung des Muskels. Scand. Arch. Physiol. 3:295-318, 1892. (Lund)

----: Die Länge und die Spannung des Muskels. Zweite Abhandlung. Scand. Arch. Physiol. 4:399-409, 1893. (Lund)

----: Die Länge und die Spannung des Muskels. Dritte Abhandlung. Scand. Arch. Physiol. 5:150-172, 1895. (Lund)

----: Die Länge und die Spannung des Muskels. Vierte Abhandlung. Scand. Arch. Physiol. 5:173-206, 1895. (Lund)

----: Zur Frage über die menschliche Arbeitskraft. Scand. Arch. Physiol. 15:122-146, 1904. (Lund)

Blount, S. G., Jr.; and Reeves, J. T.: The circulatory dynamics in pulmonary emphysema during treadmill exercise. Amer. Rev. Resp. Dis. 80:128-130, July (Part 2), 1959. (Denver)

Blum, L.: The clinical entity of anterior crural ischemia. Report of four cases. Arch. Surg. 74:59-64, Jan., 1957. (New York)

Blyth, A. W.: Observations on the ingesta and egesta of Mr. E. P. Weston during his walk of 5,000 miles in 100 days. Proc. Roy. Soc. 37:46-55, 1884.

Bobbert, A. C.: Energy expenditure in level and grade walking. J. Appl. Physiol. 15:1015-1021, Nov., 1960. (Leiden)

----: Physiological comparison of three types of ergometry. J. Appl. Physiol. 15:1007-1014, Nov., 1960. (Leiden)

Bock, Arlie V.: The circulation of a marathoner. J. Sport Med. 3:80-86, June-Sept., 1963.

----: Fatigue. Trans. Coll. Physicians Phila. 10:75-81, June, 1942. (Boston)

----: On some aspects of the physiology of muscular exercise. New Eng. J. Med. 200:638-642, Mar. 28, 1929. (Boston)

----, Vancaulaert, C.; Dill, D. B.; Fölling, A.; and Hurxthal, L. M.: Studies in muscular activity. III. Dynamical changes occurring in man at work. J. Physiol. 66:136-161, Oct. 10, 1928. (Boston)

----, ----, ----, ----, and ----: Studies in muscular activity. IV. The "steady state" and the respiratory quotient during work. J. Physiol. 66:162-164, Oct. 10, 1928. (Boston)

Bocles, Jose S.; Ehrenkranz, N. Joel; and Marks, Asher: Abnormalities of respiratory function in varicella pneumonia. Ann. Intern. Med. 60:183-195, Feb., 1964. (Miami)

Bodansky, Oscar; and Hendley, Charles D.: Effect of methemoglobinemia on the visual threshold at sea level, at high altitudes, and after exercise. J. Clin. Invest. 25:717-722, Sept., 1946. (Edgewood Arsenal and New York)

Boeckh, Eva Maria; and Haebisch, Horst: Die Dauer der elektrokardiographischen Phasen warend und nach dynamischer und statischer Arbeit im Liegen und Stehen. Zeits. Kreislaufforsch. 50:425-436, May, 1961. (São Paulo)

----, and ----: Grösse und Richtung der elektrokardiographischen Vektoren wärend und nach dynamischer und statischer Arbeit im Liegen und Stehen. Zeits. Kreislaufforsch. 50:477-488, May, 1961. (São Paulo)

Bøje, Ove: Arbeitshypoglykämie nach Glukoseeingabe. (Vorläufige Mitteilung). (Development of hypoglycemia during muscular work following ingestion of dextrose; preliminary report) (Dan). Scand. Arch. Physiol. 83:308-312, June, 1940. (Copenhagen)

----: Der Blutzuker wärend und nach körperlicher Arbeit. Scand. Arch. Physiol. 74(Suppl. 10): 1-48, 1936.

----: Energy production, pulmonary ventilation, and length of steps in well-trained runners working on a treadmill. Acta Physiol. Scand. 7:362-375, July 18, 1944. (Copenhagen)

----: Motionens profylaktiske vaerdi i det overudviklede samfund. (Prophylactic value of exercise in overdeveloped society) (Dan). Manedsskr. Prakt. Laegegern. 42:165-178, Apr., 1964.

Boeri, E.: La iperventilozione da anidride carbonica e la iperventilazione da lavoro muscolare. Tentativo di una trattazione matematica della regolazione chimica del respiro. Arch. Sci. Biol. 30:145-158, May, 1944-Dec., 1945.

Boigey, Maurice A. J.: Effets physiologiques de l'exercice. Paris Med. 39:231-235, Mar. 19, 1921. (Also in Un. Med. Canada 50:287-295, 1921.

Boigey, Maurice A. J.: Effets physiologiques de l'exercice; nécessité de son contrôle par le
    médecin hygiéniste. Rev. Hyg., 45:460-468, 1923.

----: Exercice physique et grandes fonctions. Biol. Méd. 27:321-357, May, 1937.

----: Influence de l'exercice sur les fonctions circulatoire et respiratoire. J. Méd. Franc.
    16:298-304, July, 1927.

----: Influence de l'exercice sur la sécrétion urinaire et sudorale. J. Physiol. Path. Gen. 25:
    249-253, 1927.

----: Influence de l'exercice sur le tissu glandulaire et les fonctions d'excrétion. Ann. Med.
    Phys. 31:169-175, 1938.

----: Influence générale de l'exercice sur les grandes fonctions. Arch. Méd. Pharm. Milit.
    79:411-453, 1923.

----: Influence hygiénique de l'exercice et méfaits de la sédentarité. Rev. Hyg., 45:1050-1067,
    1923.

----: Note sur la durée des perturbations cardio-vasculaires produits par l'exercice. Bull. Acad.
    Med., 3rd series. 91:220-224, Feb. 12, 1924.

----: Note sur les effets de l'exercice corporel sur l'enfant. Bull. Acad. Med., 3rd series.
    94:1026-1030, Nov. 17, 1925.

Boikan, William S.; and Gunnar, Rolf M.: Aberrant conduction in supraventricular extrasystoles elim-
    inated by exercise. Amer. Heart J. 47:626-629, Apr., 1954. (Chicago)

Bojanovský, I.; and Filip, J.: The influence of exhausting graded exercise on the level and compo-
    sition of the blood serum proteins in trained athletes. Rev. Czech. Med. 2:339-345, 1956.

Bojesen, Ejgil; and Egense, Johan: Elimination of endogenous corticosteroids in vivo: the effects of
    hepatectomy and total abdominal evisceration in the acutely adrenalectomized cat, and the effect
    of muscular exercise and insulin administration on the isolated hindquarter preparation. Acta
    Endocr. 33:347-369, Mar., 1960. (Copenhagen)

Boldero, H.: The physiology and pathology of exercise. Middlesex Hosp. J. 18:217-228, 1914-1915.

Bolt, W.; and Phlippen, R.: Die Herzleistungsreserven bei angeborenen und erworbenen Herzfehlern
    im Vergleich zur Altersnorm. Cardiologia 43:239-255, 1963. (Köln)

Bonnet, De l'exercice des fonctions considéré dans ses rapports avec l'hygiène et la thérapeutique.
    Gaz. Med. Lyon 2:189; 205, 1850.

Boothby, Walter M.: A determination of the circulation rate in man at rest and at work. The
    regulation of the circulation. Amer. J. Physiol. 37:383-417, May, 1915. (Boston)

----, and Berry, Frank B.: The effect of work on the percentage of haemoglobin and number of
    red corpuscles in the blood. Amer. J. Physiol. 37:378-382, May, 1915. (Boston)

Borelli, Giovanni Alfonso: De motu animalium. Ed. Novissima. Lugduni in Batavia, P. vander
    Aa, 1710.

Borg, Gunnar: Bestämning av motivationens inverkan på fysisk prestation. (Determination of
    motivations influencing physical work capacity) (Swed). Nord. Psykiat. T. 18:591-596, 1964.

Borg, Gunnar, and Dahlström, Hans: The perception of muscular work, a psychophysical study of
    short-time work on the bicycle ergometer. Umea (Sweden), Vetenskapliga Biblioteket, 1960.

----, and ----: (Psychophysical study of work on the bicycle ergometer) (Swed). Nord. Med.
    62:1383-1386, Sept. 17, 1959.

----, and ----: The reliability and validity of a physical work test. Acta Physiol. Scand.
    55:353-361, Aug., 1962. (Lund)

Borgatti, E.; Altilia, F.; Pascucci, E.; and Bracchetti, D.: Sulle modificazioni del flusso ematico
    locale indotte dal lavoro muscolare nell 'uomo. Boll. Soc. Ital. Biol. Sper. 39:269-273,
    Mar. 15, 1963.

Borghetti, A.; Canaletti, R.; Ferrari, S.; Greca, G.; and Novarini, A.: Studio delle modificazioni
    elettrocardiografiche in lavoro aerobico ed anaerotico e nella fase di ricupero. Gior. Clin.
    Med. 42:857-867, Aug., 1961.

Borney, G.: La portata cardiaca, a riposo e dopo sforzo, determinata con un metodo fisico indiretto
    su 100 silicotici in vario stadio. Minerva Cardioangiol. 11:707-710, Nov., 1963.

Bornstein, A.: Eine Methode zur vergleichenden Messung des Herzschlagvolumens beim Menschen.
    Pflüger Arch. ges. Physiol. 132:307-318, Apr. 26, 1910. (Hamburg)

Borský, I.; and Hubač, M.: Zmeny počtu eozinofilov v periférnej krvi po statickom a dynamickom
    zatáženi. (Changes in the eosinophil count in the peripheral blood following static and
    dynamic work loads) (Cz). Prac. Lek. 16:193-197, July, 1964.

Botelho, Stella Y.; Cander, Leon; and Guiti, Nasser: Passive and active tension-length diagrams of
    intact skeletal muscle in normal women of different ages. J. Appl. Physiol. 7:93-98, July,
    1954. (Philadelphia)

Bouhuys, A.: De bepaling von het lichamelijk arbeidsvermogen bij de mens. 1. Onderzoek von-
    gezonde personen. Nederl. T. Geneesk. 105:1877-1887, Sept. 23, 1961.

----, Hagstam, K.-E.; and Lundin, G.: Efficiency of pulmonary ventilation during rest and light
    exercise. A study of alveolar nitrogen wash-out curves in normal subjects. Acta Physiol.
    Scand. 35:289-304, Feb. 20, 1956. (Lund)

Bouisset, S.; and Monod, H.: Étude de la consommation d'oxygène et de la ventilation pulmonaire
    pour différents cas de travail dynamique du membre supérieur. J. Physiologie 53:281-282,
    Mar.-Apr., 1961.

Bour, H.: (The lipid requirements of athletes) (Fr). Bull. Soc. Sci. Hyg. Aliment. 51:63-76,
    1963.

Bourdon, Isidore: Recherches sur le mécanisme de la respiration et sur la circulation du sang.
    Paris, S. Baillière, 1820.

Bourguignon, A.; and Scherrer, J.: Influence de l'entraînement musculaire et de la fatigue sur
    la puissance critique du travail dynamique local. Comptes Rend. Soc. Biol. 154:921-924,
    May 14, 1960. (Paris)

Boussingault, Jean Baptiste Jospeh Dieudonné: Analyses comparées de l'aliment consummé et des
    excréments rendus par une tourterelle, enterprises pour rechercher s'il y a exhalation d'azote
    pendant la respiration des granivores. Ann. Chim. Phys. Sér. 3. 11:433-456, 1844.

Bovet, Daniel; and Amorico, Luigi: Effet de l'amphétamine sur une réaction conditionnée a'évitement an cours d'un exercice prolongé. Comptes Rend. Acad. Sci. 256:3901-3904, Apr. 29, 1963. (Rome)

Bowen, Wilbur P.: Changes in heart-rate, blood-pressure, and duration of systole resulting from bicycling. Amer. J. Physiol. 11:59-77, Apr., 1904. (Ann Arbor)

Boyle, Robert W.; and Scott, F. H.: Some observations on the effect of exercise on the blood, lymph and muscle in its relation to muscle soreness. Amer. J. Physiol. 122:569-584, June, 1938. (Minneapolis)

Boys, Floyd; and Curry, E. Thayer: Measurement of auditory thresholds before and after strenuous physical exercise; a preliminary report. Ann. Otol. 65:190-197, Mar., 1956. (Urbana)

Bradbury, Pamela A.; Fox, R. H.; Goldsmith, R.; and Hampton, I. F. G.: The effect of exercise on temperature regulation. J. Physiol. 171:384-396, June, 1964. (London)

Bradford, E. H.: Health of rowing men. Sanitarian 5:529-536, 1877.

Brainard, John B.: Effect of prolonged exercise on atherogenesis in the rabbit. Proc. Soc. Exper. Biol. Med. 100:244-246, Feb., 1959. (Minneapolis)

Brambilla, I.; and Cerretelli, P.: Determinazione del massimo consumo di ossigeno nel lavoro muscolare. Boll. Soc. Ital. Biol. Sper. 34:676-679, June 30, 1958.

Brandi, G.; and Brambilla, I.: Arterio-venous difference of oxygen, cardiac output and stroke volume in function of the energy consumption. Int. Zeits. angew. Physiol. 19:130-133, Nov. 28, 1961. (Modena)

----, and Soro, A.: (Research on bloodless methods of determination of the difference in arterial and venous CO_2 and on the behavior of the stroke volume during muscular work) (It). Arch. Fisiol. 62:1-12, Apr. 10, 1963.

----, and ----: Variazioni della gettata pulsatoria durante lavoro. Boll. Soc. Ital. Biol. Sper. 38:854-856, Sept. 15, 1962.

Brandis, S. A.; Gorkin, Z. D.; and Gorkin, M. Y.: Physiologische Analyse der Leibesübungen und ihre Wirkung auf die Arbeitsfähigkeit. Fiziol. Zh. 18:191-204, 1935.

----, and Pilovitskaya, V. N.: Prolonged breathing of a gas mixture high in O_2 and low in CO_2 at rest and during exercise. Fed. Proc. (Transl. Suppl.) 22:86-90, Jan.-Feb., 1963. (Donetsk, U.S.S.R.)

Brassfield, Charles R.: Peripheral chemical control of pulmonary ventilation. Proc. Soc. Exper. Biol. Med. 26:833, June, 1929. (Ann Arbor)

Braunwald, Eugene; Chidsey, Charles A.; Harrison, Donald C.; Gaffney, Thomas E.; and Kahler, Richard L.: Studies on the function of the adrenergic nerve endings in the heart. Circulation 28:958-969, Nov., 1963. (Bethesda)

----, and Kelly, Eugene R.: The effects of exercise on central blood volume in man. J. Clin. Invest. 39:413-419, Feb., 1960. (Bethesda)

Brebbia, D. R.; Goldman, R. F.; and Buskirk, E. R.: Water vapor loss from the respiratory tract during outdoor exercise in the cold. J. Appl. Physiol. 11:219-222, Sept., 1957. (Natick)

----, ----, and ----: Water vapor loss from the respiratory tract during outdoor exercise in the cold. Environ. Protect.Div. QM Res. and Devel. Center, U. S. Army. Tech. Rep. EP-57, May, 1957.

Brecher, Gerhard A.: Venous return. New York, Grune and Stratton, 1956.

Brechter, C. L.; and Forsby, N. H.: (On the influence of physical exertion on experimental rabbit atheromatosis, induced by administration of saturated fats and cholesterol-free diet) (Ger). Zeits. Ernährungswiss. 3:95-110, Oct., 1962.

Brendel, W.: (Temperature increases in man) (Ger). Hippokrates 34:45-53, Jan. 31, 1963.

Brendstrup, Per: Late edema after muscular exercise. Arch. Phys. Med. 43:401-405, Aug., 1962. (Virum, Denmark)

Brennemann, Joseph: Disparity between oral and rectal temperatures after exercise. Amer. J. Dis. Child. 66:16-20, July, 1943. (Los Angeles)

Bridge, Ezra V.; Henry, Franklin M.; Cook, Sherburne F.; Williams, O. L.; Lyons, William R.; and Lawrence, John H.: Decompression sickness; nature and incidence of symptoms during and after artificial decompression to 38,000 feet for 90 minutes with exercise during exposure. J. Aviation Med. 15:316-327, Oct., 1944. (Berkeley)

Briggs, Henry: Physical exertion, fitness and breathing. J. Physiol. 54:292-318, Dec. 7, 1920. (Edinburgh)

----: Physical exertion, fitness and breathing. J. Roy. Army Med. Corps. 37:278-301, 1921.

Briol, Auguste Pierre Adolphe Christophe: Contribution à l'étude des réactions cardio-vasculaires consécutives aux exercices physiques. Bordeaux, Delmas, 1937.

Brobeck, John R.: Hypothalamus, appetite, and obesity. Physiol. Physicians 1:1-6, Nov., 1963. (Philadelphia)

Brod, Jan: Haemodynamic basis of acute pressor reactions and hypertension. Brit. Heart J. 25:227-245, Mar., 1963. (Prague)

----, Hejl, Z.; and Ulrych, M.: Metabolic changes in the forearm muscle and skin during emotional muscular vasodilatation. Clin. Sci. 25:1-10, Aug., 1963.

Brody, Samuel: Bioenergetics and growth; with special reference to the efficiency complex in domestic animals. New York, Reinhold, 1945. (Columbia, Missouri)

Broome, T. P.; and Holt, John M.: Venous stasis and forearm exercise during venipuncture as sources of error in plasma electrolyte determinations. Canad. Med. Ass. J. 90:1105-1107, May 9, 1964. (Kingston, Ontario)

Brouha, Lucien: Effects of muscular work and heat on the cardiovascular system. Industr. Med. Surg. 29:114-120, Mar., 1960. (Newark, Del.)

Brouha, Lucien: Heat and the older worker. J. Amer. Geriat. Soc. 10:35-39, Jan., 1962.
(Newark, Del.)

----, Cannon, W. B.; and Dill, D. B.: The heart rate of the sympathectomized dog in rest
and exercise. J. Physiol. 87:345-359, Sept. 8, 1936. (Boston)

----, and Harrington, M. E.: Heart rate and blood pressure reactions of men and women during
and after muscular exercise. J. Lancet 77:79-80, Mar., 1957. (Wilmington, Del.)

----, Maxfield, Mary F.; Smith, Paul E., Jr.; and Stopps, Gordon J.: Discrepancy between heart
rate and oxygen consumption during work in the warmth. J. Appl. Physiol. 18:1095-1098,
Nov., 1963. (Wilmington, Del.)

----, and Savage, B. M.: Variability of physiologic measurements in normal young men at rest
and during muscular work. Rev. Canad. Biol. 4:131-143, 1945.

----, Smith, P. E., Jr.; Delanne, R.; and Maxfield, M. E.: Physiological reactions of men and
women during muscular activity and recovery in various environments. J. Appl. Physiol. 16:
133-140, Jan., 1961. (Wilmington, Del.)

Broun, G. O.: Blood destruction during exercise. I. Blood changes occurring in the course of a
single day of exercise. J. Exp. Med. 36:481-500, Nov., 1922. (New York)

----: Blood destruction during exercise. II. Demonstration of blood destruction in animals exercised
after prolonged confinement. J. Exp. Med. 37:113-130, Jan., 1923. (New York)

----: Blood destruction during exercise. III. Exercise as a bone marrow stimulus. J. Exp. Med.
37:187-206, Feb., 1923. (New York)

----: Blood destruction during exercise. IV. The development of equilibrium between blood
destruction and regeneration after a period of training. J. Exp. Med. 37:207-220, Feb., 1923.
(New York)

Broustet, P.; Sagardiluz, J.; Bricaud, H.; et al: La détermination des possibilités d'effort chez les
cardiaques. Arch. Mal. Coeur (57 Suppl.):56-76, 1964.

Brown, Clark E.; Huang, T. C.; Bortz, Edward L.; and McCay, Clive M.: Observations on blood
vessels and exercise. J. Geront. 11:292-297, July, 1956. (Ithaca)

Brown, Frank J.: Ballistocardiographic study of marathon runners. J. Lancet 77:89-90, Mar.,
1957. (Point Pleasant, N.J.)

Brown, J. R.; and Crowden, G. P.: Energy expenditure ranges and muscular work grades. Brit.
J. Industr. Med. 20:277-283, Oct., 1963. (London)

Browse, Norman: Observations on the activity of surgical patients. Brit. Med. J. 1:669-670,
Mar. 14, 1964. (London)

Bruce, Robert A.: Evaluation of functional capacity and exercise tolerance of cardiac patients.
I. Functional capacity. Mod. Concepts Cardiov. Dis. 25:321-326, Apr., 1956. (Seattle)

----, Blackmon, J. R.; Jones, J. W.; and Strait, G.: Exercising testing in adult normal subjects and
cardiac patients. Pediatrics (32 Suppl.):742-756, Oct., 1963. (Seattle)

----, Cobb, Leonard A.; Katsura, Shigeaki; Morledge, John H.; Andrus, W. Wyman; and Fuller,
Theodore J.: Exertional hypotension in cardiac patients. Circulation 19:543-551, Apr., 1959.
(Seattle)

Bruce, Robert A.; Cobb, Leonard A.; Morledge, John H.; and Katsura, Shigeaki: Effects of posture, upright exercise, and myocardial stimulation on cardiac output in patients with diseases affecting diastolic filling and effective systolic ejection of the left ventricle. Amer. Heart J. 61:476-484, Apr., 1961. (Seattle)

----, ----, and Williams, Robert H.: Effects of exercise and isoproterenol on free fatty acids and carbohydrates in cardiac patients. Amer. J. Med. Sci. 241:59-67, Jan., 1961. (Seattle)

----, Jones, John W.; and Strait, Gail B.: Anaerobic metabolic responses to acute maximal exercise in male athletes. Amer. Heart J. 67:643-650, May, 1964. (Seattle)

----, Lovejoy, Frank W., Jr.; Yu, Paul N. G.; and McDowell, Marion E.: Observations of cardiorespiratory performance in normal subjects under unusual stress during exercise. Arch. Industr. Hyg. Occup. Med. 6:105-112, Aug., 1952. (Rochester, N.Y.)

Brummer, Pekka: Proteinuria of effort and its significance in the diagnosis of congestive heart failure. Acta Med. Scand. 124:252-265, 1946. (Helsinki)

Bruns, O. and Roemer, G. A.: Die Einfluss angestrengter körperlicher Arbeit auf radiographische Herzgrösse, Blutdruck und Puls. Zeits. klin. Med. 94:22-48, 1922. (Göttingen)

Brunton, T. Lauder: Exercise and over-exercise. Quart. Med. J. Sheffield 7:107-135, Jan., 1898-1899.

----: On the physiological basis of physical education; address to inspectors, South-Western Polytechnic, Chelsea, April, 1905. London, Harrison and Sons, 1905.

----, and Tunnicliffe, F. W.: Remarks on the effect of resistance exercise upon the circulation in man, local and general. Brit. Med. J. 2:1073-1075, Oct. 16, 1897. (London)

Bryan, A. C.; Bentivoglio, L. G.; Beerel, F.; MacLeish, H.; Zidulka, A.; and Bates, D. V.: Factors affecting regional distribution of ventilation and perfusion in the lung. J. Appl. Physiol. 19:395-402, May, 1964. (Montreal)

Bryce, Lucy M.: March haemoglobinuria: description of the features of this condition, and report of a case. Med. J. Aust. 2:49-52, July 15, 1944.

Buchanan, Florence: The physiological significance of the pulse rate. Trans. Oxford Scientific Club. No. 34, page 35, 1909.

Bucht, H.; Ek, J.; Eliasch, H.; Holmgren, A.; Josephson, B.; and Werko, L.: The effect of exercise in the recumbent position on the renal circulation and sodium excretion in normal individuals. Acta Physiol. Scand. 28:95-100, May 30, 1953. (Stockholm)

Buchthal, Fritz; Høncke, P.; and Linhard, J.: Temperature measurements in human muscles in situ at rest and during muscular work. Acta Physiol. Scand. 8:230-258, Dec. 8, 1944. (Copenhagen)

Budnick, Thea: Untersuchungen über Blutdruck und Puls bei dosierter Arbeit und gymnastischen Uebungen. Kallmünz, M. Lassleben, 1934. (München)

Bühlmann, A.: Oxymetrie, Arbeitsversuche und Bestimmung der Arbeitsfähigkeit. Schweiz. med. Wschr. 81:374-376, Apr. 21, 1951.

Bühlmann, A.: Thoraxerweiterung und Lungenvolumzunahme bei verschiedener Arbeit und bei
vermindertem atmosphärischem Druck. Helv. Physiol. Pharmacol. Acta 8:286-296,
Oct., 1950. (Basel)

----, and Hofstetter, J. R.: Arbeitsversuche in mittlern Höhen. Helv. Physiol. Pharmacol.
Acta 9:222-226, June, 1951. (St. Moritz and Zurich)

----, and Rossier, P. H.: (Arterial blood gases and electrolytes during physical work) (Ger).
Zeits. Biol. 111:235-240, Oct., 1959.

----, Scherrer, M.; and Herzog, H.: Vorschläge zur einheitlichen Beurteilung der Arbeitsfähigkeit
durch die Lungenfunktionsprüfung. Schweiz. med. Wschr. 91:105-109, Jan. 28, 1961.
(Zurich, Bern and Basel)

Bugard, P.; Henry, M.; Plas, F.; and Chailley-Bert, P.: Les corticoïdes et l'aldosterone dans
l'effort prolongé du sportif. Indication avec les métabolismes. Rev. Path. Gen. 61:
159-175, Jan., 1961. (Paris)

Bugyi, B.: (On the mechanism of acidosis during the course of muscular effort) (Fr). Poumon
Coeur 15:1021-1023, Nov., 1959.

----: Wirkung körperlicher Anstrengungen auf die Magentätigkeit; Beiträge zu den Untersuchungs-
methoden der Magenkrankheiten. Deutsch. Zeits. Verdauungskr. 16:38-40, 1956.

Bullen, Beverly A.; Monello, Lenore F.; Cohen, Haskel; and Mayer, Jean: Attitudes towards
physical activity, food and family in obese and nonobese adolescent girls. Amer. J. Clin.
Nutr. 12:1-11, Jan., 1963. (Boston)

----, Reed, Robert B.; and Mayer, Jean: Physical activity of obese and nonobese adolescent girls
appraised by motion picture sampling. Amer. J. Clin. Nutr. 14:211-223, Apr., 1964.
(Boston)

Burch, George E.; and DePasquale, Nicholas P.: Cardiac performance in relation to blood volume.
Amer. J. Cardiol. 14:784-795, Dec., 1964. (New Orleans)

Burcq, V.: École de gymnastique de Joinville; influence des exercices sur les forces musculaires,
sur le volume et le poids du corps et la capacité pulmonaire; résumé. Gaz. Med. Paris,
6° série 4:473-475, 1822.

Bürgi, Emil: Der respiratorische Gaswechsel bei Ruhe und Arbeit auf Bergen. Leipzig, Veit and
Co., 1900. (Bern)

Burk, Dean: The free energy of glycogen-lactic acid breakdown in muscle. Proc. Roy. Soc.
104B:153-170, 1929. (London)

Burke, Hugh E.; and Mankiewicz, Edith: The pathogenesis of intrapleurally induced tuberculosis
in guinea pigs including some observations on the effects of rest and exercise. Amer. Rev.
Resp. Dis. 88:360-375, Sept., 1963. (Montreal)

Burke, W. E.; Tuttle, W. W.; Thompson, C. W.; Janney, C. D.; and Weber, R. J.: The relation
of grip strength and grip-strength endurance to age. J. Appl. Physiol. 5:628-630, Apr.,
1953. (Iowa City)

Burkhardt, W. L.; Adler, H. F.; Thometz, A. F.; Atkinson, A. J.; and Ivy, A. C.: Decompression
sickness; factors which affect incidence of bends at altitude. J.A.M.A. 133:373-377, Feb. 8,
1947. (Chicago)

Burt, J. J.; Blyth, C. S.; and Rierson, H. A.: The effects of exercise on the coagulation fibrinolysis equilibrium. J. Sport Med. 4:213-216, Dec., 1964.

----, and Martorano, J. J.: Regional variations in blood lactate concentrations. U. S. Naval Med. Field Res. Lab. 13:1-8, Aug., 1963.

Buskirk, E.; Taylor, H. L.; and Simonson, E.: Relationships between obesity and pulse rate at rest and during work in young and older men. Int. Zeits. angew. Physiol. 16:83-89, 1955.

Buskirk, E. R.; Thompson, R. H.; Lutwak, L.; and Whedon, G. D.: Energy balance of obese patients during weight reduction: influence of diet restriction and exercise. Ann. N. Y. Acad. Sci. 110:918-940, Sept. 26, 1963. (Bethesda)

----, Welch, B. E.; and Iampietro, P. F.: Variations in resting metabolism with changes in food, exercise and climate. Army Med. Nutrition Lab. Rep. 215, Oct. 14, 1957.

Busnengo, E.: (Quantitative evaluation of the ballistocardiogram after muscular work) (It). Riv. Med. Aero. 23:385-396, July-Sept., 1960.

Byck, Robert; and Hearst, Eliot: Adjustment of monkeys to five continuous days of work. Science 138:43-44, Oct. 5, 1962. (Washington)

Byford, William H.: On the physiology of exercise. Amer. J. Med. Sci., n.s. 30:32-42, July, 1855. (Evansville)

----: Physiology, pathology, and therapeutics of muscular exercise. Chicago, J. Barnet, 1858.

----: Physiology, pathology, and therapeutics of muscular exercise. Chicago Med. J., n.s. 15:357-382, 1858.

Bywaters, E. G. L.; and Dible, J. H.: Acute paralytic myohaemoglobinuria in man. J. Path. Bact. 55:7-15, Jan., 1943. (London)

Caccuri, S.; Graziani, G.; Fusco, M.; Mole, R.; and Vecchione, C.: (The Master test according to Ford and Hellerstein in normal subjects) (It). Cuore Circ. 46:121-135, June, 1962.

Cairella, M.; Francesconi, A.; and Vecchi, L.: Variazioni della clearance epatica frazionata del rosa-bengala I 131 negli sportivi (canottieri) dopo prova da sforzo. Ann. Med. Nav. 68: 941-946, Nov.-Dec., 1963.

----, Policreti, C.; Trasatti, M.; et al: Variazioni del contenuto in acido piruvico del fegato di ratti sottoposti a sforzo fisico prolungato. Ann. Med. Nav. 69:557-562, July-Aug., 1964.

Caldwell, L. S.: Relative muscle loading and endurance. Rep. 486. U. S. Army Med. Res. Lab. 1-11, July 29, 1963.

Calvy, G. L.; Cady, L. D.; Mufson, M. A.; Nierman, J.; and Gertler, M. M.: Serum lipids and enzymes. Their levels after high-caloric, high-fat intake and vigorous exercise regimen in Marine Corps recruit personnel. J.A.M.A. 183:1-4, Jan. 5, 1963. (New York)

----, Coffin, Lawrence H., Jr.; Gertler, Menard M.; and Cady, Lee D.: The effect of strenuous exercise on serum lipids and enzymes. Milit. Med. 129:1012-1016, Nov., 1964.

Camerada, P.; Congiu, M.; and Leo, P.: (Effect of muscular work on the fibrinolytic potential of the plasma) (It). Rass. Med. Sarda 62:1037-1041, Nov.-Dec., 1960.

Campbell, J. Argyll: Concerning the influence of atmospheric conditions upon the pulse rate and "oxygen debt" after running. Proc. Roy. Soc. 96B:43-59, Feb. 1, 1924. (Hampstead, Eng.)

Campbell, J. M. H.; Douglas, C. G.; Haldane, J. S.; and Hobson, F. G.: The response of the respiratory centre to carbonic acid, oxygen, and hydrogen ion concentration. J. Physiol. 46:301-318, July 18, 1913. (Oxford)

----, ----, and Hobson, F. G.: Respiratory exchange of man during and after muscular exercise. Phil. Trans. Roy. Soc. 210B:1-47, 1921.

----, Mitchell, G. O.; and Powell, A. T. W.: The influence of exercise on digestion. Guy's Hosp. Rep. 78:279-293, July, 1928.

Campos, F. A. de M.; Cannon, W. B.; Lundin, H.; and Walker, T. T.: Some conditions affecting the capacity for prolonged muscular work. Amer. J. Physiol. 87:680-701, Jan., 1929. (Boston)

Canappe, Jean: Du mouvement des muscles. Lyon, 1541; Movimento musulorum. Paris, 1546.

Cannon, W. B.: The emergency function of the adrenal medulla in pain and the major emotions. Amer. J. Physiol. 33:356-372, Feb. 2, 1914. (Boston)

----, Lewis, J. T.; and Britton, S. W.: Studies on the conditions of activity in endocrine glands. XVII. A lasting preparation of the denervated heart for detecting internal secretion, with evidence for accessory accelerator fibers from the thoracic sympathetic chain. Amer. J. Physiol. 77:326-352, July, 1926. (Cambridge)

----, and Nice, L. B.: The effect of adrenal secretion on muscular fatigue. Amer. J. Physiol. 32:44-60, May 1, 1913. (Boston)

Cannon, W. B.; and Uridil, J. E.: Studies on the conditions of activity in endocrine glands. VIII. Some effects on the denervated heart of stimulating the nerves of the liver. Amer. J. Physiol. 58:353-364, Dec., 1921. (Boston)

Cantone, A.: Effetto del lavoro muscolare sulla quantità di alimento ingerito. Arch. Sci. Biol. 48:277-284, July-Sept., 1964.

----: Physical effort and its effect in reducing alimentary hyperlipaemia. J. Sport Med. 4:32-36, Mar., 1964.

----, and Cerretelli, P.: The effect of muscular work on serum aldolase activity in trained and untrained man. Int. Zeits. angew. Physiol. 18:107-111, 1960.

----, and ----: Effect of training on proteinuria following muscular exercise. Int. Zeits. angew. Physiol. 18:324-329, 1960.

Capen, E. K.: Study of 4 programs of heavy resistance exercises for development of muscular strength. Res. Quart. 27:132-142, May, 1956.

Carbery, William J.; Toller, Walter E.; and Freiman, Alvin H.: A system for monitoring the ECG under dynamic conditions. Aerospace Med. 31:131-137, Feb., 1960. (Deer Park, N.Y. and New York)

Cardanus, Hieronymus: De subtilitate et de rerum varietate. Venezia, 1562.

Cardinet, G. H., III; Fowler, M. E.; and Tyler, W. S.: The effects of training, exercise, and tying-up on serum transaminase activities in the horse. Amer. J. Vet. Res. 24:980-984, Sept., 1963.

----, ----, and ----: Heart rates and respiratory rates for evaluating performance in horses during endurance trail ride competition. J. Amer. Vet. Med. Ass. 143:1303-1309, Dec., 15, 1963.

Cardot, H.; Régnier, J.; Santensise, D.; and Varé, P.: Influence de l'activité musculaire sur l'excitabilité corticale. Comptes Rend. Soc. Biol. 97:698-701, Aug. 26, 1927. (Lyon)

Carlens, Eric; and Dahlstrom, Gunnar: The clinical evaluation of bronchospirometry with special reference to posture and exercise. Amer. Rev. Resp. Dis. 83:202-207, Feb., 1961.

Carlin, M. Richard; Mueller, C. Barber; and White, H. L.: Effects of exercise on renal blood flow and sodium excretion in dogs. J. Appl. Physiol. 3:291-294, Nov., 1950. (St. Louis)

Carlson, Lars A.; Havel, Richard I.; Ekelung, Lars-Göran; and Holmgren, Alf: Effect of nicotinic acid on the turnover rate and oxidation of the free fatty acids of plasma in man during exercise. Metabolism 12:837-845, Sept., 1963. (Stockholm)

----, and Mossfeldt, Folke: Acute effects of prolonged, heavy exercise on the concentration of plasma lipids and lipoproteins in man. Acta Physiol. Scand. 62:51-59, Sept.-Oct., 1964. (Stockholm)

----, and Pernow, Bengt. Oxygen utilization and lactic acid formation in the legs at rest and during exercise in normal subjects and in patients with arteriosclerosis obliterans. Acta Med. Scand. 164: 39-52, May 9, 1959. (Stockholm)

Carlson, Lars A.; and Pernow, Bengt: Studies on blood lipids during exercise. I. Arterial and venous plasma concentrations of unesterified fatty acids. J. Lab. Clin. Med. 53:833-841, June, 1959. (Stockholm)

----, and ----: Studies on blood lipids during exercise. II. The arterial plasma-free fatty acid concentration during and after exercise and its regulation. J. Lab. Clin. Med. 58:673-681, Nov., 1961. (Stockholm)

----, and ----: Studies on blood lipids during exercise. III. Arterial concentration of plasma-free fatty acids during short periods of exercise in normal women and in subjects with low physical working capacity due to vasoregulatory asthenia. J. Lab. Clin. Med. 60:655-661, Oct., 1962. (Stockholm)

Carlsten, A.; Hallgren, B.; Jagenburg, R.; Svanborg, A.; and Werkö, L.: Arterial concentrations of free fatty acids and free amino acids in healthy human individuals at rest and at different work loads. Scand. J. Clin. Lab. Invest. 14:185-191, 1962. (Göteborg)

----, ----, ----, ----, and ----: Myocardial metabolism of glucose, lactic acid, amino acids and fatty acids in healthy human individuals at rest and at different work loads. Verh. deutsch. Ges. Kreislaufforsch. 27:195-196, 1961.

Carns, Marie L.; Schade, Maja L.; Liba, Marie R.; Hellebrandt, F. A.; and Harris, Chester W.: Segmental volume reduction by localized versus generalized exercise. Hum. Biol. 32:370-376, 1960. (Madison)

Carpenter, Thorne M.: Tables, factors and formulas for computing respiratory exchange and biological transformations of energy. 3rd edition. Washington, Carnegie Institute, 1939.

----, and Fox, Edward L.: The effect of muscular work upon the respiratory exchange of man after the ingestion of glucose and of fructose. I. The respiratory quotient and the mechanics of breathing. Arbeitsphysiol. 4:532-569, 1931. (Boston)

----, and ----: The effect of muscular work upon the respiratory exchange of man after the ingestion of glucose and of fructose. II. Heat production, efficiency, oxygen debt, excess respiratory quotient, and metabolism of carbohydrates. Arbeitsphysiol. 4:570-599, 1931.

Carrière, Rita; and Isler, H.: Effect of frequent housing changes and of muscular exercise on the thyroid gland of mice. Endocrinology 64:414-418, Mar., 1959. (Montreal)

Carter, A. Barham; Richards, R. L.; and Zachary, R. B.: The anterior tibial syndrome. Lancet 2:928-934, Nov. 19, 1949. (Middlesex, Oxford and Sheffield)

Cassels, Donald E.; and Morse, Minerva: Blood volume and exercise. J. Pediat. 20:352-364, Mar., 1942. (Chicago)

----, and Murrell, D. Shirley: The effect of exercise on left to right shunt of blood through a ventricular septal defect. Dis. Chest 36:73-80, July, 1959. (Chicago)

Cassinis, U.; and Adilardi, G.: Il chloro di sodio nel lavoro muscolare del soldato. Boll. Soc. Ital. Biol. Sper. 6:1034-1036, Dec., 1931. (Also in Gior. Med. Milit. 80:61-69, Feb., 1932.)

Castelfranco, M.; Ghiringelli, G.; and Piane, C.: Il consumo di ossigeno durante lavoro dei soggetti cardiopatici, prima e dopo digitalizzazione acute. Folia Cardiol. 16:45-70, Feb. 28, 1957.

Castelfranco, M.; Ghiringelli, G.; and Piane, C.: Sulle modalità di contrazione del debito di O_2 durante lavoro aerobico ed anaerobico. Folia Cardiol. 17:211-230, June 30, 1958.

Castren, O.: Urinary excretion of noradrenaline and adrenaline in late normal and toxemic pregnancy. Effect of rest, work, and reserpine treatment. Acta Pharmacol. 20(Suppl. 2): 1-98, 1963.

Casula, D.; Cherchi, P.; Fulghesu, G. and Spinazzola, A.: (Muscular work and blood coagulation) (It). Gior. Clin. Med. 42:619-638, June, 1961.

Catelli, P.; and Privitera, A.: Considerazioni sul test di Master "doppio" nel giovane sano. Cuore Circ. 47:202-210, Aug., 1963.

Cathcart, E. P.; and Burnett, W. A.: The influence of muscle work on metabolism in varying conditions of diet. Proc. Roy. Soc. 99B:405-426, May 1, 1926. (Glasgow)

----, Richardson, D. T.; and Campbell, W.: Studies in muscle activity. II. The influence of speed on the mechanical efficiency. J. Physiol. 58:355-361, Mar. 14, 1924. (Glasgow)

Cavagna, G. A.; Saibene, F. P.; and Margaria, R.: Mechanical work in running. J. Appl. Physiol. 19:249-256, Mar., 1964.

----, ----, and ----: (Simultaneous registration in 3 spatial directions of acceleration to which one is subjected during marching) (It). Boll. Soc. Ital. Biol. Sper. 36:1802-1804, Dec. 31, 1960.

----, ----, and ----: (Work completed against gravity during marching at various speeds) (It). Boll. Soc. Ital. Biol. Sper. 36:1804-1806, Dec. 31, 1960.

Cerretelli, P.; and Brambilla, I.: Cinetica della contrazione di un debito di O_2 nell'uomo. Boll. Soc. Ital. Biol. Sper. 34:679-682, July 15, 1958.

----, Cantone, A.; and Chiumello, G.: (Behavior of free fatty acids in the blood (NEFA) as a function of the duration and intensity of muscular work) (It). Boll. Soc. Ital. Biol. Sper. 37:1660-1662, Dec. 31, 1961.

----, ----, and Respighi, E.: (Quantitative and qualitative changes induced by training on proteinuria of effort) (It). Boll. Soc. Ital. Biol. Sper. 36:1276-1278, Nov. 30, 1960.

----, Piiper, J.; and Mangili, F.: Il costo energetico della corsa nei cani. Boll. Soc. Ital. Biol. Sper. 39:1806-1809, Dec. 31, 1963.

----, ----, ----, et al: Aerobic and anerobic metabolism in exercising dogs. J. Appl. Physiol. 19:25-28, Jan., 1964.

----, ----, ----, et al: Impiego del metodo della termodiluizione (T.D.M.) per la determinazione della gettata cardiaca nel cane durante lavoro. Boll. Soc. Ital. Biol. Sper. 39:2038-2040, Dec. 31, 1963.

----, ----, ----, Cuttica, F.; and Ricci, B.: Circulation in exercising dogs. J. Appl. Physiol. 19:29-32, Jan., 1964. (Milan and Göttingen)

Chaffee, William R.; Smulyan, Harold; Keighley, John F.; and Eich, Robert H.: The effect of exercise on pulmonary blood volume. Amer. Heart J. 66:657-663, Nov., 1963. (Syracuse)

Chagovets, N. R.: Izmenenie soderzhaniia limonnoĭ i shchavelouksusnoĭ kislot v myshtsakh pre razlichnykh funktsional'nykh sostoianilakh. (Changes in the content of citric and oxalic acids in muscles in various functional conditions) (Russ). Ukr. Biokhim Zh. 36:499-505, 1964.

Chaiken, Bernard H.; Whalen, Edward J.; Learner, Norman; and Smith, Nathan J.: Variants of "march hemoglobinuria". Amer. J. Med. Sci. 225:514-520, May, 1953. (Fort Dix, N.J. and Philadelphia)

Chailley-Bert, P.: Actions physiologiques des activités physiques. Rev. Prat. 7:2057-2059, July 1, 1957.

----, Labignette, P.; and Fabre-Chevalier (Mme): Contribution à l'étude des variations du cholestérol sanguin au cours des activités physiques. Presse Méd. 63:415-416, Mar. 19, 1955.

----, Plas, F.; Abou., Henry M.; and Bugard, P.: (Metabolic modifications during prolonged exertion in the athlete) (Fr). Rev. Path. Gen. 61:143-157, Jan., 1961.

----, ----, and Pallardy, G.: Le métabolisme protidique au cours de l'effort prolongé. Presse Méd. 70:705-707, Mar. 24, 1962. (Paris)

----, ----, and Talbot: Modifications de l'électrocardiogramme observées au cours d'un effort cycliste de longue durée. Arch. Mal. Coeur 49:910-915, Oct., 1956.

Chamberlain, D. A.; and Howard, Jane: The haemodynamic effects of beta-sympathetic blockage. Brit. Heart J. 26:213-217, Mar., 1964. (London)

Champigny, Odette: Influence d'une double restriction énergétique et protidique (quantitative et qualitative) sur la gestation et la lactation de la ratte. Comptes Rend. Acad. Sci. 254:1155-1157, Feb. 5, 1962. (Bellevue, Seine-et-Oise)

Chapman, Carleton B.; Baker, Orland; and Mitchell, Jere H.: Left ventricular function at rest and during exercise. J. Clin. Invest. 38:1202-1213, July, 1959. (Dallas)

----, Fisher, Joseph N.; and Sproule, Brian J.: Behavior of stroke volume at rest and during exercise in human beings. J. Clin. Invest. 39:1208-1213, Aug., 1960. (Dallas)

----, Henschel, Austin; Minckler, John; Forsgren, Arthur; and Keys, Ancel: The effect of exercise on renal plasma flow in normal male subjects. J. Clin. Invest. 27:639-644, Sept., 1948. (Minneapolis)

Chapman, Carrie E.; Hollander, A. Gerson: Tuberculosis and rehabilitation: dynamic physical restoration of patients with active disease. Calif. Med. 100:88-91, Feb., 1964. (Los Angeles and Oakland)

Chardack, William M.: Heart block treated with an implantable pacemaker. Past experience and current developments. Progr. Cardiov. Dis. 6:507-537, May, 1964. (Buffalo)

Charvát, J.; Polák, H.; and Němec, J.: The influence of stress conditions on the motility of human leukocytes. Int. Rec. Med. 170:672-677, Dec., 1957. (Prague)

Chauderon, J.: (The practical physiology of work) (Fr). Maroc Med. 42:161-176, Feb., 1963.

Chauveau, A.: Source et nature du potentiel directement utilisé dans le travail musculaire, d'après les échanges respiratoires, chez l'homme en état d'abstinence. Comptes Rend. Acad. Sci. 122: 1163-1169, May 26, 1896.

----: Du travail physiologique et de son équivalence. Paris, (Quantin), 1888 (Also in Rev. Scient., 3rd series 15:129-139, 1888.)

----, and Kaufmann: Nouveaux documents sur les relations qui existent entre le travail chimique et le travail mécanique du tissu musculaire. De l'activité nutritive et respiratiore des muscles qui functionnent physiologiquement sans produire de travail mécanique. Comptes Rend. Acad. Sci. 104:1763-1769, June 20, 1887.

----, Tissot; and DeVarigny: La destination immédiate des aliments gras, d'après la détermination, par les échanges respiratoires, de la nature du potentiel directement utilisé dans le travail musculaire chez l'homme en digestion d'une ration de graisse. Comptes Rend. Acad. Sci. 122:1169-1172, May 26, 1896.

Chavany, J. A.: La céphalée à l'effort. Presse Méd. 53:645, Nov. 24, 1945.

Chebanova, O. V.: Izmeneniia myshechnoi rabotosposobnosti v protsesse forminovaniia i narusheniia drigatel'nogo dinamicheskogo stereotipa razlichnoi slozhnosti. (Modification of muscular work capacity during the process of formation and disorders of the motor dynamic stereotype of varied complexity) (Russ). Gig. Tr. Prof. Zabol. 7:21-27, Oct., 1963.

Chevalier, Robert B.; Bowers, John A.; Bondurant, Stuart; and Ross, Joseph C.: Circulatory and ventilatory effects of exercise in smokers and nonsmokers. J. Appl. Physiol. 18:357-360, Mar., 1963. (Indianapolis)

Chevallier, P.: (The adenopathy of muscular work) (Fr). Rev. Med. Moyen Orient 18:7-10, Jan.-Feb., 1961.

Chevat, H.; Demaille, A.; and Bertrand, M.: (Renal manifestations during prolonged muscular exertion) (Fr). Lille Med. 6:847-849, Nov., 1961.

Chiavaro, A.; Dagianti, A.; Angrisani, P.; et al: Il comportamento della diffusione alveolo-capillare del CO durante sforzo muscolare progressivamente crescente in soggetti mitralici in buone condizioni emodinamiche. II. Boll. Soc. Ital. Cardiol. 8:634-638, 1963.

Chidsey, Charles A.; Harrison, Donald C.; and Braunwald, Eugene: Augmentation of the plasma nor-epinephrine response to exercise in patients with congestive heart failure. New Eng. J. Med. 267:650-654, Sept. 27, 1962. (Bethesda)

Chirico, Anna-Marie; and Stunkard, Albert J.: Physical activity and human obesity. New Eng. J. Med. 263:935-940, Nov. 10, 1960. (Philadelphia)

Christensen, B. C.: Studies on the effort syndrome. I. The patients' capacity for work and the variations in the arterial pressures and pulse rate during muscular work compared with conditions found in normals. Acta Med. Scand. 121:194-216, 1945. (Copenhagen)

----: Studies on the effort syndrome. II. The conditions of the large arteries during muscular work illustrated by oscillometric measurements. Acta Med. Scand. 121:319-332, 1945. (Copenhagen)

Christensen, Erik Hohwü: Beiträge zur Physiologie schwerer körperlicher Arbeit. I. Die Blutzucker
   währent und nach körperlicher Arbeit. Arbeitsphysiol. 4:128-153, 1931. (Copenhagen)

----: Beiträge zur Physiologie schwerer körperlicher Arbeit. II. Die Körpertemperatur während
   und unmittelbar nach schwerer körperlicher Arbeit. Arbeitsphysiol. 4:154-174, 1931.

----: Beiträge zur physiologie schwerer körperlicher Arbeit. III. Gasanalytische Methoden zur
   Bestimmung des Herzminutenvolumens in Ruhe und während körperlicher Arbeit. Arbeitsphysiol.
   4:175-202, 1931.

----: Beiträge zur Physiologie schwerer körperlicher Arbeit. IV. Die Pulsfrequenz während und
   unmittelbar nach schwerer körperlicher Arbeit. Arbeitsphysiol. 4:453-469, 1931. (Copenhagen)

----: Beiträge zur Physiologie schwerer körperlicher Arbeit. V. Minutenvolumen und Schlagvolumen
   des Herzens während schwerer körperlicher Arbeit. Arbeitsphysiol. 4:470-502, 1931.
   (Copenhagen)

----: Das Herzminutenvolumen. Ergebn. Physiol. 39:348-407, 1937. (Copenhagen)

----: Intervallarbeit und Intervalltraining. Int. Zeits. angew. Physiol. 18:345-356, 1960.

----, and Hansen, Ove: Arbeitsfähigkeit und Ernährung. Scand. Arch. Physiol. 81:160-171, 1939.

----, Hedman, Rune; and Holmdahl, Inga: The influence of rest pauses on mechanical efficiency. Acta
   Physiol. Scand. 48:443-447, Apr. 25, 1960. (Stockholm)

----, ----, and Saltin, Bengt: Intermittent and continuous running. (A further contribution to the
   physiology of intermittent work). Acta Physiol. Scand. 50:269-286, Dec. 30, 1960. (Stockholm)

----, and Högberg, P.: Physiology of skiing. Arbeitsphysiol. 14:292-303, 1950.

Christensson, B.; Gustafson, A.; and Westling, H.: The effect of saluretics on pulse rate, blood pressure
   and electrocardiogram during exercise in normal subjects. Acta Med. Scand. 175:727-734, June,
   1964. (Lund)

Christopher, Jean; and Mayer, Jean: Effect of exercise on glucose uptake in rats and men. J. Appl.
   Physiol. 13:269-272, Sept., 1958. (Boston)

Chrometzka, F.; and Witten, K. H.: Der Einfluss von Kurzund Dauerkraftleistungen auf den Stoffwechsel.
   Zeits. klin. Med. 136:378-390, 1939.

Cier, J. F.; Lacour, R.; and Cier, A.: Influence du travail musculaire sur la répartition des ions
   Na^+ et K^+ dans l'organisme du rat. Comptes Rend. Soc. Biol. 153:96-98, Apr. 30, 1959.
   (Lyon)

----, ----, and ----: (Muscular work and ionic balances in the rat) (Fr). Path. Biol. 8:1147-1154,
   June, 1960.

Cioffi, L. A.; and Imbimbo, B.: (The influence of physical activity on blood coagulation) (It). Boll.
   Soc. Ital. Biol. Sper. 37:813-817, Sept. 15, 1961.

Clapperton, J. L.: The effect of walking upon the utilization of food by sheep. Brit. J. Nutr. 18:
   39-46, 1964. (Ayr, Scot.)

Clapperton, J. L.: The energy metabolism of sheep walking on the level and on gradients. Brit. J. Nutr. 18:47-54, 1964. (Ayr, Scot.)

Clarke, R. S. J.; and Hellon, R. F.: Hyperaemia following sustained and rhythmic exercise in the human forearm at various temperatures. J. Physiol. 145:447-458, Mar. 12, 1959. (Oxford)

Class, I.: (The effect of increased physical activity on the weight of the organs of albino mice. II. Quantitative studies on the pure-bred strain "Agnes Bluhm") (Ger). Zeits. Anat. Entwicklungsgesch. 122:251-265, 1961.

Clement, F.: (Does physical activity retard the decline of the intellectual capacities? (Study of a group of particularly physically active cyclists))(Fr). Rev. Franc. Geront. 7:379-412, Oct., 1961.

Cloquet, Jules-Germain: De l'influence des efforts sur les organes renfermés dans la cavité thoracique. Paris, Mequignon-Marvis, 1820.

----: De l'influence des efforts sur les organes renfermés dans la cavité thoracique. Nouv. J. Med. Chir., Pharm. 6:309-375, 1819.

Cobb, Leonard A.; and Johnson, Willard P.: Hemodynamic relationships of anaerobic metabolism and plasma free fatty acids during prolonged, strenuous exercise in trained and untrained subjects. J. Clin. Invest. 42:800-810, June, 1963. (Seattle)

----, ----, and Bruce, Robert A.: Responses in stroke volume to upright exercise in man. (Abstract). Clin. Res. 9:84, Jan., 1961. (Seattle)

Coffman, Jay D.: Blood flow and oxygen debt repayment in exercising skeletal muscle. Amer. J. Physiol. 205:365-369, Aug., 1963. (Boston)

Cohen, B. J.; and Serrano, L. J.: The effects of exercise and confinement on growth, maze learning, and organ weights in rats. Lab. Anim. Care 13:689-696, Oct., 1963.

Cohen, Harold; and Goldberg, Cissie: Effects of physical exercise on alimentary lipaemia. Brit. Med. J. 2:509-511, Aug. 13, 1960. (Sheffield)

Cohn, E.: Ueber die Veränderung des Hemoglobins sowie des Eiweisgehaltes in Blutserum bei Muskelarbeit und Schwitzen. Zeits. Biol. 70:366-370, 1919.

Cohn, Felix: Über den Einfluss der Muskelarbeit auf den Lactacidogengehalt in der roten und weissen Muskulatur des Kaninchens. Hoppe-Seyler Zeits. physiol. Chem. 113:253-262, Apr. 5, 1921. (Frankfurt)

Collett, Mary E.; and Liljestrand, G.: The minute volume of the heart in man during some different types of exercise. Scand. Arch. Physiol. 45:29-42, 1924.

Comroe, Julius H., Jr.: The effects of direct chemical and electrical stimulation of the respiratory center in the cat. Amer. J. Physiol. 139:490-498, Aug., 1943. (Philadelphia)

----: The hyperpnea of muscular exercise. Physiol. Rev. 24:319-339, July, 1944. (Philadelphia)

----: The location and function of the chemoreceptors of the aorta. Amer. J. Physiol. 127:176-191, Aug., 1939. (Philadelphia)

----, and Schmidt, Carl F.: The part played by reflexes from the carotid body in the chemical regulation of respiration in the dog. Amer. J. Physiol. 121:75-97, Jan., 1938. (Philadelphia)

Comroe, Julius H. , Jr. ; and Schmidt, Carl F. : Reflexes from the limbs as a factor in the hyperpnea of muscular exercise. Amer. J. Physiol. 138:536-547, Feb. , 1943. (Philadelphia)

Conard, V. ; and Franckson, J. R. M. : Influence de l'effort musculaire sur l'assimilation glucidique chez l'homme normal. Comptes Rend. Soc. Biol. 151:2228-2230, 1957. (Bruxelles)

----, and ----: Variations de la consommation du glucose au cours de l'effort musculaire. Arch. Int. Physiol. 68:374-376, Mar. , 1960. (Bruxelles)

Congiu, L. ; and Liguori, G. : Modificazioni del polso arterioso in conseguenza del lavoro muscolare nell'uomo. Boll. Soc. Ital. Biol. Sper. 33:236-238, Mar. , 1957.

Connell, A. M. ; Cooper, J. ; and Redfearn, J. W. : The contrasting effects of emotional tension and physical exercise on the excretion of 17-ketogenic steroids and 17-ketosteroids. Acta Endocr. 27:179-194, Feb. , 1958. (Surrey, Eng.)

Consiglio, G. C. ; Dattino, R. ; and Marzetti, L. : Il reogramma periferico in donne normali a termine di gravidanza, a riposo e dopo sforzo. Quad. Clin. Ostet. Ginec. 18:1070-1074, Dec. , 1963.

Consolazio, C. Frank; Konishi, Frank; Ciccolini, Robert V. ; Jamison, Jay M. ; Sheehan, Edward J. ; and Steffen, William F. : Food consumption of military personnel performing light activities in a hot desert environment. Metabolism 9:435-442, May, 1960. (Denver)

----, Matoush, LeRoy O. ; Nelson, Richard A. ; Isaac, Gerhard J. : and Hursh, Laurence M. : Effect of octacosanol, wheat germ oil, and vitamin E on performance of swimming rats. J. Appl. Physiol. 19:265-267, Mar. , 1964. (Denver)

----, ----, ----, Torres, Juan B. ; and Isaac, Gerhard J. : Environmental temperature and energy expenditures. J. Appl. Physiol. 18:65-68, Jan. , 1963. (Denver)

----, Nelson, Richard A. ; Matoush, LeRoy O. ; Harding, Richard S. ; and Canham, John E. : Nitrogen excretion in sweat and its relation to nitrogen balance requirements. J. Nutr. 79:399-406, Apr. , 1963. (Denver)

Cook, Charles D. ; Mead, Jere; and Orzalesi, Marcello M. : Static volume-pressure characteristics of the respiratory system during maximal efforts. J. Appl. Physiol. 19:1016-1022, Sept. , 1964. (Boston)

Cook, F. ; and Pembrey, M. S. : Observations on the effects of muscular exercise upon man. J. Physiol. 45:429-446, Feb. 5, 1913. (London)

Cook, S. F. ; Williams, O. L. ; Lyons, W. R. ; and Lawrence, J. H. : A comparison of altitude and exercise with respect to decompression sickness. War Med. 6:182-187, Sept. , 1944. (Berkeley)

Cooper, E. A. : The work of ventilating the lungs on exertion. Quart. J. Exp. Physiol. 46:13-21, Jan. , 19 61. (Birmingham, Eng.)

Cooper, Eric L. ; O'Sullivan, John; and Hughes, E. : Athletics and the heart: an electrocardiographic and radiological study of the response of the healthy and diseased heart to exercise. Med. J. Aust. 1:569-579, Apr. 17, 1937. (Melbourne)

Cope, Otis M. : The effect of exercise on ventricular minute-output time. Amer. J. Physiol. 94:140-143, July, 1930. (Omaha)

Cordero, Narciso: On the alveolar CO_2 tension following vigorous muscular exercise. Amer. J. Physiol. 77:91-99, June, 1926. (St. Louis)

Cornelius, C. E.; Burnham, L. G.; and Hill, H. E.: Serum transaminase activities of
thoroughbred horses in training. J. Amer. Vet. Med. Ass. 142:639-642, Mar. 15,
1963. (Davis and Imperial Beach, Calif.)

Correa Castillo, H.: Flebotrombosis de la pierna por esfuerzo. Arch. Soc. Cir. Hosp. 14:
551-552, Sept., 1944.

Cortes, Felix M.: Acute atrial overloading. A response to stress. Amer. J. Med. Sci.
246:443-450, Oct., 1963. (Philadelphia)

Coster, A. de; Levarlet, M.; Conard, V.; and Franckson, J. R. M.: Influence de l'effort musculaire
sur les lactates, le pH et les acides gras plasmatiques. Comptes Rend. Soc. Biol. 106:
1937-1939, Feb. 28, 1962. (Brussels)

Cotes, J. E.: Continuous versus intermittent administration of oxygen during exercise to patients
with chronic lung disease. Lancet 1:1075-1077, May 18, 1963. (Penarth)

----: Exercise limitation in health and disease. Brit. Med. Bull. 19:31-36, Jan., 1963. (Penarth)

----: The role of body temperature in controlling ventilation during exercise in one normal subject
breathing oxygen. J. Physiol. 129:554-563, Sept. 28, 1955. (Penarth)

----: Role of oxygen, carbon dioxide and lactic acid in ventilatory response to exercise in patients
with mitral stenosis. Clin. Sci. 14:317-328, May, 1955. (Penarth)

----, Pisa, Z.; and Thomas, A. J.: Effect of breathing oxygen upon cardiac output, heart rate,
ventilation, systemic and pulmonary blood pressure in patients with chronic lung disease. Clin.
Sci. 25:305-321, Oct., 1963. (Penarth)

Cotton, T. F.; Rapport, D. L.; and Lewis, Thomas: After effects of exercise on pulse rate and systolic
blood pressure in cases of "irritable heart". Heart 6:269-284, May 20, 1917. (Hampstead)

Courtice, F. C.; and Douglas, C. G.: The effects of prolonged muscular exercise on the metabolism.
Proc. Roy. Soc. 119B:381-439, Mar. 2, 1936. (Oxford)

----, ----, and Priestley, J. G.: Adrenaline and muscular exercise. Proc. Roy. Soc. 127B:288-297,
July 4, 1939. (Oxford)

Cowan, C. R.; and Solandt, O. M.: The duration of the recovery period following strenuous muscular
exercise, measured to a base line of steady, mild exercise. J. Physiol. 89:462-466, June 3, 1937.
(Toronto)

Crabbé, J.; Riondel, A. M.; and Mach, E.: Contribution a l'etudes des réactions corticosurrénaliennes.
Modifications du taux des 17-OH corticostéroïdes plasmatiques à la suite d'un effort physique
(compétition d'aviron). Acta Endocr. 22:119-124, June, 1956. (Geneva)

Craig, Albert B., Jr.: Regulation of respiration in exercise and breath holding. Ann. N. Y. Acad.
Sci. 109:901-907, June 24, 1963. (Rochester)

----, and Babcock, Stuart A.: Alveolar CO_2 during breath holding and exercise. J. Appl. Physiol.
17:874-876, Nov., 1962. (Rochester)

Craig, Albert B., Jr.; Halstead, Lauro S.; Schmidt, Gerhard H.; and Schnier, Brian R.: Influences of exercise and O_2 on breath holding. J. Appl. Physiol. 17:225-227, Mar., 1962. (Rochester)

Craig, F. N.: Effects of atropine, work and heat on heart rate and sweat production in man. J. Appl. Physiol. 4:826-833, May, 1952. (Army Chemical Center, Md.)

----: Pulmonary ventilation during exercise and inhalation of carbon dioxide. J. Appl. Physiol. 7:467-471, Mar., 1955. (Army Chemical Center, Md.)

----, and Cain, S. M.: Breath holding after exercise. J. Appl. Physiol. 10:19-25, Jan., 1957. (Army Chemical Center, Md.)

----, and Cummings, E. G.: Breath holding during exercise. J. Appl. Physiol. 13:30-34, July, 1958. (Army Chemical Center, Md.)

----, and ----: Breathing in brief exercise. J. Appl. Physiol. 15:583-588, July, 1960. (Army Chemical Center, Md.)

----, and ----: Breathing in brief exercise. U. S. Army Chem. Warfare Techn. Rep. CWLR 2364:1-22, Apr., 1960.

----, and ----: Slowing of the heart at the beginning of exercise. J. Appl. Physiol. 18:353-356, Mar., 1963. (Army Chemical Center, Md.)

----, ----, and Blevins, W. V.: Regulation of breathing at the beginning of exercise. J. Appl. Physiol. 18:1183-1187, Nov., 1963. (Edgewood Arsenal, Md.)

Crampton, E. W.: Nutrient-to-calorie ratios in applied nutrition. J. Nutr. 82:353-365, Mar., 1964. (Quebec)

Crane, Chilton: Deep venous thrombosis in the leg following effort or strain. New Eng. J. Med. 246:529-533, Apr. 3, 1952. (Boston)

Creutzfeldt, Werner; Husten, Maria; and Haager, Klara: Zur histologischen Funktionsdiagnostik der Nebennieren. (Untersuchungen am Meerschweinchen beim Schwimmtraining und im Hungerversuch). Beitr. path. Anat. 113:428-449, Dec. 30, 1953. (Freiburg i. Br.)

Crile, George W.; Glasser, Otto; and Quiring, Daniel P.: Shock exhaustion and restoration; the underlying principle and practical application in war. Proc. Interstate Postgrad. Med. Ass. N. Amer. 18:157-160, 1942.

Critz, Jerry B.; and Merrick, Arthur W.: Serum glutamic-oxalacetic transaminase levels after exercise in men. Proc. Soc. Exper. Biol. Med. 109:608-610, Mar., 1962. (Columbia)

----, and ----: Transaminase changes in rats after exercise. Proc. Soc. Exper. Biol. Med. 115: 11-14, Jan., 1964. (Columbia and Vermillion, S.D.)

Croft, Phyllis G.; and Richter, D.: Muscular activity and cholinesterase. J. Physiol. 102: 155-169, Sept. 30, 1943. (London)

Cronin, R. F. Patrick; and Macintosh, Donald J.: The effect of induced hypoxia on oxygen uptake during muscular exercise in normal subjects. Canad. J. Biochem. Physiol. 40:717-726, June, 1962. (Montreal)

Cropp, Gerd J. A.; and Comroe, Julius H., Jr.: Role of mixed venous blood P_{CO_2} in respiratory
control. J. Appl. Physiol. 16:1029-1033, Nov., 1961. (San Francisco)

Crowden, G. P.: The effect of duration of work on the efficiency of muscular work in man.
J. Physiol. 80:394-408, Feb. 28, 1934. (London)

Cumming, Gordon R.: The heart and physical exercise. Canad. Med. Ass. J. 88:80-85, Jan.
12, 1963. (Winnipeg)

----, and Cumming, P. M.: Working capacity of normal children tested on a bicycle ergometer.
Canad. Med. Ass. J. 88:351-355, Feb. 16, 1963. (Winnipeg)

----, and Danzinger, R.: Bicycle ergometer studies in children. II. Correlation of pulse rate with
oxygen consumption. Pediatrics 32:202-208, Aug., 1963. (Winnipeg)

----, and Edwards, A. H.: Indirect measurement of left ventricular function during exercise.
Canad. Med. Ass. J. 89:219-221, Aug. 3, 1963. (Winnipeg)

Cureton, Thomas K., Jr.: Postexercise blood pressures in maximum exertion tests and relationships
to performance time, oxygen intake, oxygen debt, and peripheral resistance. J. Lancet
77:81-82, Mar., 1957. (Urbana)

----, and Phillips, E. E.: Physical fitness changes in middle-aged men attributable to equal eight-
week periods of training, non-training and re-training. J. Sport Med. 4:87-93, June, 1964.

----, and Sterling, L. F.: Factor analyses of cardiovascular test variables. J. Sport Med. 4:1-24,
Mar., 1964.

Currie, J. A.: The heart in muscular exercise. Guy's Hosp. Gaz. 35:113, 1921.

Dabney, Joe M.: Energy balance and obesity. A short review. Ann. Intern. Med. 60: 689-699, Apr., 1964. (Oklahoma City)

Dacso, Michael M.; Luczak, Aleksander, K.; Haas, Albert; and Rusk, Howard A.: Bracing and rehabilitation training. Effect on the energy expenditure of the elderly hemiplegic; preliminary report. Postgrad. Med. 34:42-47, July, 1963. (New York City)

Dahlbäck, O.; Dahn, I.; and Westling, H.: Hemodynamic observations in coarctation of the aorta, with special reference to the blood pressure above and below the stenosis at rest and during exercise. Scand. J. Clin. Lab. Invest. 16:339-346, 1964. (Lund)

Dahlstrom, H.; and Ihrman, K.: A clinical and physiological study of pregnancy in a material from northern Sweden. V. The results of work tests during and after pregnancy. Acta Soc. Med. Upsala. 65:305-314, 1960.

Dalderup, L. M.; Pappie, A. B.; De Vaagd, N.; and Siemelink, R.: Electrocardiographic changes in healthy young men after exercise. Lancet 2:1345, Dec. 19, 1964. (Wageningen and The Hague)

Dambax, Alexis: De l'entraînement. Paris, Thèse numéro 257, 1866.

Damoiseau, J.; Deroanne, R.; and Petit, J. M.: Consommation maximale d'oxygène aux différents ergomètres. J. Physiologie 55:235-236, Mar.-Apr., 1963. (Liège)

----, Deroanne, R.; and Petit, J. M.: Influence des modalités d'exécution des exercises musculaires sur la valeur de la consommation maximum d'O_2. Arch. Int. Physiol. 71:275-277, Mar., 1963. (Liege)

---- Petit, J. M.; Belge, G.; and Collée, G.: Méthode simplifiée de mesure de la consommation maximum d'O_2. Arch. Int. Physiol. 70:131-132, Feb., 1962. (Liège)

----, ----, Namur, M.; and Lagneaux, D.: Régime ventilataire stable au cours de l'exercise musculaire prolongé chez l'individu sain. Arch. Int. Physiol. 69:310-326, May, 1961. (Liège)

D'Anaya, Manuel: De l'influence de l'exercice sur l'homme. Paris, Thèse numéro 293, vol. 612, 1858.

Danzinger, Rudolph G.; and Cummings, Gordon, R.: Effects of chlorothiazide on working capacity of normal subjects. J. Appl. Physiol. 19:636-638, July, 1964. (Winnipeg)

Darling, R. C.; Johnson, R. E.; Pitts, G. C.; Consolazio, F. C.; and Robinson, P. F.: Effects of variations in dietary protein on the physical well being of men doing manual work. J. Nutr. 28:273-281, Oct., 1944. (Boston)

----, and Shea, Ethel: The effect of a short period of strenuous exercise on hemoconcentration. Arch. Phys. Med. 32:392-396, June, 1961. (New York City)

Davidson, Ronald J.: Exertional haemoglobinuria: a report on three cases with studies on the haemolytic mechanism. J. Clin. Path. 17:536-540, Sept., 1964. (Dundee)

Davies, C. T. M.; and Copland, J. G.: Pulse counting during heavy exercise using new electrodes for displaying the electrocardiogram. J. Appl. Physiol. 19:325, Mar., 1964. (Edinburgh)

Davies, C. T. M.; Drysdale, H. C.; and Passmore, R.: Does exercise promote health?
Lancet 2:930-932, Nov. 2, 1963. (Edinburgh)

----, and Harris, E. A.: Heart rate during transition from rest to exercise, in relation to
exercise tolerance. J. Appl. Physiol. 19:857-862, Sept., 1964. (Edinburgh)

Davis, Elwood Craig; and Logan, Gene Adams: Biophysical values of muscular activity,
with implications for research. Dubuque, Iowa, W. C. Brown and Co., 1961.

Dawson, Percy M.: Effect of physical training and practice on the pulse rate and blood pressures
during activity and during rest, with a note on certain acute infections and on the distress
resulting from exercise. Amer. J. Physiol. 50:443-479, Dec., 1919. (Madison)

----, and Hellebrandt, Frances A.: The influence of aging in man upon his capacity for physical
work and upon his cardio-vascular responses to exercise. Amer. J. Physiol. 143:420-427,
Mar., 1945. (Durham and Madison)

Dearborn, George Van Ness: Some relations of exercise to nutrition. Boston Med. Surg. J.
178:458-467, Apr. 4, 1918. (Cambridge)

Dearnaley, E. J.: Estimates of endurance under risky conditions. J. Gen. Psychol. 68:243-250,
Apr., 1963. (Manchester)

De Coster, A.; Messin, R.; and Denolin, H.: Acide lactique, pouls et électrocardiogramme au cours de
l'ergospirométrie. Poumon Coeur 19:633-639, 1963.

De Crinis, K.; Redisch, W.; and Steele, J. M.: Vascular effects of nylidrine hydrochloride during
exercise. Proc. Soc. Exp. Biol. Med. 102:29-31, Oct., 1959. (New York)

Defares, J. G.; Derksen, H. E.; and Duyff, J. W.: Cerebral blood flow in the regulation of
respiration. Acta Physiol. Pharmacol. Neerl. 9:327-360, Oct., 1960. (Leiden)

De France, F.-J.-F.: De l'entraînement. Paris, 1859.

Dejours, Pierre: Chemoreflexes in breathing. Physiol. Rev. 42:335-358, July, 1962. (Paris)

----: Control of respiration by arterial chemoreceptors. Ann. N. Y. Acad. Sci. 109:682-695,
June 24, 1963.

----: Exercice musculaire. Chapter 19 in Physiologie, Charles Kayser (editor). Paris, Editions
Médicales Flammarion, 1963.

----: La régulation de la ventilation au cours de l'exercice musculaire chez l'homme. J.
Physiologie 51:163-261, Mar.-Apr., 1959. (Paris)

----: La régulation de la ventilation au cours de l'exercice musculaire chez l'homme. J.
Physiologie 51:929-935, Sept.-Oct., 1959. (Paris)

----: The regulation of breathing during muscular exercise in man. A neuro-humoral theory.
In: The regulation of human respiration, D. J. C. Cunningham and B. B. Lloyd, editors.
Blackwell, Oxford, 1963.

Dejours, Pierre: La regulation de la ventilation au cours de l'exercise musculaire chez l'homme. Lyon Méd. 91:1165-1169, Dec. 20, 1959.

----, Bechtel-Labrousse, Ivette; Lefrançois, R.; and Raynaud, Jeanne: Etude de la mécanique ventilatoire au cours de l'exercice musculaire. J. Physiologie 53:318-319, Mar.-Apr., 1961. (Paris)

----, ----, ----: Etude du contrôle de la fréquence cardiaque et de la ventilation au cours des exercices passif et actif chez l'homme. Comptes Rend. Acad. Sci. 252:2012-2014, Mar. 27, 1961. (Paris)

----, Flandrois, P., Lefrançois, R.; and Teillac, A.: Etude de la régulation de la ventilation au cours de l'exercice musculaire chez l'homme. J. Physiologie 53:321-322, Mar.-Apr., 1961.

----, Girard, F.; Labrousse, Y.; and Teillac, A.: Etude de la régulation de la ventilation de repos chez l'homme en haute altitude. Rev. Franc. Etud. Clin. Biol. 4:115-127, 1959.

----, Kellogg, Ralph H.; and Pace, Nello: Regulation of respiration and heart rate response in exercise during altitude acclimatization. J. Appl. Physiol. 18:10-18, Jan., 1963. (Berkeley, San Francisco, Big Pine)

----, Labrousse, Y.; Raynaud, Jeanne; Girard, F.; and Teillac, A.: Stimulus oxygène de la ventilation au repos et au cours de l'exercice musculaire, à basse altitude (50 m.) chez l'homme. Rev. Franc. Etud. Clin. Biol. 3:105-123, 1958.

----, Lefrançois, R.; Flandrois, R.; and Teillac, A.: Autonomie des stimulus ventilatoires oxygène, gaz carbonique et neurogenique de l'exercice musculaire. J. Physiologie 52:63-64, Jan.-Feb., 1960. (Paris)

----, Teillac, A.: Caractères des variations de la ventilation pulmonaire au cours de l'exercice musculaire dynamique chez l'homme. Etude expérimentale et théorique. Rev. Franc. Etud. Clin. Biol. 8:439-444, May, 1963.

de la Camp: Experimentelle Studien über die acute Herzdilatation. Zeits. klin. Med. 51:1-79, 1904.

De Lanne, René: Répercussions des activités musculaires sur la fonctionnement renal. Acta Belg. Arte Méd. Pharm. Milit. 110:611-620, Dec., 1957.

----: Variation provoquées dans le sang veineux par l'activité musculaire. Bruxelles, Presses académiques européennes, 1957.

----, Barnes, J. R.; and Brouha, L.: Changes in osmotic pressure and ionic concentrations of plasma during muscular work and recovery. J. Appl. Physiol. 14:804-808, Sept., 1959. (Wilmington)

----, ----, ----: Hematological changes during muscular activity and recovery. J. Appl. Physiol. 15:31-36, Jan., 1960. (Wilmington)

----, ----, ----, and Massart, F.: Changes in acid-base balance and blood gases during muscular activity and recovery. J. Appl. Physiol. 14:328-332, May, 1959. (Wilmington)

Delfosse, Jean: Diètetique de l'effort. Acta Belg. Arte Méd. Pharm. Milit. 110:589-596, Dec., 1957.

Deloff, L.; Pudelski, J.; Próby wysilkowe w ocenie wydolności narzad i addechowo-krazeniowego. (The effort test in the evaluation of the respiratory and circulatory system) (Pol). Pol. Tyg. Lek. 18:1256-1260, Aug. 19, 1963.

Delucchi, José Raúl: Effects of total ventilation by obstructing blood vessels and by muscular effort. J. Aviation Med. 14:23-27, Feb., 1943.

Dempsey, J. A.: Relationship between obesity and treadmill performance in sedentary and active young men. Res. Quart. Amer. Ass. Health Phys. Educ. 35:288-297, Oct., 1964.

Dempster, J. H.: Respiration: an historical account. Detroit Med. J. 13:320-327, 1913.

De Nayer, P.; and Ostyn, M.: Lichamelijk inspanning en adoptatie der bijnieven. Acta Belg. Arte Med. Pharm. Milit. 110:621-630, Dec., 1957.

Denolin, H.: La fonction pulmonaire au cours de l'effort. Acta Belg. Arte Med. Pharm. Milit. 110:521-572, Dec., 1957.

Derevenco, P.; and Derevenco, Vera: Experimental data on neuroendocrine regulation during physical exertion. Rumanian Med. Rev. 5:141-142, 1961. (Cluj)

----, and ----: Die Wirkung einiger Substanzen mit zentralem Effect auf die Freisetzung von Corticotropin nach physischer Anstrengung. Endokrinologie 45:25-33, Sept., 1963. (Cluj)

Deshayes, Jean Louis: Essai médical sur les avantages de l'exercice. Paris, Thèse numéro 164, vol. 149, 1819.

Desroches, Harry F.; Kimbrell, Gordon M.; and Allison, Julian T.: Effect of age and experience on bar pressing and activity in the rat. J. Geront. 19:168-172, Apr., 1964. (Mountain Home and Knoxville)

Dettling, Georges-Edouard: Le corps humain; anatomie et physiologie. Influence de l'exercice sur l'organisme. Paris, O. Doin, 1905.

----: Le corps humain: anatomie et physiologie, influence de l'exercice sur l'organisme. Troisième édition. Paris, G. Doin, 1931.

Deutsch, Felix: Die Herzgrössenschwankungen, speziell die deminatio cordis, unmitterlbar nach sportlichen Leistungen, Arbeitsphysiol. 2:215-232, Oct. 21, 1929. (Wien)

Devlin, H. B.: The management of osteoporosis: a treatment regime and its results. J. Irish Med. Ass. 54:135-140, May, 1964.

Devlin, James G.: The effect of training and acute physical exercise on plasma insulin-like activity. Irish J. Med. Sci. 6th series:423-425, Sept., 1963. (Dublin)

Dexter, L.; Whittenberger, J. L.; Haynes, F. W.; Goodale, W. T., Gorlin, R.; and Sawyer, C. G.: Effect of exercise on circulatory dynamics of normal individuals. J. Appl. Physiol. 3:439-453, Feb., 1951. (Boston)

De Young, Vernon R.; Rice, Hugh, A.; and Steinhaus, Arthur H.: Studies in the physiology of exercise. VII. The modification of colonic motility induced by exercise and some indications of a nervous mechanism. Amer. J. Physiol. 99:52-63, Dec., 1931.

Dickinson, Sylvia: The dynamics of bicycle pedalling. Proc. Roy. Soc. 103B:225-233,
    Aug. 1, 1928. (London)

----: The efficiency of bicycle pedalling, as affected by speed and load. J. Physiol. 67:242-255,
    June 7, 1929.

Diczfalusy, E.; Cassmer, O.; and Ullmark, R.: Assessment of the functional reserve capacity of
    the adrenal cortex in healthy subjects following exhaustive exercise. J. Clin. Endocr. 22:
    78-86, Jan., 1962. (Stockholm)

Di Giovanni, Cleto, Jr.; and Chambers, Randall, M.: Physiologic and psychologic aspects of the
    gravity spectrum. (Concluded). New Eng. J. Med. 270:134-139, Jan. 16, 1964.
    (Philadelphia and Johnsvilla)

Dill, David B.: Blood changes in exercise. J. Lancet 56:313-315, 1931.

----: Comparative physiology of oxygen transport. J. Sport Med. 3:191-200, Dec., 1963.

----: The economy of muscular exercise. Physiol. Rev. 16:263-291, Apr., 1936. (Boston)

----: Effects of physical strain and high altitudes on heart and circulation. Amer. Heart J. 23:
    441-454, Apr., 1942. (Cambridge)

----: The influence of age on performance as shown by exercise tests. Pediatrics 32(Suppl.):737-741,
    Oct., 1963. (Bloomington)

----: The nature of fatigue. Personnel 9:113-116, 1933.

----: The nature of fatigue. Geriatrics 10:474-478, Oct., 1955. (Army Chemical Center, Md.)

----: Symposium on exercise fitness tests: their physiological basis and clinical application to
    pediatrics. Historical introduction: personal reminiscences. Pediatrics 32(Suppl.):653-655,
    Oct., 1963. (Bloomington)

----: Symposium on work and the heart. Introduction. Amer. J. Cardiol. 14:729-730, Dec.,
    1964. (Bloomington)

----, Bock, Arlie; Behnke, A. R., Thompson, Arthur H.; Keys, Ancel; Sneidman, George I.; and
    Wickhorst, Frank H.: Symposium on war medicine: Fatigue. Clinics 2:1126-1154, Feb.,
    1944. (Fort Knox, Boston, Bethesda, Carlisle, Minneapolis, etc.)

----, Horvath, S. M.; and Craig, F. N.: Responses to exercise as related to age. J. Appl. Physiol.
    12:195-196, Mar., 1958. (Army Chemical Center, Md., and Iowa City)

----, Robinson, S.; Balke, Bruno; and Newton, J. L.: Work tolerance: age and altitude. J.
    Appl. Physiol. 19:483-488, May, 1964. (Bloomington)

----, ----, and Newton, J. L.: Work tolerance: age and altitude. Rep. 63-33. U. S.
    Civil Aeromed. Res. Inst. 1-8, Dec., 1963.

----, and Sacktor, B.: Exercise and the oxygen debt. J. Sport Med. 2:66-72, June, 1962.

----, Talbott, J. H.; and Edwards, H. T.: Studies in muscular activity. VI. Response of several
    individuals to a fixed task. J. Physiol. 69:267-305, May, 1930.

Dimond, E. Grey: Marked electrocardiogram changes after exercise. Dis. Chest 39:225, Feb., 1961. (La Jolla)

Döbeln, Wilhelm von: Dehydration and physical performance of human subjects. (Abstract). Acta Physiol. Scand. 25(Suppl. 89):16, 1951. (Stockholm)

----: Human standard and maximal metabolic rate in relation to fatfree body mass. Acta Physiol. Scand. 37(Suppl. 126):3-78, 1956. (Stockholm)

----: Maximal oxygen intake, body size, and total hemoglobin in normal man. Acta Physiol. Scand. 38:193-199, Dec. 31, 1956. (Stockholm)

----: A single bicycle ergometer. J. Appl. Physiol. 7:222-224, Sept., 1954. (Stockholm)

Dolgin, Peter: Die optimale Kontraktionsgeschwindigkeit kleiner Muskeln. Arbeitsphysiol. 2:205-214, Oct., 21, 1929. (Dortmund)

----, and Lehmann, Gunther: Ein Beitrag zur Physiologie der statisschen Arbeiten. Arbeitsphysiol. 2:248-252, Oct. 21, 1929, (Dortmund)

Doll, E.; König, K.; and Reindell, H.: Das Verhalten der arteriellen Sauerstoffspannung und anderer arterieller blutgasanalytischer Daten in Ruhe und während körperlicher Belastung. Pflüger Arch. ges. Physiol. 271:283-295, July 7, 1960. (Freiburg)

Donald, David E.; Milburn, Sidney E.; and Shepherd, John T.: Effect of cardiac denervation on the maximal capacity for exercise in the racing greyhound. J. Appl. Physiol. 19:849-852, Sept., 1964. (Rochester, Minn. and Elk Point, S.D.)

----, and Shepherd, John T.: Changes in heart rate on intravenous infusion in dogs with chronic cardiac denervation. Proc. Soc. Exp. Biol. Med. 113:315-317, June, 1963. (Rochester, Minn.)

----, ----: Initial cardiovascular adjustment to exercise in dogs with chronic cardiac denervation. Amer. J. Physiol. 207:1325-1329, Dec., 1964. (Rochester, Minn.)

----, ----: Response to exercise in dogs with cardiac denervation. Amer. J. Physiol. 205:393-400, Aug., 1963. (Rochester, Minn.)

----, ----: Sustained capacity for exercise in dogs after complete cardiac denervation. Amer. J. Cardiol. 14:853-859, Dec., 1964. (Rochester, Minn.)

Donald, Kenneth W.: Exercise and heart disease; a study in regional circulation. Brit. Med. J. 1:985-994, Apr. 18, 1959. (Edinburgh)

----: Exercise studies in heart disease. Mod. Conc. Cardiov. Dis. 28:529-534, June, 1959. (Edinburgh)

----, Bishop, J. M.; Cumming, G.; and Wade, O. L.: The effect of exercise on cardiac output and circulatory dynamics of normal subjects. Clin. Sci. 14:37-73, Feb., 1955. (Birmingham, Engl.)

----, ----, and Wade, O. L.: Changes in the oxygen content of axillary venous blood during leg exercise in patients with rheumatic heart disease. Clin. Sci. 14:531-551, Aug., 1955. (Birmingham, Engl.)

Donald, Kenneth W.; Bishop, J. M.; and Wade, O. L.: A study of minute to minute changes of arterio-venous oxygen content difference, oxygen uptake and cardiac output and rate of achievement of a steady state during exercise in rheumatic heart disease. J. Clin. Invest. 33:1146-1167, Aug., 1954. (Birmingham, Engl.)

----, Gloster, J.; Harris, E. A.; Reeves, J.; and Harris, P.: The production of lactic acid during exercise in normal subjects and in patients with rheumatic heart disease. Amer. Heart J. 62:494-510, Oct., 1961. (Birmingham, Engl.)

----, Wormald, P. N.; Taylor, S. H.; and Bishop, J. M.: Changes in the oxygen content of femoral venous blood and leg blood flow during leg exercise in relation to cardiac output response. Clin. Sci. 16:567-591, Aug., 1957. (Birmingham, Engl.)

Donaldson, Henry Herbert: On the influence of exercise on weight of the central nervous system of the albino rat. J. Comp. Neurol. 21:129-137, Apr. 15, 1911. (Philadelphia)

----: Summary of data for the effects of exercise on the organ weights of the albino rat: comparison with similar data from the dog. Amer. J. Anat. 56:57-70, Jan., 1935. (Philadelphia)

Donati, G.: Il lavoro fisico a l'emozione nella patogenesi del "cuore di guerra". Gior. Med. Milit. 94:345-370, Sept.-Oct., 1947.

Donkerlo, W. T.: Radioelectrocardiografie tijdens inspanning. (Radioelectrocardiography during exertion) (Dutch). Nederl. T. Geneesk. 108:385-387, Feb. 22, 1964.

Donnet, Vincent; Duflot, Jean-Claude; Jacquin, Michel; and Pruneyre, Andrée: Le muscle qui se contracte est-il soustrait aux interventions vaso-motrices nerveuses ou pharmacodynamiques? J. Physiologie 56:339, May-June, 1964. (Marseilles)

----, ----, ----, and Rioux, G.: Le muscle en travail "échappe-t-il" comme le soutient Rein, aux influences vasomotrices nerveuses et pharmacodynamiques? Comptes Rend. Soc. Biol. 158:591-594, July 20, 1964. (Marseilles)

Dop, G. H.: Maatschappelijke aspecten. (Work time and rest time, social aspects) (Dutch). T. Soc. Geneesk. 41:626-628, Oct. 11, 1963.

Dornhorst, A. C.: Hyperaemia induced by exercise and ischemia. Brit. Med. Bull. 19:137-140, May, 1963. (London)

----, and Whelan, R. F.: The blood flow in muscle following exercise and circulatory arrest: the influence of reduction in effective blood pressure, of arterial hypoxia and of adrenaline. Clin. Sci. 12:33-40, Feb., 1953. (London)

Dorris, Ronald, J.; and Stunkard, Albert J.: Physical activity: performance and attitudes of a group of obese women. Amer. J. Med. Sci. 233:622-628, June, 1957. (Syracuse and New York City)

Douglas, Claude Gordon: Die Regulation der Atmung beim Menschen. Ergebn. Physiol. 14:338-430, 1914. (Oxford)

----, and Haldane, J. S.: The capacity of the air passages under varying physiological conditions. J. Physiol. 45:235-238, Oct. 22, 1912. (Oxford)

Douglas, Claude Gordon; and Haldane, J. S.: The effects of previous forced breathing and oxygen inhalation on the distress caused by muscular work. J. Physiol. 39:i-iv, June 26, 1909. (Abstract) (Oxford)

----, ----: Investigations by the carbon monoxide method on the oxygen tension of arterial blood. Skand. Arch. Physiol. 25:169-182, 1911. (Oxford)

----, ----: The regulation of the general circulation rate in man. J. Physiol. 56:69-100, Feb. 14, 1922. (Oxford)

----, ----: The regulation of normal breathing. J. Physiol. 38:420-440, June 15, 1909. (Oxford)

----, ----: The regulation of the general circulation rate in man. J. Physiol. 56:69-100, Feb. 14, 1922. (Oxford)

----, ----, Henderson, Yandell; and Schneider, E. C.: Physiological observations made on Pike's Peak, Colorado, with special reference to low barometric pressures. Phil. Trans. 203B:185-318, 1913. (Oxford)

Downey, John A.; and Darling, Robert C.: Effect of salicylates on elevation of body temperature during exercise. J. Appl. Physiol. 17:323-325, Mar., 1962. (New York City)

----, ----: Effects of salicylates on exercise metabolism. J. Appl. Physiol. 17:665-668, July, 1962. (New York City)

Dransfeld, B.; and Mellerowicz, H.; Der Sauerstoffpuls während einer Leistung von 1 Watt/kg Körpergewicht. Zeits. Kreislaufforsch. 49:901-906, Oct., 1959.

Drews, A.: Röntgenologische Herzflächenbestimmungen bei Gesunden und Herzkranken in Ruhe und nach Belastung. Zeits. Kreislaufforsch. 51:622-628, June, 1962.

----, and Rosenkranz, K.-A.: Kreislauf und Atmung bei Doppelbeinamputierten während körperlicher Belastung. Zeits. Kreislaufforsch. 51:611-621, June, 1962.

Dripps, Robert D.; and Comroe, Julius H., Jr.: The effect of the inhalation of high and low oxygen concentrations on respiration, pulse rate, ballistocardiogram, and arterial oxygen saturation (oximeter) of normal individuals. Amer. J. Physiol. 149:277-291, May 1, 1947. (Philadelphia)

----, ----: The respiratory and circulatory response of normal man to inhalation of 7/6 and 10.4 per cent CO_2 with a comparison of maximal ventilation produced by severe muscular exercise, inhalation of CO_2 and maximal voluntary hyperventilation. Amer. J. Physiol. 149:43-51, Apr., 1947. (Philadelphia)

Dryerre, Henry; Millar, N. G.; and Ponder, Eric: An investigation into the size of human erythrocytes before and after exercise. Quart. J. Exp. Physiol. 16:69-86, 1926. (Edinburgh)

Drysdale, H. C.: Exercise and health. Nurs. Times 60:965-966, July 24, 1964.

Duchênne-Marullaz, P.; Vacher, J.; and Talvard, J.: Modifications de l'ammoniémie veineuse au cours de la contraction musculaire. Comptes Rend. Soc. Biol. 158:1510-1513, 1964. (Riem)

Dudley, Donald L.; Holmes, Thomas H.; Martin, C. J.; and Ripley, Herbert S.: Changes in respiration associated with hypnotically induced emotion, pain, and exercise. Psychosom. Med. 26:46-57, Jan.-Feb., 1964. (Seattle)

----, Martin, C. J.; and Holmes, Thomas H.: Psychophysiologic studies of pulmonary ventilation. Psychosom. Med. 26:645-660, Nov.-Dec., 1964. (Seattle)

Duffie, Edward R., Jr.; and Adams, Forrest, H.: The use of the working capacity test in the evaluation of children with congenital heart disease. Pediatrics 32(Suppl.):757-768, Oct., 1963. (Los Angeles)

Dufour, François-Etienne: Sur l'exercice; considéré comme moyen de conserver la santé. Paris, Thèse numéro 196, vol. 195, 1825.

Dulong: Sur la chaleur animale. Ann. Chim. Phys. Sér. 3, 1:440-455, 1841.

Dunér, H.; and Pernow, B.: Histamine and leukocytes in blood during muscular work in man. Scand. J. Clin. Lab. Invest. 10:394-396, 1958. (Stockholm)

Dunlop, J. C.; Paton, D. Nöel; Stockman, R.; and Maccadam, Ivison: On the influence of muscular exercise, sweating, and massage on the metabolism. J. Physiol. 22:68-91, Sept. 1, 1897. (Edinburgh)

Duperray, Bernard; and Pachéco, Henri: Influence du travail musculaire et du régime alimentaire sur le métabolisme du cholestérol chez le rat. Comptes Rend. Acad. Sci. 257:2549-2551, Oct. 21, 1963.

Dupuy, G.; and Fabre, Henri: Les modifications phonocardiographiques consécutives a l'activité musculaire. J. Physiologie 51:456-457, May-June, 1959. (Bordeaux)

Durand, J.; Donato, L.; Parker, J. O.; Rochester, D. F.; and Cournand, A.: (Attempted separate measurement of the volumes of blood present in the 2 ventricles during the different phase of the cardiac cycle in stable conditions and during moderate muscular exercise) (Fr). Arch. Sci. Physiol. 15:55-78, 1961.

----, ----, ----, ----, ----: Modifications du volume et du débit des deux ventricules chez l'homme normal au début de l'effort. J. Physiologie 52:88-90, Jan.-Feb., 1960. (New York)

Durnin, J. V. G. A.: Food intake and energy expenditure of elderly people. Geront. Clin. 4: 128-133, 1962.

----, and Mikulicic, V.: The influence of graded exercises on the oxygen consumption, pulmonary ventilation and heart rate of young and elderly men. Quart. J. Exp. Physiol. 41:442-452, Oct., 1956. (Glasgow)

Dydenko, H. H.: Zming bilkovykh fraktsii syrovatky krovi sobak pry m'iazoïï diial'nosti riznoi intensyvnosti. (Changes in the protein fractions of the blood serum in dogs during muscle activity of varying intensity) (Uk). Fiziol. Zh. 10:55-60, Jan.-Feb., 1964.

Dzhuganian, R. A.: Issledovanie funktsional'nogo sostoianiia nadpochechnikov u detei srednego shkol'nogo voznasta pri zaniatiiakh fizicheskimi uprazhneniiami. (Functional study of the adrenal glands in secondary school age children during physical exercise) (Russ). Pediatriia 43:77-81, Feb., 1964.

Eason, R. G.: Relation between effort, tension level, skill, and performance efficiency in a
    perceptual-motor task. Percept. Motor Skills 16:297-317, Apr., 1963.

Ebert, Richard V.; and Stead, Eugene A., Jr.: Demonstration that in normal man no reserves of
    blood are mobilized by exercise, epinephrine, and hemorrhage. Amer. J. Med. Sci. 201:
    655-664, May, 1941. (Boston)

----, and ----: An error in measuring changes in plasma volume after exercise. Proc. Soc.
    Exper. Biol. Med. 46:139-141, Jan., 1941. (Boston)

Eckstein, Richard W.: Effect of exercise and coronary artery narrowing on coronary collateral
    circulation. Circ. Res. 5:230-235, May, 1957. (Cleveland)

Editorial: Bodily exercise. J.A.M.A. 175:801-802, Mar. 4, 1961.

----: Emotion, exercise, and the adrenal cortex. Brit. Med. J. 2:496-497, Aug. 23, 1958.

----: The fuel of muscular exercise. Lancet 2:276-277, Sept. 5, 1959.

----: Physical activity and myocardial infarction. Nutr. Rev. 19:221-222, July, 1961.

----: Physical activity of obese girls. Nutr. Rev. 21:108-109, Apr., 1963.

----: Renal response to exercise. Brit. Med. J. 2:1281-1282, Nov. 22, 1958.

Edwards: Note sur l'exhalation et l'absorption de l'azote dans la respiration. Ann. Chim. Phys.
    22:35-43, 1823.

Edwards, Edward A.; Cohen, Norman R.; and Kaplan, Marshall M.: Effect of exercise on the
    peripheral pulses. New Eng. J. Med. 260:738-741, Apr. 9, 1959. (Boston)

Edwards, H. T.; Hochrein, M.; Dill, D. B.; and Henderson, L. J.: Das physikalisch-chemische
    System des Blutes in seiner Beziehung zu Atmung und Kreislauf. III. Mitteilung: über die
    Ionenverteilung in Ruhe und Arbeit. Naunyn Schmiedeberg Arch. exp. Path. 143:161-169,
    1929. (Boston)

----, Richards, T. K.; and Dill, D. B.: Blood sugar, urine sugar and urine protein in exercise.
    Amer. J. Physiol. 98:352-356, Sept., 1931. (Cambridge)

----, Thorndike, A., Jr.; and Dill, D. B.: The energy requirement in strenuous muscular exercise.
    New Eng. J. Med. 213:532-535, Sept. 12, 1935. (Cambridge)

Efimoff, W. W.; and Arschawski, I. A.: Die Einwirkung der Hyperventilation bei sehr schwerer
    Arbeit auf die Erholung. Arbeitsphysiol. 2:253-260, Oct. 21, 1929. (Moscow)

----, and Samitschkina, D. S.: Zur Biochemie der Ermüdung. Einwirkung der Gewerbearbeit
    und der Erholung auf die Alkalireserve und den Gehalt an Phosphor im Blut nach Untersuchungen
    an Spinnerinnen. Arbeitsphysiol. 2:341-346, Dec. 20, 1929. (Moscow)

Egeberg, O.: Changes in the activity of antihemophilic A factor (F. VIII) and in the bleeding
    time associated with muscular exercise and adrenalin infusion. Scand. J. Clin. Lab.
    Invest. 15:539-549, 1963. (Oslo)

Egeberg, O.: The effect of muscular exercise on hemostasis in von Willebrand's disease.
Scand. J. Clin. Lab. Invest. 15:273-283, 1963. (Oslo)

----: On the nature of the blood antihemophilic A factor (AHA = F. VIII) increase associated with muscular
exercise. Scand. J. Clin. Lab. Invest. 15:202-203, 1963. (Oslo)

Eggleton, Marion Grace: Muscular exercise. London; Kegan, Paul, Trench, Trubner and Co., Ltd.;
1936.

Eichholtz, F.: Ermudungsbekampfung; über Stimulantien. Deutsch. med. Wschr. 67:1355,
Dec. 12, 1941.

Eichna, Ludwig W.; Horvath, Steven M.; and Bean, William B.: Cardiac asystole in normal young
men following physical effort. Amer. Heart J. 33:254-262, Feb., 1947. (Ft. Knox)

----, ----, and ----: Post-exertional orthostatic hypotension. Amer. J. Med. Sci. 213:641-654,
June, 1947. (Ft. Knox)

Ejrup, B.: Tonoscillography after exercise as an early diagnostic method in organic peripheral
arterial disease. Acta Med. Scand. 138(Suppl. 239):347-355, 1950. (Stockholm)

Ejsmont, W.: The influence of physical stress on the level of cholesterol in blood of seafarers.
Bull. Inst. Mar. Med. Gdansk 15:199-205, 1964.

Ekelund, L. G.; and Holmgren, A.: Circulatory and respiratory adaptation, during long-term, non-
steady state exercise, in the sitting position. Acta Physiol. Scand. 62:240-255, Nov., 1964.
(Stockholm)

Eliasch, Harald; Wade, Geoffrey; and Werkö, Lars: The effects of work on pulmonary circulation
in mitral stenosis. Circulation 5:271-278, Feb., 1952. (Stockholm)

Eliseo, A.; and Grieco, B.: Lavoro muscolare e consumo di ossigeno in soggetti sani sottoposti
a trattamento con 2, amino-6, metil-6, eptanolo cloridrato. Folia Med. 47:750-759,
Aug., 1964.

Elliott, John B.: Exercise as a physiological necessity. New Orleans Med. Surg. J. 10:498-508,
Jan., 1883. (New Orleans)

Elmqvist, Ada; and Rydin, Håkan: The influence of muscular exercise on the tolerance of digitalis
in guinea-pigs. Acta Physiol. Scand. 15:63-69, Feb. 28, 1948. (Stockholm)

Embden, Gustav: Neue Untersuchungen über die Tätigkeits-Substanzen der quergestreiften Muskulatur
und den Chemismus der Muskelkontraktion. Klin. Wschr. 6:628-631, Apr. 2, 1927.
(Frankfurt)

----, and Adler, Erich: Über die Phosphorsäureverteilung in der weissen und roten Muskulatur des
Kaninchens. Hoppe-Seyler Zeits. physiol. Chem. 113:201-222, Apr. 5, 1921. (Frankfurt)

----, and Grafe, Eduard: Über den Einfluss der Muskelarbeit auf die Phosphorsäureausscheidung.
Hoppe-Seyler Zeits. physiol. Chem. 113:108-137, Mar. 30, 1921. (Frankfurt)

----, ----, and Schmitz, Ernst: Über Steigerung der Leistungsfähigkeit durch Phosphatzufuhr.
Hoppe-Seyler Zeits. physiol. Chem. 113:67-107, Mar. 30, 1921. (Frankfurt)

Embden, Gustav; and Isaac, S.: Über den Einfluss der Phosphorvergiftung auf den Lactacidogengehalt des Kaninchenmuskels. Hoppe-Seyler Zeits. physiol. Chem. 113:263-270, Apr. 5, 1921. (Frankfurt)

----, and Laquer, Fritz: Über die Chemie des Lactacidogens. III. Hoppe-Seyler Zeits. physiol. Chem. 113:1-9, Mar. 25, 1921. (Frankfurt)

----, Schmitz, Ernst; and Meincke, Peter: Uber den Einfluss der Muskelarbeit auf den Lactacidogengehalt der quergestreiften Muskulatur. Hoppe-Seyler Zeits. physiol. Chem. 113:10-66, Mar. 25, 1921. (Frankfurt)

----, and Zimmermann, Margarete. Über die Chemie des Lactacidogens. IV. Mitteilung. Hoppe-Seyler Zeits. physiol. Chem. 141:225-232, Dec. 31, 1924. (Frankfurt)

Engelhardt, Hugo T.; and Sodeman, William A.: Syncope on exertion: relationship to coronary artery disease. Ann. Intern. Med. 22:225-233, Feb., 1945. (New Orleans)

Engels, Josef; and Nieske, Ludwig: Über das Verhalten des arteriellen Druckes während körperlicher Arbeit. Zeits. ges. exp. Med. 110:81-91, Feb. 10, 1942. (Köln)

Enschedé, F. A.; and Jongbloed, J.: The physical condition of top-skaters during training. Int. Zeits. angew. Physiol. 20:252-257, Feb., 1964.

Eranko, Olavi; and Harkonen, Matti: Distribution and concentration of adrenaline and noradrenaline in the adrenal medulla of the rat following depletion induced by muscular work. Acta Physiol. Scand. 51:247-253, Feb.-Mar., 1961. (Helsinki)

----, and ----: Effect of muscular work and denervation on histochemically demonstrable acid phosphatase activity in the adrenal medulla of the rat. Ann. Med. Exp. Fenn. 40:129-133, 1962. (Helsinki)

----, and ----: Long-term effects of muscular work on the adrenal medulla of the mouse. Endocrinology 69:186-187, July, 1961. (Helsinki)

----, Karvonen, M. J.; and Räisänen, L.: Long-term effects of muscular work on the adrenal medulla of the rat. Acta Endocrinol. 39:285-287, Feb., 1962. (Helsinki)

Erez, V. P.: Vliianie dlitel'nykh zaniatiĭ fizicheskoi kul'turoĭ na funktsiiu sistemy gipofiz-kora nadpochechnikov u pozhilykh liudeĭ. (Effect of prolonged physical exercise on the adreno-cortical-pituitary activity in the aged) (Russ). Ter. Arkh. 36:15-19, Mar., 1964.

Erickson, Lester; Simonson, Ernst; Taylor, Henry Longstreet; Alexander, Howard; and Keys, Ancel: The energy cost of horizontal and grade walking on the motor-driven treadmill. Amer. J. Physiol. 145:391-401, Jan., 1946. (Minneapolis)

Erikson, H.: The respiratory gaseous exchange after a short burst of exercise. Acta Physiol. Scand. 40:182-195, Oct. 10, 1957. (Swarthmore)

----: The respiratory response to acute exercise of Eskimoes and white. Acta Physiol. Scand. 41:1-11, Nov. 26, 1957. (Point Barrow)

Ernst, E.; and Mies, H.: Weitere Untersuchungen über den Einfluss des "Lezithins" auf den Erholungsvorgang. München. med. Wschr. 102:713-716, Apr. 8, 1960. (Koln)

Eronin, F. T.: Vliianie razlichnykh pit'evykh rezhimov na diurez v usloviiakh vysokoi temperatury vozdukha i fizicheskoĭ nagruzki. (Effect of various drinking patterns on diuresis under the condition of high air temperature and physical load) (Russ). Fiziol. Zh. SSSR Sechenov. 49:1249-1253, Oct., 1963.

Errebo-Knudsen, E.: Diabetes mellitus and exercise; a physiopathologic study of muscular work in patients with diabetes mellitus. (Trans. by Einar Christensen; thesis) Copenhagen, 1948.

Escobar Del Rey, F.; and Morreale De Escobar, G.: Studies on the peripheral disappearance of thyroid hormone. II. The effect of swimming for two hours on the I^{131} distribution in thyroidectomized, 1-thyroxine maintained rats after the injection of I^{131} labeled 1-thyroxine. Acta Endocr. 23: 393-399, Dec., 1956. (Leiden)

----, and ----: Studies on the peripheral disappearance of thyroid hormone. III. The effect of running for 12 hours on the I^{131} distribution in thyroidectomized, 1-thyroxine maintained rats after the injection of I^{131}-labeled 1-thyroxine. Acta Endocr. 23:400-406, Dec., 1956. (Leiden)

Eskildsen, P.; Gøtzsche, H.; and Hansen, A. Tybjaerg: Measuring of the intra-arterial blood pressure during exercise. Acta Med. Scand. 138(Suppl. 239):245-250, 1950. (Copenhagen)

Essex, Hiram E.: Response of coronary circulation to exercise, to certain drugs and to anoxic stresses. J. Aviation Med. 21:456-460, Dec., 1950. (Rochester, Minn.)

----, Herrick, J. F.; Baldes, Edward J.; and Mann, Frank C.: Effects of exercise on the coronary blood flow, heart rate and blood pressure of trained dogs with denervated and partially denervated hearts. Amer. J. Physiol. 138:687-697, Apr., 1943. (Rochester, Minn.)

----, ----, ----, and ----: Influence of exercise on blood pressure, pulse rate and coronary blood flow of the dog. Amer. J. Physiol. 125:614-623, Mar., 1939. (Rochester, Minn.)

Ettinger, G. H.; and Jeffs, Doreen: Effects in the dog of infusion of adrenal cortical extract on exercise tolerance, blood constituents, and adrenal cortex. Endocrinology 32:351-355, Apr., 1943. (Kingston, Ont.)

Euler, Curt von; and Söderberg, Ulf: Medullary chemosensitive receptors. J. Physiol. 118:545-554, Dec. 30, 1952. (Stockholm)

----, and ----: Slow potentials in the respiratory centres. J. Physiol. 118:555-564, Dec. 30, 1952. (Stockholm)

Euler, U. S. von; and Liljestrand, G.: The regulation of respiration during muscular work. Acta Physiol. Scand. 12:268-278, Nov. 26, 1946. (Stockholm)

----, and ----: The regulation of the blood pressure with special reference to muscular work. Acta Physiol. Scand. 12:279-300, Nov. 26, 1946. (Stockholm)

Evans, W. O.: A titration schedule on a treadmill. J. Exper. Anal. Behav. 6:219-221, Apr., 1963.

Evers, H.: The physiology of respiration and circulation in muscular exercise. Univ. Durham Coll. Med. Gaz. 14:93-99, 1913-1914.

Ewerhardt, F. H.: Physical exercise. In: Glasser, O., ed. Medical physics. Chicago, Year Book, 1944. Vol. 1. pa. 1040-1043. (St. Louis)

Fabre, Henri: Les troubles et les accidents cardiaques consécutifs aux excès sportifs. J. Méd. Bordeaux 136:244-247, Feb., 1959. (Bordeaux)

----, and Fabre R.: Les répercussions circulatoires de l'effort; étude expérimentale sur l'homme. J. Physiologie 44:645-654, 1952. (Bordeaux)

----, Linquette, Y.; and Rougier, G.: Modifications électrocardiographiques consécutives a l'apnéa volontaire avec ou sans effort. (Résultats complémentaires). J. Physiologie 49:149-150, Jan.-Mar., 1957. (Bordeaux)

----, and Rougier, G.: Les répercussions circulatoires de l'effort; étude expérimentale sur le chien. J. Physiologie 44:655-661, 1952. (Bordeaux)

Fabre, R.; Fabre, Henri; Dervillée, E.; and Chemin, P.: Modifications électrocardiographiques consécutives à une activité musculaire intense poursuivie jusqu' a épuisement. J. Physiologie 56:345-346, May-June, 1964. (Bordeaux)

Fabricius ab Aquapendente, Hieronymus: De motu locali animalium secundum totum. Patavii, J. B. de Martin, 1618.

Fahri, L. E.; and Rahn, H.: Gas stores of the body and the unsteady state. J. Appl. Physiol. 7:472-484, Mar., 1955. (Rochester)

Fanfani, M.: Le alterazioni istopatologiche del miocardio correlate con le modificazioni dell'elettrocardiogramma in conigli sottoposti a sforzo e a spavento. Atti Soc. Ital. Cardiol. 16:232-234, 1954.

Farez, Demosthène Camille: Sur l'exercice, son influence sur l'économie animale dans l'état de santé et dans l'état de maladie. Paris, Thèse Numero 222, vol. 176, 1822.

Farneti, P.; Boccardi, S.; and Colombo, I.: L'apparato muscolare nel vecchio. Aspetti di patologia e di terapia. Gior. Geront. 33(Suppl.):171, 1964.

Farquharson, Robert: The influence of athletic sports on health. Lancet 1:513-515, Apr. 9; 1:545-546, Apr. 16, 1870. (Rugby)

Faugère, P. J.: Les réactions cardiovasculaires sous l'influence des exercices physiques. Bordeaux, Samie, 1943.

Faulkner, J. A.: Effect of cardiac conditioning on the anticipatory, exercise, and recovery heart rates of young men. J. Sport Med. 4:79-86, June, 1964. (Boston)

Fechner, G. T.: Ueber den Gang der Muskelübung. Ber. Verh. Sachs. Ges. Wissensch., Leipzig 9:Math. phys. Kl. 113-120, 1857.

Federici, Ernest E.; Lerner, A. Martin; and Abelmann, Walter H.: Observations on the course of Coxsackie A-9 myocarditis in C3H mice. Proc. Sox. Exper. Biol. Med. 112:672-676, Mar., 1963. (Boston)

Fedorova, G. P.: Vliianie myshechnoi deiatel'nosti razlichnoi dlitel'nosti na soderzhanie NAD i NAD-N v myshtsakh, pecheni i krovi. (Effect of muscular activity of various durations on the content of NAD and NAD-N in the muscle, liver and blood) (Russ). Ukr. Biokhim. Zh. 36:119-125, 1964.

Fehler, Hans Werner Rudolf Herbert: Der Einfluss von Ruhe und Bewegung auf den alimentären
Alkoholspiegel des Blutes. Berlin, Kühn, 1939. (Berlin)

Fellows, Gladys; Goldsmith, Grace A.; Luenzman, Lenore; Sammons, Louise; Williams, Clara B.;
and Zimmerman, Beulah W.: Effect of physical exercise upon the complex reaction time and
auditory acuity. Amer. J. Physiol. 77:402-408, July, 1926. (Madison)

Felman, A. L.: Immediate effects of exercise on apparent limb mass and circumference. Int.
Zeits. angew. Physiol. 20:38-44, 1963.

Fendler, K.; Telegdy, G.; and Endröczi, E.: Effect of chronic stress on the oxytocic and antidiuretic
activity of the hypophysis in the rat. Acta Physiol. Acad. Sci. Hung. 24:287-292, 1964.

Fenicia, M.: La glicemia nel sangue arterioso e venoso dei vasi, femorali durante il lavoro dei gruppi
muscolari dell'arto corréspondente. Riv. Pat. Sper. 16:445-459, 1936.

Fenn, Wallace O.: A quantitative comparison between the energy liberated and the work performed
by the isolated sartorius muscle of the frog. J. Physiol. 58:175-203, Dec. 28, 1923. (Manchester
and London)

----: The relation between the work performed and the energy liberated in muscular contraction.
J. Physiol. 58:373-395, May 23, 1924. (Manchester and London)

----, and Craig, Albert B., Jr.: Effect of CO_2 on respiration using a new method of administering
CO_2. J. Appl. Physiol. 18:1023-1024, Sept., 1963. (Rochester, N.Y.)

Ferreira, Affonso L.; Goncalves, Renato Pinto; and Lison, Lucien: Influence de l'exercice forcé
sur les mitoses de l'épithélium cornéen chez le rat. Comptes Rend. Acad. Sci. 252:4058-4059,
June 19, 1961. (Sao Paulo)

Ferrero, C.; Leupin, A.; Moret, P.; and Cuénod, C.-L.: Oscillographie artérielle de la jambe;
changements de volumes et contours sphygmiques aprés effort. Cardiologia 30:126-133, 1957.
(Geneva)

Fick, Adolf: Mechanische Arbeit und Wärmeentwickelung bei der Muskelthätigkeit. Leipzig, 1882.

----: Ueber die Messung des Blutquantums in den Herzventrikeln. Sitzungsb. physik. med. Ges.
Würzburg, 1870. p. 16.

----: Untersuchungen über Muskelarbeit. Basel, H. Georg, 1867.

----, and Wislicenus, J.: On the origin of muscle power. London, Edinburgh & Dublin
Philosoph. Mag. Fourth series (supplement) 31:485-503, June, 1866.

----, and ----: Ueber die Entstehung der Muskelkraft. Zurich Vierteljahrsschr. 10:317-348,
1865. (Also in Ann. Sci. Nat. (Zool.) 10:257-279, 1868.)

Fidanza, F.; Mancini, M.; and Cioffi, L. A.: (Blood lipid and coagulation picture in man in
relation to diet and physical activity) (It). Minerva Med. 51:1183-1188, Apr. 7, 1960. (Naples)

Figueiredo Magalhães, B.; and Mesquita, Q. H. de: Velocidade sanguínea e prova de esforço.
Rev. Clín. São Paulo 16:117-120, Aug., 1944.

Filipova, G. G.: Zmina rukhovykh kharchovykh (Kharchoz-dobuval'nykh) umovnykh refleksiv u sobak pid vplyvom dynamichnogo navantazhennia. (Changes in motor alimentary (food-procuring) conditioned reflex in dogs under the influence of dynamic stress) (Uk). Fiziol. Zh. 9:443-450, Aug.-Sept., 1963.

Filippova, E. A.; and Zernov, N. G.: Dispansernoe nabliudenie nad det'mi s funktsional'nymi serdechno-sosudistymi izmeneniiami. (Dispensary observation on children with functional cardiovascular changes) (Russ). Vop. Okhr. Materin. Dets. 8:55-59, June, 1963.

Filley, Giles F.; MacIntosh, Donald J.; and Wright, George W.: Carbon monoxide uptake and pulmonary diffusing capacity in normal subjects at rest and during exercise. J. Clin. Invest. 33:530-539, Apr., 1954. (Trudeau, N.Y.)

Fischer, Ernst: Volume changes of heart and of skeletal muscle during and after activity. (Abstract) Amer. J. Physiol. 113:42-43, Sept., 1935. (Rochester, N.Y.)

Fischl, R.: Ueber Abhärtung. Fortschr. Med. 28:1575-1581, 1910.

Fisher, A. Murray; and Bernstein, Alan: March hemoglobinuria; a case report. Bull. Johns Hopkins Hosp. 67:457-461, Dec., 1940. (Baltimore)

Fishman, Alfred P.; Fritts, Harry W., Jr.; and Cournand, André: Effects of acute hypoxia and exercise on the pulmonary circulation. Circulation 22:204-215, Aug., 1960. (New York)

Fitzgerald, Mabel Purefoy; and Haldane, John Scott: The normal alveolar carbonic acid pressure in man. J. Physiol. 32:486-494, July 13, 1905. (Oxford)

Flandrois, R.: La consommation maximale d'oxygène. Presse Méd. 69:1267-1269, June 10, 1961. (Paris)

Fleisch, A. O.: Elektrokardiographie während Belastung unter direkter Kontrolle am Sichtgerät. Cardiologia 40:235-244, 1962. (Mammern, Switz.)

----: (Effort tests of average duration in the healthy subject) (Fr). Poumon Coeur 15:883-889, Nov., 1959.

----: Gefahren und Grenzen des Arbeitsversuches im Elektrokardiogram. Schweiz. med. Wschr. 92:456-460, Apr. 14, 1962. (Mammern, Switz.)

Fleming, Ralph G.; and Kinsman, J. Murray: March hemoglobinuria, with 2 case reports. Southern Med. J. 38:739-742, Nov., 1945. (Durham, N.C. and Louisville)

Fletcher, J. G.: Maximal work production in man. J. Appl. Physiol. 15:764-768, Sept., 1960. (London)

Fletcher, W. Morley: The influence of oxygen upon the survival respiration of muscle. J. Physiol. 28:354-359, Sept. 12, 1902. (Cambridge, Eng.)

----: Lactic acid formation, survival respiration and rigor mortis in mammalian muscle. J. Physiol. 47:361-380, Dec. 19, 1913. (Cambridge, Eng.)

----: The osmotic properties of muscle, and their modifications in fatigue and rigor. J. Physiol. 30:414-438, Feb. 25, 1904. (Cambridge, Eng.)

Fletcher, W. Morley: The relation of oxygen to the survival metabolism of muscle. J. Physiol. 28:474-498, Dec. 15, 1902. (Cambridge, Eng.)

----: The survival respiration of muscle. J. Physiol. 23:10-99, June 10, 1898. (Cambridge, Eng.)

----, and Hopkins, F. Gowland: Lactic acid in amphibian muscle. J. Physiol. 35:247-309, Mar. 27, 1907. (Cambridge, Eng.)

----, and ----: The respiratory process in muscle and the nature of muscular motion. Croonian Lecture. Proc. Roy. Soc. 89B:444-467, Mar. 1, 1917.

Flint, Austin, Jr.: The influence of excessive and prolonged muscular exercise upon the elimination of effete matters from the kidneys; based on an analysis of the urine passed by Mr. Weston, while walking one hundred miles in twenty-one hours and thirty-nine minutes. New York Med. J. 12:280-289, Oct., 1870. (New York)

----: The influence of long-continued muscular exercise on the composition of the urine. Med. Gaz. 5:211-213, Oct. 1, 1870. (New York)

----: Relations of urea to muscular exercise. Practitioner 6:250-253, Apr., 1871. (New York)

----: Supplementary remarks on the physiological effects of severe and protracted muscular exercise, with special reference to its influence upon the excretion of nitrogen. J. Anat. & Physiol. 11:109-117, 1876-1877.

Fodstad, D. O.: Ventilatory response to muscular exercise in patients with cardiac dyspnea. Scand. J. Clin. Lab. Invest. 8:104-107, 1956. (Oslo)

Fogel'son, L. I.; and Iazburskis, B. I.: Radioeléktrokardiografiia kak metod issledovaniia deiatel'nosti serdtsa vo vremia proizvodstvennoi raboty. (Radioelectrocardiography as a method of determining cardiac activity during the performance of work) (Russ). Kardiologiia 4:67-73, July-Aug., 1964.

----, Lebedeva, O. V.; Malysheva, L. G.; et al: Trudosposobnost'bol'nykh khronicheskimi zabolevaniiami legkikh. (The work capacity of patients with chronic lung diseases) (Russ). Ter. Arkh. 35:26-33, June, 1963.

Foldes, F. F.; Monte, A. P.; Brunn, H. M., Jr.; and Wolfson, B.: The influence of exercise on the neuromuscular activity of relaxant drugs. Canad. Anaesth. Soc. J. 8:118-127, Mar., 1961.

Ford, Amasa B.: The energy cost of work. Phys. Ther. Rev. 40:859-862, Dec., 1960. (Cleveland)

Fornoza, A.: Modifications of the hemogramme in swimmers and gymnasts by physical exercise and the Finnish bath, Sauna. J. Sport Med. 4:37-42, Mar., 1964.

Forssander, C. A.: Alveolar air changes following inhalation of carbon dioxide during exercise, and calculation of cardiac output. J. Appl. Physiol. 8:509-512, Mar., 1956. (Montreal)

Forssman, Olof; and Bergman, Halvar: Cytotoxic factor in a patient with sudden death occurring during exercise. Acta Allerg. 18:471-473, 1963. (Karlskogattospital, Swed.)

Foster, Glenn L.: The effects of exercise on respiratory exchange and peripheral blood flow. Med. Arts & Sci. 10:145-151, Fourth Quarter, 1956. (Los Angeles)

----, and Reeves, T. Joseph: Hemodynamic responses to exercise in clinically normal middle-aged men and in those with angina pectoris. J. Clin. Invest. 43:1758-1768, Sept., 1964. (Birmingham, Ala.)

Foster, Ruth C.; Brouwer, Stephen W.; and Kurtz, Chester M.: Thrombosis of the inferior vena cava following physical exertion. J.A.M.A. 117:2167-2168, Dec. 20, 1941. (Madison)

Foster, Wilfred L.: The relation of exercise to adolescent heart development. Arch. Pediat. 26:814-817, Nov., 1909. (Brooklyn)

Fothergill, H. J.: Strain in its relation to the circulatory organs. Brit. Med. J. 1:281, 1873.

Fouré, G. C. F.: Sur l'influence de l'exercice sur l'économie animale dans l'etat de santé et de maladie. Paris, Thèse Numero 3, volume 69, 1808.

Fowler, P. B. S.; and Guz, A.: Blood pressure during exercise and the effect of hexamethonium. Brit. Heart J. 16:1-7, Jan., 1954. (London)

Fowler, William M., Jr.; Chowdhury, Sudhir R.; Pearson, Carl M.; Garoner, Gerald; and Bratton, Robert: Changes in serum enzyme levels after exercise in trained and untrained subjects. J. Appl. Physiol. 17:943-946, Nov., 1962. (Los Angeles)

----, and Gardner, Gerald W.: The relation of cardiovascular tests to measurements of motor performance and skills. Pediatrics 32(Suppl.):778-789, Oct., 1963. (Los Angeles)

Fox, Samuel M., III; and Skinner, James S.: Physical activity and cardiovascular health. Amer. J. Cardiol. 14:731-746, Dec., 1964. (Washington)

Fracchia, P.; and Antognetti, R. M.: L'azione della fatica muscolare sull'attività perossidasica leucocitaria dei soggetti normali. Gazz. Int. Med. Chir. 68(Suppl.):3114-3121, Dec. 31, 1963.

Frade Fernández, M. M.: Comportamiento circulatorio en reposo y en esfuerzo de los subalimentados. Medicina (Madrid) (part 2) 11:1-16, July, 1943.

Franck, C.; Grandpierre, R.; Santenoise, D.; and Stankoff, E.: Modifications de l'excitabilité des centres respiratoires chez les aviateurs en état de fatigue. Comptes Rend. Soc. Biol. 139:835-836, June 30, 1945. (Nancy)

Frank, A.; and Husten, M.: Experimentelle Untersuchungen zur Frage der Arbeitshypertrophie des Herzens nach Milzexstirpation. Zeits. ges. exp. Med. 119:450-456, 1952.

Frank, Otto: Thermodynamik des Muskels. Ergebn. Physiol. 3(Pt. 2):349-514, 1904. (München)

Franklin, Dean L.; Ellis, Richard M.; and Rushmer, R. F.: Aortic blood flow in dogs during treadmill exercise. J. Appl. Physiol. 14:809-812, Sept., 1959. (Seattle)

----, and Van Citters, Robert L.: Stroke volume changes in baboons during spontaneous activity and exercise. Amer. J. Cardiol. 12:816-821, Dec., 1963. (La Jolla)

Franseen, Elizabeth B.; Finesinger, Jacob E.; and Watkins, Arthur L.: The response of psychoneurotic patients and women to brisk submaximal exercise. Arch. Phys. Med. 30:219-233, Apr., 1949. (Boston)

Fraser, H. F.; Jones, B. E.; Rosenberg, D. E.; and Thompson, A. K.: Effects of addiction to intravenous heroin on patterns of physical activity in man. Clin. Pharmacol. Ther. 4:188-196, Mar.-Apr., 1963. (Lexington, Ky.)

Fraser, T. R.: The effects of rowing on circulation as shown by examination with the sphygmograph. J. Anat. & Physiol. 3:127-130, 1868-1869.

Freedman, M. E.; Snider, G. L.; Brostoff, P.; Kimelblot, S.; and Katz, L. N.: Effects of
    training on response of cardiac output to muscular exercise in athletes. J. Appl. Physiol.
    8:37-47, July, 1955. (Chicago)

Freedman, M. H.; and Connell, G. E.: The heterogeneity of gamma-globulin in post-exercise
    urine. Canad. J. Biochem. 42:1065-1097, July, 1964. (Toronto)

Freiman, Alvin H.; Tolles, William; Carbery, William J.; Ruesegger, Paul; Abarquez, Ramon F.;
    and Ladue, John S.: The electrocardiogram during exercise. Amer. J. Cardiol. 5:506-515,
    Apr., 1960. (New York)

Frenkel, Marcel: The effect of insulin and potassium in myasthenia gravis. Arch. Neurol. 9:
    447-457, Nov., 1963. (Chicago)

Frenkl, R.; and Csalay, L.: The effect of regular muscular activity on adrenocortical function in
    rats. J. Sport Med. 2:207-211, Dec., 1962.

----, ----, and Makara, G.: The effect of regular muscular activity on gastric acid secretion and
    on the development of experimental ulcer in the albino rat. Acta Physiol. Acad. Sci. Hungary
    22:203-208, 1962.

----, ----, ----, et al: The effect of regular muscle activity on the histamine sensitivity of
    the rat. Acta Physiol. Acad. Sci. Hungary 25:199-202, 1964.

----, ----, ----, et al: L'effet de l'activité musculaire régulière sur la sensibilité à la sérotonine
    des rats. Med. Exp. 10:190-194, 1964.

----, ----, ----, et al: Rendszeres izomtevékenység hatása patkányok serotonin-érzékenységére.
    (Effect of systematic muscular activity on the serotonin sensitivity in rats) (Hun). Kiserl.
    Orvostud. 16:391-393, Aug., 1964.

Frick, M. Heikki; Konttinen, Aarne; and Sarajas, H. S. Samuli: Effects of physical training on
    circulation at rest and during exercise. Amer. J. Cardiol. 12:142-147, Aug., 1963. (Helsinki)

----, and Somer, Tino: Base-line effects on response of stroke volume to leg exercise in the supine posi-
    tion. J. Appl. Physiol. 19:639-643, July, 1964. (Helsinki)

Friedberg, Charles K.: Physical effort and emotion in acute coronary thrombosis. (Editorial)
    Circulation 27:855-857, May, 1963. (New York)

----, Jaffe, Harry L.; Pordy, Leon; and Chesky, Kenneth: The two-step exercise electrocardiogram.
    A double-blind evaluation of its use in the diagnosis of angina pectoris. Circulation 26:1254-1260,
    Dec., 1962. (New York)

Friedberg, Samuel J.; Harlan, W. R., Jr.; Trout, D. L.; and Estes, E. Harvey, Jr.: The effect of exer-
    cise on the concentration and turnover of plasma nonesterified fatty acids. J. Clin. Invest. 39:
    215-220, Jan., 1960. (Durham, N.C.)

----, Sher, Paul B.; Bogdonoff, Morton D.; and Estes, E. Harvey, Jr.: The dynamics of plasma free
    fatty acid metabolism during exercise. J. Lipid Res. 4:34-38, Jan., 1963. (Durham, N.C.)

Friedberg, Samuel J.; Sreter, F. A.; and Friedman, C. L.: The effect of vasopressin and aldosterone on the distribution of water, sodium, and potassium and on work performance in old rats. Gerontologia 7:65-76, 1963.

Friedrich, Heinrich: Erträglichkeitsgrenze für wechselnde Raumtemperatur und -feuchte bei Ruhe und Arbeit. Pflüger Arch. ges. Physiol. 250:182-191, July 20, 1948. (Frankfurt)

Friehoff, Franzjosef: Der Gasaustausch bei gesunden Männern unter Ruhebedingungen und während körperlicher Arbeit. Pflüger Arch. ges. Physiol. 270:431-444, Mar. 11, 1960. (Bochum)

Friehoff, F.: (The normal alveolar-arterial P_{O2} gradient at rest and during exercise) (Fr). Poumon Coeur 16:987-992, Nov., 1960.

Fries, E. Corinne: Some physiologic effects of passive and active exercise. I. The cardiovascular response to graded exercises. Arch. Phys. Ther. 25:540-545, Sept., 1944. (Madison)

----: Some physiologic effects of passive and active exercise. II. Training effects on strength of specific muscle groups. Arch. Phys. Ther. 25:546-549, Sept., 1944. (Madison)

Froeb, H. F.; and Kim, B. M.: Changes in pH and pCO_2 in the pulmonary circulation during CO_2 breathing and exercise. Med. Thorac. 19:306-316, 1962.

Frohman, Charles E.; Latham, L. K.; Warner, K. A.; Brosius, C. O.; Beckett, P. G. S.; and Gottlieb, J. S.: Motor activity in schizophrenia; effect on plasma factor. Arch. Gen. Psychiat. 9:83-88, July, 1963. (Detroit)

Frucht, Adolf Henning: Die Grenzen der menschlichen Leistungs-fähigkeit im Sport. Berlin, Akademie-Verlag, 1960.

Frumerie, Karl: Über das Verhältnis des Ermüdungsgefühls zur CO_2-Abgabe bei statischer Muskelarbeit. Scand. Arch. Physiol. 30:409-440, 1913. (Stockholm)

Fugazza, Jeanne: Contribution à l'étude de la noradrénaline cérébrale. J. Physiologie 55(Suppl. 8): 1-76, Sept.-Oct., 1963. (Paris)

Fujioka, H.; Sumida, T.; and Nagamori, M.: (Inhibitory effects of L-aspartic acid salts against fatigue resulting from march) (Jap). Nat. Def. Med. J. 10:525-528, Nov., 1963.

Full, Fritz: Zur Frage der Leistungssteigerung durch perorale Kalktherapie bei Leibesübungen. Zeits. ges. phys. Ther. 41:98-104, Aug. 12, 1931.

----, and Lehmann, Gunther: Der Energieverbrauch beim Hantelstossen. Pflüger Arch. ges. Physiol. 201:611-619, 1923. (Berlin)

Furberg, C.; and Ringqvist, T.: Effekt av penicillin på fysisk arbetsförmaga och på upplevelsen av trötthet under arbete. (Effect of penicillin on the physical capacity for work and on the experience of fatigue during work) (Sw). Avensk. Lakartidn. 60:2650-2655, Sept. 11, 1963.

Furbetta, D.; Bufalari, A.; and Arcelli, M.: (Behavior of blood and tissular fluid exchange in relation to work) (It). Folia Med. 42:1299-1312, Nov., 1959.

----, ----, and ----: (Study on muscular work. Behavior of electrical resistance) (It). Folia Med. 43:934-944, Oct., 1960.

Furusawa, K.: Muscular exercise, lactic acid and the supply and utilization of oxygen. Part
    IX. Muscular activity and carbohydrate metabolism in the normal individual. Proc. Roy.
    Soc. 98B:65-76, May 1, 1925.

----: Muscular exercise, lactic acid and the supply and utilization of oxygen. Part X. The
    oxygen intake during exercise while breathing mixtures rich in oxygen. Proc. Roy. Soc.
    98B:287-289, July 1, 1925.

----: Muscular exercise, lactic acid and the supply and utilization of oxygen. Part XIII. The
    gaseous exchanges of restricted muscular exercise in man. Proc. Roy. Soc. 99B:155-166,
    Jan. 1, 1926.

----, Hill, A. V.; Long, C. N. H.; and Lupton, H.: Muscular exercise and oxygen requirement.
    Part VIII. Proc. Roy. Soc. 97B:167-176, Dec. 1, 1924.

----, ----, and Parkinson, J. L.: The dynamics of "sprint" running. Proc. Roy. Soc. 102B:29-42,
    Aug. 1, 1927.

----, ----, and ----: The energy used in "sprint" running. Proc. Roy. Soc. 102B:43-50, Aug. 1,
    1927.

Furuya, Hideo; Yamakure, Katsumaro; Minamitani, Kazutoshi; Yamanaka, Yoshitada; Kitamura, Kazuo;
    and Yamakawa, Kunio: The clinical evaluation of the exercise-test by the use of radioelectrocardio-
    graph. Jap. Heart J. 4:81-91, Jan., 1963. (Tokoyo)

Gabagni, R.; Angelino, P. F.; and Lixi, M.: Il comportamento del consumo di ossigeno sotto sforzo nei cardiaci. Minerva Med. 49:1277-1284, Apr. 4, 1958.

Gaisböck, F.: Zur Physiologie und Pathologie der Leibesübungen. Zeits. Hyg. Infektionskr. 112: 576-600, Sept. 15, 1931. (Innsbruck)

Galdston, Morton; and Wollack, A. C.: Oxygen and carbon dioxide tensions of alveolar air and arterial blood in healthy young adults at rest and after exercise. Amer. J. Physiol. 151: 276-281, Dec., 1947. (Army Chemical Center, Md.)

Galletti, P. M.: Les échanges respiratoires pendant l'exercice musculaire. Helv. Physiol. Pharmacol. Acta 17:34-61, Apr., 1959. (Lausanne)

----, Haab, P.; May, P.; and Fleisch, A.: L'état d'équilibre des échanges respiratoires pendant l'exercice musculaire. J. Physiologie 48:548-553, May-June, 1956. (Lausanne)

Gambill, Earl E.; and Hines, Edgar A., Jr.: Blood pressure in arm and thigh of man. IV. Blood pressure in exercised extremities. Amer. Heart J. 28:782-785, Dec., 1944. (Rochester, Minn.)

Gander, M.: Arbeitskapazität und totaler Hämoglobingehalt im Alter von über 40 Jahren. Helv. Med. Acta 31:669-695, Dec., 1964. (Zürich)

Gandevia, Bryan: Ventilatory response to exercise and the results of a standardized exercise test in chronic obstructive lung disease. Amer. Rev. Resp. Dis. 88:406-408. Sept., 1963.

Ganslen, R. V.; Balke, Bruno; Nagle, F. J.; and Phillips, E. E.: Effects of some tranquilizing, analeptic and vasodilating drugs on physical work capacity and orthostatic tolerance. Aerospace Med. 35:630-633, July, 1964. (Oklahoma City)

Gant, F. J.: Physiological observations in the case of W. Gale, during his walk of 4,000 quarters of a mile in 4,000 consecutive ten minutes; a period of twenty-eight days. Med. Exam. 2:982, 1877. (London)

Garbus, Joel; Highman, Benjamin; and Altland, Paul D.: Serum enzymes and lactic dehydrogenase isoenzymes after exercise and training in rats. Amer. J. Physiol. 207:467-472, Aug., 1964. (Bethesda)

Gardner, Ernest; and Jacobs, John: Joint reflexes and regulation of respiration during exercise. Amer. J. Physiol. 153:567-579, June, 1948. (Detroit)

Gardner, G. W.; Bratton, R.; Chowdhury, S. R.; et al: Effect of exercise on serum enzyme levels in trained subjects. J. Sport Med. 4:103-110, June, 1964.

Gardner, Horace T.; Rovelstad, Randolph A.; Moore, Douglas J.; Streitfeld, Franklin A.; and Knowlton, Marjorie: Hepatitis among American occupation troops in Germany: a follow-up study with particular reference to interim alcohol and physical activity. Ann. Intern. Med. 30:1009-1019, May, 1949. (Washington)

Gardner, Kenneth D., Jr.: "Athletic pseudonephritis" - alteration of urine sediment by athletic competition. J.A.M.A. 161:1613-1617, Aug. 25, 1956. (Philadelphia)

Garimoldi, M.; Pradella, F.; Ginesu, F.; et al: La valutazione del lavoro aerobico massimo coi diversi tipi di ergometro. Gior. Ital. Tuberc. 18:226-242, Nov.-Dec., 1964.

Garlind, T.; Goldberg, L.; Graf, K.; Perman, E. S.; Strandell, T.; and Strom, G.: Effect of ethanol on circulatory, metabolic, and neurohormonal function during muscular work in men. Acta Pharmacol. Toxicol. 17:106-114, 1960. (Stockholm)

Gaskell, W. H.: On the tonicity of the heart and blood-vessels. J. Physiol. 3:48-75, 1882. (Cambridge, Eng.)

Gasser, H. S.; and Hartree, W.: The inseparability of the mechanical and thermal responses in muscle. J. Physiol. 58:396-404, May 23, 1924. (London and Cambridge, Eng.)

----, and Hill, A. V.: The dynamics of muscular contraction. Proc. Roy. Soc. 96B:398-437, Aug. 1, 1924. (London)

----, and Meek, Walter J.: A study of the mechanisms by which muscular exercise produces acceleration of the heart. Amer. J. Physiol. 34:48-71, Apr., 1914. (Madison)

Gattuso, C.; Ciriminna, A.; and Bardino, M.: Influenza degli ormoni corticosurrenali sui fenomeni di proteosintesi e di proteolisi durante il lavoro, in relazione all'età. Sicilia Sanit. 1:71-73, July-Sept., 1963.

Gauer, Otto H.: Volume changes of the left ventricle during blood pooling and exercise in the intact animal. Their effects on left ventricular performance. Physiol. Rev. 35:143-155, Jan., 1955. (Durham, N.C.)

Gayet, R.: Sur les mécanismes d'adaptation de l'organisme dans l'exercice musculaire. Rev. Prat. Biol. 28:161-166, 1935.

Geddes, L. A.; Partridge, M.; and Hoff, H. E.: An EKG lead for exercising subjects. J. Appl. Physiol. 15:311-312, Mar., 1960. (Houston)

Gemmill, Chalmers L.; and Riberio, B. A.: A study of the phosphates and creatine in blood of man after strenuous muscular exercise. Sunti Congr. Internaz. Fisiol. 14 Congr. 1932, p. 98.

Gemzell, Carl A.; Robbe, Hjördis; and Ström, Gunnar: Total amount of haemoglobin and physical working capacity in normal pregnancy and puerperium (with iron medication). Acta Obstet. Gynec. Scand. 36:93-136, 1957. (Stockholm)

George, J. C.; and Vallyathan, N. V.: Effect of exercise on free fatty acid levels in the pigeon. J. Appl. Physiol. 19:619-622, July, 1964. (Baroda)

George, William K.; George, William D., Jr.; Smith, John P.; Gordon, Fallon T.; Baird, Elwood E.; and Mills, Gordon C.: Changes in serum calcium, serum phosphate and red-cell phosphate during hyperventilation. New Eng. J. Med. 270:726-728, Apr. 2, 1964. (Galveston)

Georgiyev, V. I.: Changes in efferent impulsation in the nerves to some vascular regions during muscular exertion. Fiziol. Zh. SSSR Sechenov 47:1517-1524, 1961.

Georgopoulos, A. J.; Proudfit, W. L.; and Page, Irvine H.: Effect of exercise on electrocardiograms of patients with low serum potassium. Circulation 23:567-572, Apr., 1961. (Cleveland)

Geppert, J.; and Zuntz, N.: Ueber die Regulation der Atmung. Pflüger Arch. ges. Physiol. 42: 189-245, 1888.

Gerheim, E. B.; and Miller, A. T., Jr.: The influence of brief periods of strenuous exercise on the blood platelet count. Science 109:64-65, Jan. 21, 1949. (Chapel Hill, N.C.)

Gerking, S. D.; and Robinson, Sid: Decline in the rates of sweating of men working in severe heat. Amer. J. Physiol. 147:370-378, Oct., 1946. (Bloomington, Ind.)

Gersten, Jerome W.; Brown, Isadore; Speck, Louise; and Grueter, Barbara: Comparison of tension development and circulation in biceps and triceps in man. Amer. J. Phys. Med. 42:156-165, Aug., 1963. (Denver)

Gesell, Robert: The chemical regulation of respiration. Physiol. Rev. 5:551-595, Oct., 1925. (Ann Arbor)

Gessler, H.: Die Ökonomie der menschlichen Muskelarbeit. II. Mitteilung. Deutsch. Arch. klin. Med. 157:36-45, Sept., 1927. (Heidelberg)

Geuens, L.: Contribution à l'etude des modifications de éléments figurés du sang, au repos et après l'effort. Acta Belg. Arte Med. Pharm. Milit. 110:601-610, Dec., 1957.

----: Etude sur quelques modifications du sang au cours d'exercices physiques. Acta Belg. Arte Med. Pharm. Milit. 109:155-163, Sept.-Dec., 1956.

Gey, G. O., Jr.; and Kennard, D. W.: Work and power capacity of normal mice and those suffering from muscular dystrophy, measured during stationary swimming. Nature 202:264-266, Apr. 18, 1964. (Cambridge, Eng.)

Gfeller, G.; and Roux, J. L.: L'atteinte cardiaque dans la myotonie atrophique de Steinert. Cardiologia 42:200-205, 1963. (Geneva)

Ghiringhelli, G.; and Bosisio, E.: Contributo alla conoscenza della fisiologia respiratoria, in condizioni di riposo e di lavoro muscolare, in soggetti di sesso femminile in eta giovanile. Arch. Fisiol. 57:82-101, July 30, 1957.

----, and ----: Rapporti tra valori degli indici spirometrici di riposo, della ventilazione polmonare massima da lavoro esauriente e del massimio lavoro aerobico in un gruppo di soggetti sani di varia età e sesso. Riv. Med. Aero. 19:619-637, Oct.-Dec., 1956.

----, ----, and Repaci, M.: Contributo alla conoscenza della fisiologia respiratoria, in condizioni di riposo e di lavoro muscolare, nei soggetti in età presenile e senile. Riv. Med. Aero. 19:486-510, July-Sept., 1956.

Ghiringhelli, L.; and Molina, C.: Catalasi e anossia anossica secondaria a lavoro eseguita in anaerobiosi. Med. Lavoro 43:463-467, Dec., 1952.

Gilat, Tuvia; Shibolet, Shlomo; and Sohar, Ezra: The mechanism of heatstroke. J. Trop. Med. Hyg. 66:204-212, Aug., 1963. (Tel-Hashomer, Israel)

Gilbert, Robert; Auchincloss, J. Howard, Jr.; and Epifano, Leonard: Exercise performance as part of a cardiac evaluation. Amer. J. Med. 34:452-460, Apr., 1963. (Syracuse)

----, and Lewis, J. K.: The effect of exercise on the plasma volume of patients with heart failure. Circulation 2:402-408, Sept., 1950. (San Francisco)

Gillespie, J. R.; Tyler, W. S.; and Eberly, V. E.: Blood pH, O_2, and CO_2 tensions in exercised control and emphysematous horses. Amer. J. Physiol. 207:1067-1072, Nov., 1964. (Davis, Calif.)

Gillespie, R. D.: The relative influence of mental and muscular work on the pulse-rate and blood-pressure. J. Physiol. 58:425-432, May 23, 1924. (Glasgow)

----, Gibson, C. R., Jr.; and Murray, D. S.: The effect of exercise on pulse rate and blood-pressure. Heart 12:1-22, June, 1925. (Glasgow)

Gilligan, D. Rourke; and Altschule, M. D.: March hemoglobinuria in a woman. New Eng. J. Med. 243:944-948, Dec. 14, 1950. (Boston)

----, and Blumgart, Herrman L.: March hemoglobinuria. Studies of the clinical characteristics, blood metabolism and mechanism: with observations on three new cases, and review of the literature. Medicine 20:341-395, Sept., 1941. (Boston)

Gini, C.: (The influence of exercise on the evolution of organs. A sub-Lamarck theory of evolution) (Fr). Acta Genet. Med. 10:312-315, July, 1961.

Giuntini, C.; Lewis, M. L.; Luis, A. Sales; and Harvey, R. M.: A study of the pulmonary blood volume in man by quantitative radiocardiography. J. Clin. Invest. 42:1589-1605, Oct., 1963. (New York)

Giusti, C.: (Auriculoventricular conduction in the electrocardiogram after exercise) (It). Cuore Circ. 45:193-203, Aug., 1961.

----: (The influence of muscular exertion on changes in right ventricular conduction) (It). Cuore Circ. 44:89-102, Apr., 1960.

Glatzel, H.; and Rettenmaier, G.: Die Blutzuckerregulation nach einer Konzentratnahrung bei Muskelarbeit. Schweiz. Zeits. Sportmed. 11:126-140, 1963.

Gleason, William L.; Bacos, James M.; Miller, D. Edmond; and McIntosh, Henry D.: A major pitfall in the interpretation of the central blood volume. (Abstract) Clin. Res. 7:227, Apr., 1959. (Durham, N.C.)

Glover, W. E.; and Shanks, R. G.: Forearm blood flow during prolonged intra-arterial infusions of adrenaline, and the effects of intra-arterial adrenaline on post-exercise hyperaemia. J. Physiol. 167:268-279, July, 1963. (Belfast)

Gobbato, F.; Turchetto, P.; Coltro, L.; et al: Velocità dell'ondo sfigmica e distensibilità delle arterie durante esercizio muscolare. Minerva Cardioangiol. 12:251-256, July, 1964.

Götze, W.; and Kofes, A.: Über Radio-Elektrencephalographie. (Eine Methode aum Studium des Einflusses körperlicher Belastungen auf die Hirnfunktion.) Zeits. ges. exp. Med. 126:439-443, Dec. 15, 1955. (Berlin)

Goff, L. G.; and Bartlett, R. G., Jr.: Elevated end-tidal CO_2 in trained underwater swimmers. J. Appl. Physiol. 10:203-206, Mar., 1957. (Bethesda)

----, Brubach, H. F.; and Specht, H.: Measurements of respiratory responses and work efficiency of underwater swimmers utilizing improved instrumentation. J. Appl. Physiol. 10:197-202, Mar., 1957. (Bethesda)

Goff, L. G.; Brubach, H. F.; Specht, H.; and Smith, N.: Effect of total immersion at various temperatures on oxygen uptake at rest and during exercise. J. Appl. Physiol. 9:59-61, July, 1956. (Bethesda)

----, Frassetto, Roberto; and Specht, H.: Oxygen requirements in underwater swimming. J. Appl. Physiol. 9:219-221, Sept., 1956. (Bethesda)

Goiffon, R.; and Chauvois, L.: Quelques modifications de l'équilibre acide-base des urines après l'exercice physique. Comptes Rend. Soc. Biol. 100:330-332, Feb. 2, 1929.

Golden, Abner: Syncope associated with exertional dyspnea and angina pectoris. Amer. Heart J. 28:689-698, Dec., 1944. (Atlanta)

Golder, Werner: Körperbau und Leistungsfahigkeit. Arzt u. Sport 12:2-3, Jan., 1936. (Berlin)

Golding, L. A.; and Barnard, J. R.: The effect of d-amphetamine sulfate on physical performance. J. Sport Med. 3:221-224, Dec., 1963.

Goldman, R. F.; Bullen, B.; and Seltzer, C.: Changes in specific gravity and body fat in overweight female adolescents as a result of weight reduction. Ann. N. Y. Acad. Sci. 110:913-917, Sept. 26, 1963. (Natick and Boston)

----, and Iampietro, P. F.: Energy cost of load carriage. J. Appl. Physiol. 17:675-676, July, 1962. (Natick)

Goldner, Fred, Jr.; and Burr, Robert Edward: Work and the heart: anticipation and ergonometry. Amer. J. Med. Sci. 246:192-199, Aug., 1963. (Nashville)

Goldspink, G.: The combined effects of exercise and reduced food intake on skeletal muscle fibers. J. Cell. Comp. Physiol. 63:209-216, Apr., 1964. (Dublin)

Goldstein, Jack E.; and Cogan, David G.: Exercise and the optic neuropathy of multiple sclerosis. Arch. Ophthal. 72:168-170, Aug., 1964. (Boston)

Goldstein, M. S.: Humoral nature of hypoglycemia in muscular exercise. Amer. J. Physiol. 200: 67-70, Jan., 1961. (Chicago)

Gollnick, Philip D.; and Hearn, George R.: Lactic dehydrogenase activities of heart and skeletal muscle of exercised rats. Amer. J. Physiol. 201:694-696, Oct., 1961. (Pullman, Wash.)

Gonţea, Iancu; Şuţescu, P.; and Dumitrache, S.: The influence of a hot microclimate on protein requirements during labour. Rumanian Med. Rev. 5:162-164, 1961.

----, ----, and ----: Investigations on protein requirements of man during labour. Rumanian Med. Rev. 4:94-96, July-Sept., 1960.

Gontzea, I.; Dumitrache, S.; and Schutzescu, P.: (Studies on the mechanism of increased nitrogen excretion in the urine under the influence of muscular work) (Ger). Int. Zeits. angew. Physiol. 19:7-17, 1961.

----, Şutzesco, P.; and Dumitrache, S.: Influence de l'adaptation à l'effort sur le bilan azoté chez l'homme. Arch. Sci. Physiol. 16:127-138, 1962. (Bucarest)

----, ----, and ----: (Protein requirements of the man at work; influence of physical exertion on nitrogen balance) (Fr). Arch. Sci. Physiol. 13:99-108, 1959.

Gontzea, I.; Şutzescho, P.; and Dumitrache, S.: Recherches sur le besoin en protéines de l'homme au cours de l'activité musculaire. Arch. Sci. Physiol. 16:97-120, 1962. (Bucarest)

Gontzea, J.; and Schutzescu, P.: (Nitrogen loss with sweat in muscular work) (Ger). Int. Zeits. angew. Physiol. 20:90-110, 1963.

----, ----, and Dumitrache, S.: (Studies on the protein requirement of man during physical work in a hot environment) (Ger). Int. Zeits. angew. Physiol. 18:248-263, 1960.

González Cruz, A.: Modificaciones de la presión venosa con el esfuerzo en personas sanas de edad geriátrica. Med. Esp. 32:124-149, Aug., 1954.

González Deleito, F.: Corazón y ejercicios físicos. Rev. Esp. Med. Cir. 10:194-201, 1927.

Good, J. Mason: Observations on the treadwheel. London Med. & Phys. J. 50:205-208, Sept., 1823.

Goor, H. van; and Mosterd, W. L.: Gas exchange during and after muscular work. Proc. Kon. Ned. Akad. Wet. (Biol. Med.) 64:96-98, 1961.

Gordon, Burgess: Effect of exercise on the circulation, sugar metabolism, and other factors. Northwest Med. 25:376-379, July, 1926. (Philadelphia)

Gorlin, Richard; Krasnow, Norman; Levine, Herbert J.; and Messer, Joseph V.: Effect of exercise on cardiac performance in human subjects with minimal heart disease. Amer. J. Cardiol. 13:293-300, Mar., 1964. (Boston)

Goudemand, M.; Foucaut, M.; Habay, D.; and Parquet-Gernez, A.: Les variations du taux de facteur 8 au cours de l'exercice musculaire. Essai d'interprétation. Ann. Inst. Pasteur Lille 14:203-215, 1963.

----, ----, ----, and ----: Les variations du taux de facteur VIII au cours de l'exercice musculaire. Essai d'interprétation. Nouv. Rev. Franc. Hemat. 4:315-319, Mar.-Apr., 1964. (Lille, France)

Gough, J.; and Galpin, O. P.: Paroxysmal heart block on exertion. Brit. Med. J. 1:1359, May 23, 1964. (Manchester)

Goule, Adrian Gordon; and Dye, J. A.: Exercise and its physiology. New York, Barnes, 1932.

Gould, M. K.; and Rawlinson, W. A.: Biochemical adaptation as a response to exercise. 1. Effect of swimming on the levels of lactic dehydrogenase, malic dehydrogenase and phosphorylase in muscles of 8-, 11- and 15-week-old rats. Biochem. J. 73:41-44, Sept., 1959. (Melbourne)

Graham, John: A plea for the continuation of outdoor sports in middle and advanced life. Med. News 61:403-404, Oct. 8, 1892. (Philadelphia)

Graham, Pamela; Kahlson, G.; and Rosengren, Elsa: Histamine formation in physical exercise, anoxia and under the influence of adrenaline and related substances. J. Physiol. 172:174-188, Aug., 1964. (Lund)

Granath, A.; Jonsson, B.; and Strandell, T.: Circulation in healthy old men, studied by right heart catheterization at rest and during exercise in supine and sitting position. Acta Med. Scand. 176:425-446, Oct., 1964. (Stockholm)

Granath, A.; Jonsson, B.; and Strandell, T.: Studies on the central circulation at rest and during exercise in the supine and sitting body position in old men. Preliminary report. Acta Med. Scand. 169:125-126, Jan., 1961. (Stockholm)

----, and Strandell, T.: Relationships between cardiac output, stroke volume and intracardiac pressures at rest and during exercise in supine position and some anthropometric data in healthy old men. Acta Med. Scand. 176:447-466, Oct., 1964. (Stockholm)

Grande, F.; Monagle, J. E.; Buskirk, E. R.; and Taylor, H. L.: Body temperature responses to exercise in man on restricted food and water intake. J. Appl. Physiol. 14:194-198, Mar., 1959. (Minneapolis)

Grandjean, E.: (Muscle fatigue from a physiological viewpoint) (Ger). Med. Welt 31:1587-1590, July 30, 1960.

----: Die physiologischen Grundlagen des Muskeltrainings. Schweiz. Zeits. Sportmed. 4:1-5, 1956. (Zürich)

----: Thermorégulation et effort physique. Schweiz. Zeits. Sportmed. 4:65-80, 1956. (Zürich)

----, and Abelin, T.: Die Wirkung von Nikotin auf die Schwimmleistungen und Atheromatose cholesterinbelasteter Ratten. Schweiz. Zeits. Sportmed. 12:132-144, 1964.

Grandpierre, R.: Régulation locale de la circulature peripherique au cours du travail musculaire. Acta Belg. Arte Med. Pharm. Milit. 110(Part 2):337-344, Dec., 1957.

----, Tabusse, L.; and Perles, R.: Recherche d'un test d'aptitude à l'effort: l'épreuve de l'Escabeau. Rev. Méd. Nancy 82:865-871, Aug.-Sept., 1957.

Grant, R. T.: Observations on the blood circulation in voluntary muscle in man. Clin. Sci. 3:157-173, Apr. 28, 1938. (London)

Gray, Irving; and Beetham, William P., Jr.: Changes in plasma concentration of epinephrine and norepinephrine with muscular work. Proc. Soc. Exp. Biol. Med. 96:636-638, Dec., 1957. (Natick)

Gray, James: Muscular activity during locomotion. Brit. Med. Bull. 12:203-209, Sept., 1956. (Cambridge, Eng.)

Gray, John S.: The multiple factor theory of the control of respiratory ventilation. Science 103: 739-744, June 28, 1946.

----: Pulmonary ventilation and its physiological regulation. Springfield, Charles C. Thomas, 1950.

----, and Masland, R. L.: Studies on altitude decompression sickness. II. The effects of altitude and of exercise. J. Aviation Med. 17:483-485, Oct., 1946. (Randolph Field)

Graybiel, Ashton: Auricular fibrillation in an asymptomatic young man. Effects of exercise, digitalization, atropinization and the restoration of normal rhythm. Amer. J. Cardiol. 14:828-836, Dec., 1964. (Pensacola)

Great Britain, War Office: Elementary anatomy and physiology for those studying physical training. London, 1915.

Greco, A.: Comportamento della frequenza cardiaca dopo prova dello step-test e dopo prova del massimo rendimento in soggetti allenati e non allenati. Gaz. Int. Med. Chir. 69:670-673, Apr. 15, 1964.

----: La prova dello sforzo massimo nella valutazione dell'atleta. Gaz. Int. Med. Chir. 69: 309-313, Feb. 15, 1964.

----: Rapporto fra sistole meccanica e sistole elettrica nella prova dello sforzo massimo. Gaz. Int. Med. Chir. 68:2877-2882, Dec. 31, 1963.

----: Reazioni della funzione renale all'attività fisica. Gaz. Int. Med. Chir. 69:596-601, Mar. 31, 1964.

----: Ricerche sperimentali sull'affaticamento. Effetto del lavoro fisico sul contenuto in sostanze ad alto potere energetico del miocardio nel ratto. Gaz. Int. Med. Chir. 69:1163-1166, June 30, 1964.

----: Ricerche sperimentali sull'affaticamento. La somministrazione di ATP nei ratti sottoposti a sforzofisico. Gaz. Int. Med. Chir. 69:795-798, Apr. 30, 1964.

Gregg, Donald E.; Sabiston, David C.; and Theilen, Ernest D.: Performance of the heart: changes in left ventricular end-diastolic pressure and stroke work during infusion and following exercise. Physiol. Rev. 35:130-136, Jan., 1955. (Washington)

Gréhant; and Quinquaud: Recherches expérimentales sur la mésure du volume du sang qui traverse les poumons en un temps donné. Comptes Rend. Soc. Biol. Eighth series 3:159-160, Mar. 27, 1886.

Grimby, Gunnar: Exercise in man during pyrogen-induced fever. Scand. J. Clin. Lab. Invest. 14(Suppl. 67):1-112, 1962. (Göteborg, Swed.)

----, and Nilsson, Nils Johan: Cardiac output during exercise in pyrogen-induced fever. Scand. J. Clin. Lab. Invest. 15(Suppl. 69):44-61, 1963. (Göteborg, Swed.)

----, ----, and Sanne, H.: Cardiac output during exercise in patients with varicose veins. Scand. J. Clin. Lab. Invest. 16:21-30, 1964. (Göteborg)

----, ----, and ----: Serial determination of cardiac output during prolonged exercise. Scand. J. Clin. Lab. Invest. 15(Suppl. 76):52, 1963. (Göteborg)

----, and Söderholm, B.: Energy expenditure of men in different age groups during level walking and bicycle ergometry. Scand. J. Clin. Lab. Invest. 14:321-328, 1962. (Göteborg)

Grinschpun, S.; and Awad, S.: Insuficiencia cardíaca de etiología poco común. Rev. Méd. Chile 72:829-832, Sept., 1944.

Grober, J.: Einwirkungdauernder körperlicher Leistung auf das Herz. Wien. med. Wschr. 63: 441-449, 1913.

Grodins, Fred S.: Analysis of factors concerned in regulation of breathing in exercise. Physiol. Rev. 30:220-239, Apr., 1950. (Chicago)

----, and Morgan, Donald P.: Regulation of breathing during electrically-induced muscular work in anesthetized dogs following transection of spinal cord. Amer. J. Physiol. 162:64-73, July, 1950. (Chicago)

Groetschel, H.: Herzschäden durch Kohlenoxyd und Zusätzliche körperliche Belastung. Arch. Gewerbepath. Gewerbehyg. 10:223-237, 1940.

Grollman, Arthur: The cardiac output of man in health and disease. Springfield, Charles C. Thomas, 1932.

----: The determination of the cardiac output of man by the use of acetylene. Amer. J. Physiol. 88:432-443, Apr., 1929. (Baltimore)

----: The effect of variation in posture on the output of the human heart. Amer. J. Physiol. 86: 285-301, Sept., 1928. (Baltimore)

----: Physiological variations in the cardiac output of man. XIII. The effect of mild muscular exercise on the cardiac output. Amer. J. Physiol. 96:8-15, Jan., 1931. (Baltimore)

----, Proger, S.; and Dennig, H.: Zur Bestimmung des Minutenvolumens mit der Azetylenmethode bei Arbeit, bei normalen und kranken Menschen. Naunyn Schmiedeberg Arch. exp. Path. 162:463-471, 1931. (Heidelberg)

Gross, R. E.; and Mittermaier, R.: Untersuchungen über das Minutenvolumen das Herzens. Pflüger Arch. ges. Physiol. 212:136-149, Feb. 27, 1926. (Freiburg)

Grossman, Milton; Weinstein, William W.; and Katz, Louis N.: The use of the exercise test in the diagnosis of coronary insufficiency. Ann. Intern. Med. 30:387-397, Feb., 1949. (Chicago)

Gruber, Charles M.: Further studies on the effect of adrenalin upon muscular fatigue. Amer. J. Physiol. 43:530-544, July, 1917. (Albany)

----: Studies in fatigue. III. The fatigue threshold as affected by adrenalin and by increased arterial pressure. Amer. J. Physiol. 33:335-355, Feb., 1914. (Boston)

Gruber, M.: Einfluss der Uebung auf Gaswechsel. Zeits. Biol., n. F. 10:466-491, 1891-1892.

Gsell, D.; Von Hahn, H. P.; and Schaub, M.C.: Serum and muscle creatine in exercised ageing rats. Gerontologia 9:42-51, 1964.

Guarnieri, E.; and Bianucci, G.: Effeti dell'attività muscolare intensa sulla lipidemia in soggetti allenati e non allenati. I. Modificazioni degli acidi grassi non esterificati e dei trigliceridi del plasma. Riv. Crit. Clin. Med. 64:31-44, Feb., 1964.

Gubner, Richard: Determinants of ischemic electrocardiographic abnormalities and chest pain. Part II. The exercise electrocardiogram test. J. Occup. Med. 3:110-120, Mar., 1961. (New York)

Gubser, A.; Pircher, L.; and Amsler, H. A.: (Normal values of the blood pressure and pulse rate in various age groups during rest, orthostatism and light exertion) (Ger). Schweiz. Zeits. Sportmed. 11:17-31, 1963.

Gudbrandsen, C. O.: The effect of physical exercise on cholesterol-induced atherosclerosis in rabbits. USAF Arctic Aeromed. Lab. TR 60-2:1-85, Feb., 1961.

Gudz', P. Z.: Morfologicheskie izmeneniia v myshtsakh i nervakh konechnosteĭ v usloviiakh "peretrenirovannosti". (Eksperimental'no-morfologicheskoĭ issledovanie). (Morphological changes in muscles and nerves of the extremities under conditions of "overtraining" (experimental morphological research) (Russ). Arkh. Anat. 45:55-63, July, 1963.

Guerrant, N. B.; and Dutcher, R. Adams: The influence of exercise on the growing rat in the presence and absence of vitamin B_1. J. Nutr. 20:589-598, Dec., 1940. (Pennsylvania State College)

Güttler, Flemming; Petersen, F. Bonde; and Kjeldsen, K.: The influence of phenformin on blood lactic acid in normal and diabetic subjects during exercise. Diabetes 12:420-423, Sept.-Oct., 1963. (Hillerød, Den.)

Gugger: Ein Wort über die jetzige Vernachlässigung der Leibesübungen, ihre Folgen, und einige Mittel zu ihre Beseitigung. Oest. med. Wschr. 1846, pp. 1-12.

Guild, Ruth; and Rapport, David: Calorigenic action of methylene blue during muscular exercise. Proc. Soc. Exp. Biol. Med. 34:459-461, May, 1936. (Boston)

Guild, W. R.: Fitness for adults. J. Sport Med. 3:101-104, June-Sept., 1963.

Guimaraes, J. P.; Motta, M. C.; and Ballini, I.: The effect of muscular stress on the metastatic spread of the Yoshida sarcoma. Hospital (Rio) 64:967-972, Oct., 1963.

Gullbring, B.; Holmgren, A.; Sjöstrand, T.; and Strandell, T.: The effect of blood volume variations on the pulse rate in supine and upright positions and during exercise. Acta Physiol. Scand. 50:62-71, Sept. 30, 1960. (Stockholm)

Gumener, P. I.; Dadashev, R. S.; and Sapozhnikov, V. S.: Metodika avtomaticheskogo mekhano-khronometrazha fizichestoĭ raboty. (Method for automatic mechanochronometry of physical work) (Russ). Gig. Sanit. 29:58-62, Feb., 1964.

Gup, Alex M.; and Briggs, G. W.: Elevated sweat sodium and chloride in adult without cystic fibrosis. Arch. Intern. Med. 112:699-701, Nov., 1963. (Denver)

Guy, Chester C.; and Wichowski, W. A.: Rupture of blood vessels by strenuous physical exertion. Amer. J. Surg. 85:418-423, Mar., 1953. (Chicago)

Guyton, Arthur C.; Douglas, Ben H.; Langston, Jimmy B.; and Richardson, Travis Q.: Instantaneous increase in mean circulatory pressure and cardiac output at onset of muscular activity. Circ. Res. 11:431-441, Sept., 1962. (Jackson, Miss.)

Haab, P.: Étude de la reproductibilité des mesures des échanges gazeux respiratoires lors de l'état d'équilibre à l'exercice musculaire. Rev. méd. Nancy 82:872-879, Aug.-Sept., 1957.

Häggendal, Jan: The presence of conjugated adrenaline and noradrenaline in human blood plasma. Acta Physiol. Scand. 59:255-260, Nov., 1963. (Güteborg)

Hahn, F. V. von: Die Oberflächenaktivität des Harnes bei physicher und psychischer Alteration. Arbeitsphysiol. 2:298-340, 1930. (Hamburg)

Haig, Alexander: The effect of exercise on the excretion of urea: a contribution to the physiology of fatigue. Lancet 1:610-615, Mar. 7, 1896. (London)

Hajdu, István; and Korényi, Zoltán: The volume changes of the suprarenal cortex and medulla in exercise and after the injection of certain substances. Arch. Int. Pharmacodyn. 67:373-389, June 30, 1942. (Budapest)

Halberg, F.; Frank, G.; Harner, R.; Matthews, J.; Akker, Harriet; Gravem, H.; and Melby, J.: The adrenal cycle in men on different schedules of motor and mental activity. Experientia 17:282-284, June 15, 1961. (Minneapolis, Palo Alto and Little Rock)

Haldane, John Scott: Hygiène du travail sous terre et sous l'eau. Ann. Hyg. Publ. 11:102-127, 1909. (Oxford)

----: A new form of apparatus for measuring the respiratory exchange of animals. J. Physiol. 13: 419-430, 1892.

----, Meakins, J. C.; and Priestley, J. G.: The respiratory response to anoxaemia. J. Physiol. 52:420-432, May 20, 1919. (Oxford and Taplow)

----, and Pembrey, M. S.: An improved method of determining moisture and carbonic acid in air. London, Edinburgh & Dublin Phil. Mag. & J. Sci., fifth series 29:306-331, Apr., 1890.

----, and Poulton, E. P.: The effects of want of oxygen on respiration. J. Physiol. 37:390-407, 1908.

----, and Priestley, J. G.: The regulation of the lung-ventilation. J. Physiol. 32:225-266, May 9, 1905. (Oxford)

----, and ----: Respiration. Second edition. Oxford, Clarendon Press, 1935. (Oxford)

----, and Smith, J. Lorrain: The oxygen tension of arterial blood. J. Physiol. 20:497-520, Dec. 3, 1896. (Oxford and Belfast)

----, and ----: The physiological effects of air vitiated by respiration. J. Path. Bact. 1:168-186, 1893. (Oxford)

Hall, F. G.; and Wilson, J. W.: Effects of physical activity and of simulated altitudes on pulmonary ventilation, maximal inspiratory (peak) flow and pressure in relation to oxygen requirements. J. Aviation Med. 15:160-166, June, 1944.

Hall, Victor E.: The relation of heart rate to exercise fitness: an attempt at physiological interpretation of the bradycardia of training. Pediatrics 32(Suppl.):723-729, Oct., 1963. (Los Angeles)

Halliday, John A.: Blood flow in the human calf after prolonged walking. Amer. Heart J.
60:110-115, July, 1960. (Belfast)

Halonen, Pentti I.; and Konttinen, Aarne: Effect of physical exercise on some enzymes in the
serum. Nature 193:942-944, Mar. 10, 1962. (Helsinki)

Hamar, N.; Szazados, I.; Szücs, E.; et al: Über die Stereotypen der Leistungsdisposition. Int.
Zeits. angew. Physiol. 20:271-280, Feb. 21, 1964.

Hamer, J.; Grandjean, T.; Melendez, L.; and Sowton, G. E.: Effect of propranolol (Inderal) in
angina pectoris: preliminary report. Brit. Med. J. 2:720-723, Sept. 19, 1964. (London)

Hammar, Sten; and Öbrink, Karl Johan: The inhibitory effect of muscular exercise on gastric
secretion. Acta Physiol. Scand. 28:152-161, 1953. (Uppsala)

Hammond, E. Cuyler: Smoking in relation to mortality and morbidity. Findings in first thirty-four
months of follow-up in a prospective study started in 1959. J. Nat. Cancer Inst. 32:1161-1188,
May, 1964. (New York)

Hancock, W.; Whitehouse, A. G. R.; and Haldane, John Scott: The loss of water and salts through
the skin, and the corresponding physiological adjustments. Proc. Roy. Soc. 105B:43-59,
Jan., 1930. (Oxford)

Hanninen, A.; Peltonen, T.; and Hirvonen, L.: Response of blood pressure to sucking and tilting
in the newborn premature infant. Ann. Paediat. Fenn. 10:92-98, 1964.

Hannisdahl, B.: Der Einfluss von Muskelarbeit auf die Blutsenkung. Arbeitsphysiol. 11:165-174, 1940.

Hanse, E.: Zum Vergleich des Energieumsatzes beim Radfahren und beim Treppensteigen. Arbeitsphysiol.
7:299-307, 1933.

Hansen, Emanuel: Atmung und Kreislauf bei körperlicher Arbeit. In: Handbuch der normalen und
pathologischen Physiologie. Editors: A. Bethe, G. v. Bergmann, G. Embden and A. Ellinger.
Berlin, Julius Springer, 1931. Vol. 15, part 2.

Hansen, O. H.; and Maggio, M.: Static work and heart rate. Int. Zeits. angew. Physiol. 18:
242-247, 1960.

Hansen, Ole Evald: Intermitterende, partielt hjerteblok hos toptraenet idraetsmand. Nord. Med.
62:1386-1388, Sept. 17, 1959. (Stockholm)

Hanson, John S.; and Tabakin, Burton S.: Carbon monoxide diffusing capacity in normal male
subjects, age 20-60, during exercise. J. Appl. Physiol. 15:402-404, May, 1960.
(Burlington, Vt.)

Hanson, John S.; and Tabakin, Burton S.: Electrocardiographic telemetry in skiers. Anticipatory
and recovery heart rate during competition. New Eng. J. Med. 271:181-185, July 23, 1964.
(Burlington, Vt.)

----, and ----: Simultaneous and rapidly repeated cardiac output determinations by dye-dilution
method. J. Appl. Physiol. 19:275-278, Mar., 1964. (Burlington, Vt.)

Haralambrie, G.: La valeur de certaines constantes biochimiques du sérum chez les sportifs en régime d'entraînement intense. Acta Biol. Med. German. 13:30-39, 1964.

Hardin, Robert A.; Shumacker, Harris B., Jr.; and Su, Chien Sheng: Studies on portal venous oxygen saturation. Arch. Surg. 87:831-835, Nov., 1963. (Indianapolis)

Hardinge, Mervyn G.; and Peterson, Donald I.: The effect of forced exercise on body temperature and amphetamine toxicity. J. Pharmacol. Exp. Ther. 145:47-51, July, 1964. (Loma Linda, Calif.)

----, and ----: The effects of exercise and limitation of movement on amphetamine toxicity. J. Pharmacol. Exp. Ther. 141:260-265, Aug., 1963. (Loma Linda, Calif.)

Hargrove, W. O., Jr.; and Wise, L. J., Jr.: A laboratory study of urinary changes following exercise. Bull. Tulane Med. Fac. 17:9-18, Nov., 1957. (New Orleans)

Härkönen, M.; Kontinen, E.; Kormano, M.; and Niemi, M.: Effect of heavy muscular work on the morphology and histochemistry of the rat testis. Acta Endocr. 43:311-320, June, 1963. (Helsinki)

----, Kormano, M.; and Kontinen, E.: Effect of heavy muscular work on hypothalamo-hypophysial neurosecretion in the rat. Ann. Med. Exp. Fenn. 42:17-21, 1964.

Harpuder, Karl; Lowenthal, Milton; and Blatt, Stanley: Peripheral and visceral vascular effects of exercise in the erect position. J. Appl. Physiol. 11:185-188, Sept., 1957. (New York)

Harris, E. A.: Exercise-tolerance tests. Lancet 2:409-411, Aug. 23, 1958.

----, and Porter, B. B.: On the heart rate during exercise, the oesophageal temperature and the oxygen debt. Quart. J. Exp. Physiol. 43:313-319, July, 1958. (Edinburgh)

----, and Thomson, J. G.: The pulmonary ventilation and heart rate during exercise in healthy old age. Clin. Sci. 17:349-359, 1958. (Edinburgh)

Harris, Morgan; Berg, W. E.; Whitaker, D. M.; and Twitty, V. C.: The relation of exercise to bubble formation in animals decompressed to sea level from high barometric pressures. J. Gen. Physiol. 28:241-251, Jan. 20, 1945. (Palo Alto)

Harris, Peter; Bateman, Mary; and Gloster, Josephine: The metabolism of glucose during exercise in patients with rheumatic heart disease. Clin. Sci. 23:561-569, Dec., 1962. (Birmingham, Eng.)

----, ----, and ----: Relations between the cardiorespiratory effects of exercise and the arterial concentration of lactate and pyruvate in patients with rheumatic heart disease. Clin. Sci. 23:531-543, Dec., 1962. (Birmingham, Eng.)

----, Jones, J. Howel; Bateman, M.; Chlouverkakis, C.; and Gloster, J.: Metabolism of the myocardium at rest and during exercise in patients with rheumatic heart disease. Clin. Sci. 26:145-156, Feb., 1964.

Harrison, Donald C.; Braunwald, Eugene; Glick, Gordon; Mason, Dean T.; Chidsey, Charles A.; and Ross, John, Jr.: Effects of beta adrenergic blockage on the circulation, with particular reference to observations in patients with hypertrophic subaortic stenosis. Circulation 29: 84-98, Jan., 1964. (Bethesda)

----, Goldblatt, Allan; and Braunwald, Eugene: Studies on cardiac dimensions in intact, unanesthetized man. I. Description of techniques and their validation. II. Effects of respiration. III. Effects of muscular exercise. Circ. Res. 13:448-467, Nov., 1963. (Bethesda)

Harrison, Tinsley R.; Harrison, W. G.; Calhoun, J. A.; and Marsh, J. P.: Congestive heart failure XVII. The mechanism of dyspnea on exertion. Arch. Intern. Med. 50:695-720, 1932.

Harrison, W. G., Jr.; Calhoun, J. Alfred; and Harrison, T. R.: Afferent impulses as a cause of increased ventilation during muscular exercise. Amer. J. Physiol. 100:68-73, Mar., 1932. (Nashville)

Hart, J. S.; and Jansky, L.: Thermogenesis due to exercise and cold in warm - and cold-acclimated rats. Canad. J. Biochem. 41:629-634, Mar., 1963. (Ottawa)

Hartman, Frank A.; and Griffith, Fred R., Jr.: Changes in the blood sugar and blood gases during exercise. Proc. Soc. Exp. Biol. Med. 21:561-565, May, 1924. (Buffalo)

----, Waite, F. H.; and McCordock, H. A.: The liberation of epinephrine during muscular exercise. Amer. J. Physiol. 62:225-241, 1922.

Hartmann, Eugen; and Jokl, Ernst: Untersuchungen an Sportsleuten. I. Veränderungen des morphologischen Blutbildes. Arbeitsphysiol. 2:452-460, Mar., 25, 1930. (Breslau)

Hartman, F.: (Fatigue and exhaustion) (Ger). Deutsch. Med. J. 12:260-264, Apr. 20, 1961.

Hartree, W.; and Hill, A. V.: The anaerobic processes involved in muscular activity. J. Physiol. 58:127-137, Dec. 28, 1923. (Manchester and Cambridge, Eng.)

----, and ----: The effect of hydrogen-ion concentration on the recovery process in muscle. J. Physiol. 58:470-479, May 23, 1924. (Cambridge and London, Eng.)

----, and ---: The heat production of muscles treated with caffein or subjected to prolonged discontinuous stimulation. J. Physiol. 58:441-454, May 23, 1924. (Cambridge and London, Eng.)

----, and ----: The regulation of the supply of energy in muscular contraction. J. Physiol. 55: 133-158, May 24, 1921. (Cambridge and Manchester, Eng.)

Hartwell, Alfred S.; Burrett, John B.; Graybiel, Ashton; and White, Paul D.: The effect of exercise and of four commonly used drugs on the normal human electrocardiogram with particular reference to T wave changes. J. Clin. Invest. 21:409-417, July, 1942. (Boston)

Hartwell, Edward Mussey: On the physiology of exercise. Boston Med. & Surg. J. 116:297-302, Mar. 24; 321-324, Mar. 31, 1887. (Baltimore)

Harvey, Réjane M.; Smith, William M.; Parker, John O.; and Ferrer, M. Irene: The response of the abnormal heart to exercise. Circulation 26:341-362, Sept., 1962. (New York)

Hasan, J.; Laamanen, A.; and Niemi, M.: Effect of thermal stress and muscular exercise, with and without insulin hypoglycaemia, on the body temperature, perspiration rate, and electrolyte and lactate content of sweat. Acta Physiol. Scand. 31:131-136, July 18, 1954. (Helsinki)

Hashimoto, Y.; and Kobernick, S. D.: Enzyme histochemistry of rabbit aorta, in spontaneous lesions and after acute exercise. Proc. Soc. Exp. Biol. Med. 115:212-215, Jan., 1964. (Detroit)

Hasselbalch, K. A.: Neuträlitatsregulation und Reizbarkeit des Atemzentrums in ihren Wirkungen auf die Kohlensäurespannung des Blutes. Biochem. Zeits. 46:403-439, 1912. (Copenhagen)

----, and Lundsgaard, C.: Blutreaktion und Lungen ventilation. Scand. Arch. Physiol. 27:13-31, 1912. (Copenhagen)

Hastings, A. Baird; and Steinhaus, Arthur H.: A new chart for the interpretation of acid-base changes and its application to exercise. Amer. J. Physiol. 96:538-540, Mar., 1931. (Chicago)

Hatai, Shinkishi: On the influence of exercise on the growth of organs in the albino rat. Anat. Rec. 9:647-665, Aug., 1915. (Philadelphia)

Hatch, F. T.; Hamerman, D.; and Ziporin, Z. Z.: Urinary excretion of mucoproteins and adrenal corticosteroids during rest and exercise. Relation to urine volume and physical fitness. J. Appl. Physiol. 9:465-468, Nov., 1956. (Denver)

----, ----, ----, Haynes, R. C., Jr.; and Harding, R. S.: Biochemical changes in stress. III. Effects of exercise in infantry soldiers. Army Med. Nutrition Lab. Rep. 182:1-17, June 4, 1956.

Hatzfeld, C.; Brille, D.; and Chiche, P.: Étude spirographique de la fonction respiratoire dans le rétrécissement mitral. II. Étude des réactions a l'effort. Rev. Franc. Etud. Clin. Biol. 3: 345-356, Apr., 1958.

Haufrect, Fred: Induction of labor by exercise. Obstet. Gynec. 7:462-465, Apr., 1956. (Houston)

Havard, R. E.; and Reay, G. A.: The influence of exercise on the inorganic phosphates of the blood and urine. J. Physiol. 61:35-48, Mar. 18, 1926. (Cambridge, Eng.)

Havel, Richard J.; Carlson, Lars A.; Ekelund, Lars-Göran; and Holmgren, Alf: Turnover rate and oxidation of different free fatty acids in man during exercise. J. Appl. Physiol. 19:613-618, July, 1964. (Stockholm and San Francisco)

----, Naimark, Arnold; and Borchgrevink, Christian F.: Turnover rate and oxidation of free fatty acids of blood plasma in man during exercise: studies during continuous infusion of palmitate-1-C^{14}. J. Clin. Invest. 42:1054-1063, July, 1963. (San Francisco)

Havel, V.: Die Beeinflussung der Arbeitsmenge durch scheinbare Veränderung des Zeitablaufs. Acta Biol. Med. German. 12:459-474, 1964.

Hawk, P. B.: On the morphological changes in the blood after muscular exercise. Amer. J. Physiol. 10:384-400, Mar. 1, 1904. (Philadelphia)

Hawking, Frank; Adams, Winston, E.; and Worms, Michael J.: The periodicity of microfilariae. VII. The effect of parasympathetic stimulants upon the distribution of microfilariae. Trans. Roy. Soc. Trop. Med. Hyg. 58:178-194, Mar., 1964. (London and British Guiana)

Hawley, E.: Dietary scales and standards for measuring a family's nutritive needs. Bull. U. S. Dept. Agric. No. 8, 1927.

Hayasaka, E.; and Inawashiro, R.: Studies on the effect of muscular exercise in beri-beri; the influences of muscular exercise upon circulatory apparatus, with special reference to its dynamic function as well as utilisation and supply of oxygen in beri-beri. (Cause of hypertrophy and dilatation of the heart in beri-beri and relaxation of peripheral blood vessels). Tohoku J. Exp. Med. 12:29-61, Dec., 1928.

Haynes, B.: The heart in industry: supplement. Med. J. Aust. 2:53-57, July 11, 1964.

Hayward, Graham W.; and Knott, J. M. S.: The effect of exercise on lung distensibility and respiratory work in mitral stenosis. Brit. Heart J. 17:303-311, July, 1955. (London)

Hazard, R.; Cheymol, J.; Chabrier, P.; and Drouin, H.: Action des sels d'ammonium quaternaires dérivés de la strychnine et de son aminoxyde sur la contractilité musculaire. J. Physiologie 49:198-202, Jan.-Mar., 1957. (Paris)

Hazelwood, Robert L.; and Ullrick, William C.: Glycogen mobilization and work in the rat heart. Amer. J. Physiol. 200:999-1003, May, 1961. (Boston)

Hearn, George R.: Succinic dehydrogenase and aldolase activities of skeletal muscle of exercised rats. J. Lancet 77:80, Mar., 1957. (New Brunswick, N.J.)

----, and Gollnick, P. D.: Effects of exercise on the adenosinetriphosphatase activity in skeletal and heart muscle of rats. Int. Zeits. angew. Physiol. 19:23-26, 1961.

----, and Wainio, Walter W.: Aldolase activity in the heart and skeletal muscle of exercised rats. Amer. J. Physiol. 190:206-208, Aug., 1957. (New Brunswick, N.J.)

----, and ----: Succinic dehydrogenase activity of the heart and skeletal muscle of exercised rats. Amer. J. Physiol. 185:348-350, May, 1956. (New Brunswick, N. J.)

Hearnshaw, G. R.; Kershaw, W. E.; Brewster, D. J.; and Leytham, G. W. H.: The effect of schistosomiasis upon activity and growth in mice. Ann. Trop. Med. Parasit. 57:481-498, Dec., 1963. (Liverpool)

Heath, Clark W.: The relation of physical exertion to the resistance of red blood cells to laking. Amer. J. Physiol. 139:569-573, Aug., 1943. (Boston)

Heaton, F. W.; and Hodgkinson, A.: External factors affecting diurnal variation in electrolyte excretion with particular reference to calcium and magnesium. Clin. Chim. Acta 8:246-254, Mar., 1963. (Leeds)

Hebbelinck, M.: The effect of a moderate dose of ethyl alcohol on human respiratory gas exchange during rest and muscular exercise. Arch. Int. Pharmacodyn. 126:214-218, June 1, 1960. (Oslo)

----: The effects of a small dose of ethyl alcohol on certain basic components of human physical performance. I. The effect of cardiac rate during muscular work. Arch. Int. Pharmacodyn. 140:61-67, Nov., 1962. (Helsinki)

----: Influence of muscular exercise upon the metabolism of radioactive ethyl alcohol in mice. Arch. Int. Pharmacodyn. 119:495-496, Apr. 1, 1959. (Ghent)

----: Influence of muscular work on the blood alcohol concentration in man. Arch. Int. Pharmacodyn. 119:521-523, Apr. 1, 1959. (Helsinki)

Hedlund, Sven; Nylin, Gustav; and Regenström, Olaf: The behaviour of the cerebral circulation during muscular exercise. Acta Physiol. Scand. 54:316-324, Mar.-Apr., 1962. (Stockholm)

Hedvall, Bertel: Zur Kenntnis der Ermüdung und der Bedeutung der Übung für die Leistungsfähigkeit des Muskels. Scand. Arch. Physiol. 32:115-197, 1915. (Helsinki)

Heidorn, G. H.: Pulse pressure response to a standard exercise stress. Circulation 18:249-255, Aug., 1958. (Altoona, Pa.)

Heim, E.: The electrocardiogram of long distance runners (studied in 100 Olympic long distance ski runners). Schweiz. Zeits. Sportmed. 6:1-72, 1958. (Bern)

Heinen, W.; Loosen, H.; and Schmitz-Dräger, H. G.: Die Beziehungen zwischen Herzfrequenz und QT-Dauer im Verlaufe einer Trainingsperiode. Zeits. Kreislaufforsch. 41:375-379, May, 1952. (Köln)

Heiss, F.; and Lendel, E.: Beitrag zur Einwirkung der Leibesübungen auf die Drüsen mit innerer Sekretion. Fermentforsch. 22:509-517, 1931.

Helander, E. A. S.: Influence of exercise and restricted activity on the protein composition of skeletal muscle. Biochem. J. 78:478-482, Mar., 1961. (Göteborg)

----: Myocardial protein composition and its relation to functional activity of varying degree. Cardiologia 41:94-100, 1962. (Göteborg)

Hellebrandt, Frances A.: Studies on albuminuria following exercise. I. Its incidence in women and its relationship to the negative phase in pulse pressure. Amer. J. Physiol. 101:357-364, July, 1932. (Madison)

----, Brogdon, Elizabeth; and Hoopes, Sara L.: The disappearance of digestive inhibition with the repetition of exercise. Amer. J. Physiol. 112:442-450, July, 1935. (Madison)

----, ----, and Kelso, L. E. A.: Studies on albuminuria following exercise. II. Its relationship to the speed of doing work. Amer. J. Physiol. 101:365-375, July, 1932. (Madison)

----, Houtz, Sara Jane; Hockman, Donald E.; and Partridge, Miriam J.: Physiologic effects of simultaneous static and dynamic exercise. Amer. J. Phys. Med. 35:106-117, Apr., 1956. (Chicago)

Helmer, Oscar M.: Renin activity in blood from patients with hypertension. Canad. Med. Ass. J. 90:221-225, Jan. 25, 1964. (Indianapolis)

Henderson, Lawrence J.: Das Gleichgewicht zwischen Basen und Säuren im tierischen Organismus. Ergebn. Physiol. 8:254-325, 1909. (Cambridge, Mass.)

----: The theory of neutrality regulation in the animal organism. Amer. J. Physiol. 21:427-448, May 1, 1908. (Cambridge, Mass.)

Henderson, Yandell: The volume curve of the ventricles of the mammalian heart, and the significance of this curve in respect to the mechanics of the heart-beat and the filling of the ventricles. Amer. J. Physiol. 16:325-367, July 2, 1906. (New Haven)

----, and Barringer, Theodore B., Jr.: The conditions determining the volume of the arterial blood-pressure. Amer. J. Physiol. 31:288-299, Feb. 1, 1913. (New Haven)

----, and ----: The relation of venous pressure to cardiac efficiency. Amer. J. Physiol. 31:352-369, Mar. 1, 1913. (New Haven)

Henderson, Yandell; and Haggard, Howard W.: The maximum of human power and its fuel. From observations on the Yale University Crew, Winner of the Olympic Championship, Paris, 1924. Amer. J. Physiol. 72:264-282, Apr., 1925. (New Haven)

----, ----, and Dolley, Frank S.: The efficiency of the heart, and the significance of rapid and slow pulse rates. Amer. J. Physiol. 82:512-524, Nov., 1927. (New Haven)

Henning, Ulf: Tierexperimentelle Untersuchungen zur Erzeugung eines Herztodes durch Überanstrengung in der Lauftrommel. Zeits. Kreislaufforsch. 46:25-39, Jan., 1957. (Würzburg)

Henri, G.: (Consequences of certain occupational activities on the circulatory system and the extent of pressure variations) (Fr). Arch. Mal. Prof. 23:161-163, Mar., 1962.

Henrotte, J. G.; Coquelet, M. L.; and Traverse, P. M. de: Influence du mode de vie sur la composition des protéines sériques chez les Indiens de Madras. Acta Trop. 20:279-281, 1963.

Henry, C.: Une proposition paradoxale de la physiologie comparée des sports. Comptes Rend. Soc. Biol., 10th series 1:678-681, 1894.

Henry, Franklin M.: Effects of exercise and altitude on the growth and decay of aviator's bends. J. Aviation Med. 27:250-259, June, 1956. (Berkeley)

----: Oxygen requirement of walking and running. Res. Quart. 24:169-175, May, 1953.

----: The role of exercise in altitude pain (aviators' bends). Amer. J. Physiol. 145:279-284, Jan., 1946. (Berkeley)

Henschel, Austin; De La Vega, Frederick; and Taylor, Henry Longstreet: Simultaneous direct and indirect blood pressure measurements in man at rest and work. J. Appl. Physiol. 6:506-508, Feb., 1954. (Minneapolis)

Hensley, John C.; McWilliams, Paul C.; and Oakley, Glenda E.: Physiological capacitance: a study in physiological age determination. J. Geront. 19:317-321, July, 1964. (Los Alamos, N.M.)

Hepps, Sanford A.; Roe, Benson B.; and Rutkin, Burton B.: Coronary blood flow in the intact conscious dog: studies with miniature electromagnetic flow transducers. J. Thorac. Cardiov. Surg. 46:783-794, Dec., 1963. (San Francisco)

Herbst, Robert: Der Gasstoffwechsel als Mass der körperlichen Leistungsfahigkeit. I. Mitteilung. Die Bestimmung des Sauerstoffaufnahmevermögens beim Gesunden. Deutsch. Arch. klin. Med. 162:33-50, Nov., 1928. (Berlin and Königsberg)

----: Der Gasstoffwechsel als Mass der körperlichen Leistungsfähigkeit. II. Mitteilung. Untersuchungen bei Emphysem, chronischer Bronchitis und Asthma bronchiale. Deutsch. Arch. klin. Med. 162:129-143, Dec., 1928. (Königsberg)

----: Der Gasstoffwechsel als Mass der körperlichen Leistungsfähigkeit. III. Mitteilung. Untersuchungen an Herzkranken. Deutsch. Arch. klin. Med. 162:257-279, Dec., 1928. (Königsberg)

----: Sport und Herz in Physiologie und Pathologie. Aerztl. Wschr. 11:877-880, Oct. 5, 1956.

Herman, Robert H.; and McDowell, Milton K.: Hyperkalemic paralysis (adynamia episodica hereditaria). Report of four cases and clinical studies. Amer. J. Med. 35:749-767, Dec., 1963. (Washington)

Hermann, L.: Ueber den Stoffverbrauch bei der Arbeit. Berlin. klin. Wschr. 5:199-207, 1868.

Herrick, J. F.; Grindlay, John H.; Baldes, Edward J.; and Mann, Frank C.: Effect of exercise on the blood flow in the superior mesenteric, renal and common iliac arteries. Amer. J. Physiol. 128:338-344, Jan., 1940. (Rochester, Minn.)

Hertig, Bruce A.; and Sargent, Frederick, II: Acclimatization of women during work in hot environments. Fed. Proc. 22:810-813, May-June, 1963. (Pittsburgh and Urbana)

Hervé, L.; Kunstmann, L.; and Kunstmann, G.: Las reacciones presoras al esfuerzo y al frio en los miembros inferiores y superiores de los sujetos normales. Rev. Méd. Chile 81:192-201, Apr., 1953.

Herxheimer, Herbert; and Kost, Richard: Über den Einfluss der Kohlensäureatmung auf den Gasstoffwechsel bei Kranken, Gesunden und Trainierten. Naunyn Schmiedeberg Arch. exp. Path. 165:101-110, 1932. (Berlin)

Hess, George H.; and Fultz, David A.: Damaging effects of strenuous exercise. U. S. Armed Forces Med. J. 7:369-378, Mar., 1956. (Fort Lewis, Wash.)

Hess, P.; and Seusing, J.: (The effect of tread frequency and pedal pressure on the oxygen uptake in studies with the ergometer) (Ger). Int. Zeits. angew. Physiol. 19:468-475, 1963.

Hesser, Carl Magnus: Central and chemoreflex components in the respiratory activity during acid-base displacements in the blood. Acta Physiol. Scand. 18(Suppl. 64):5-69; appendix, 1949. (Stockholm)

Hettinger, T.: (Histological and chemical changes in skeletal musculature due to muscle training and testosterone) (Ger). Aerztl. Forsch. 13:570-574, Nov. 10, 1959.

----: Die Leistungsfähigkeit des Menschen und deren Messung. München. med. Wschr. 103:1860-1864, Sept. 29, 1961. (Mülheim/Meiderich AG)

Hetzel, K. S.; and Long, C. N. H.: The metabolism of the diabetic individual during and after muscular exercise. Proc. Roy. Soc. 99B:279-306, Mar. 1, 1926.

Heusner, A.: Enregistrement de longue durée de la température centrale chez le rat libre de ses mouvements: influence d'un facteur nycthéméral et de l'activité. J. Physiologie 51:476-477, May-June, 1959. (Strasbourg)

Heusner, William W., Jr.; and Bernauer, Edmund M.: Relationship between level of physical condition and pH of antecubital venous blood. J. Appl. Physiol. 9:171-175, Sept., 1956. (Urbana, Ill.)

Heymans, Corneille; Bouckaert, J. J.; and Handovsky, H.: Sensibilité des sinus carotidiens aux excitants chimiques et modification réflexes du débit sanguin dans l'artère femorale. Comptes Rend. Soc. Biol. 119:542-545, 1935. (Ghent)

Heymans, Corneille; Bouckaert, J. J.; and Regniers, P.: Le sinus carotidien et la zone homologue cardio-aortique. Paris, G. Doin et Cie, 1933.

----, ----, and Samaan, A.: Influences des variations de la teneur du sang en oxygène et en CO_2 sur l'excitabilité réflexe et directe des elements centraux et peripheriques des nerfs cardiorégulateurs. Arch. Int. Pharmacodyn. 48:457-487, 1934. (Ghent)

----, Jacob, J.; and Liljestrand, G.: Regulation of respiration during muscular work as studied on the perfused isolated head. Acta Physiol. Scand. 14:86-101, Sept. 30, 1947. (Stockholm)

----, and Neil, E.: Reflexogenic areas of the cardiovascular system. London, Churchill, 1958. (Ghent and London)

Hickam, John B.; and Cargill, Walter H.: Effect of exercise on cardiac output and pulmonary arterial pressure in normal persons and in patients with cardiovascular disease and pulmonary emphysema. J. Clin. Invest. 27:10-23, Jan., 1948. (Atlanta, Ga. and Durham, N.C.)

----, Pryor, W. W.; Page, E. B.; and Atwell, R. J.: Respiratory regulation during exercise in unconditioned subjects. J. Clin. Invest. 30:503-516, May, 1961. (Durham, N.C.)

Highman, Benjamin; and Altland, Paul D.: Effects of exercise and training on serum enzyme and tissue changes in rats. Amer. J. Physiol. 205:162-166, July, 1963. (Bethesda)

Hill, Archibald Vivian: The absolute mechanical efficiency of the contraction of an isolated muscle. J. Physiol. 46:435-469, Aug. 18, 1913. (Cambridge, Eng.)

----: The air-resistance to a runner. Proc. Roy. Soc. 102B:380-385, Feb. 1, 1928.

----: Die Beziehungen zwischen der Wärmebildung und den im Muskel stattfindenen chemische Prozessen. Ergebn. Physiol. 15:340-479, 1916. (Cambridge, Eng.)

----: The dimensions of animals and their muscular dynamics. Proc. Roy. Instn. Great Britain 34:450-473, 1950. (Also in Sci. Progr. Twent. Cent. 38:209-230, 1950.)

----: The dynamic constants of human muscle. Proc. Roy. Soc. 128B:263-274, Feb. 15, 1940.

----: The effect of load on the heat of shortening of muscle. Proc. Roy. Soc. 159:297-318, Jan. 14, 1964. (London)

----: The efficiency of bicycle pedalling. J. Physiol. 82:207-210, Sept. 19, 1934. (London)

----: The efficiency of mechanical power development during muscular shortening and its relation to load. Proc. Roy. Soc. 159:319-324, Jan. 14, 1964. (London)

----: The energy degraded in the recovery processes of stimulated muscles. J. Physiol. 46: 28-80, Mar. 3, 1913. (Cambridge, Eng.)

----: The maximum work and mechanical efficiency of human muscles, and their most economical speed. J. Physiol. 56:19-41, Feb. 14, 1922. (Manchester, Eng.)

----: The mechanics of voluntary muscle. Lancet 2:947-951, Nov. 24, 1951. (London)

Hill, Archibald Vivian: The mechanism of muscular contraction. Physiol. Rev. 2:310-341,
Apr., 1922.

----: Muscular activity. Baltimore, Williams and Wilkins Company, 1926. (16th Herter
Lecture at Johns Hopkins)

----: Muscular activity in man from the engineering aspect. Sci. Progr. Twent. Cent. 22:
630-640, 1928.

----: Muscular exercise. Proc. Roy. Instn. Great Britain 24:23-38, 1925. (Also in Nature 112:
77-84, 1923.)

----: Muscular movement in man: the factors governing speed and recovery from fatigue. The
George Fuher Baker non-resident Lecture. New York, McGraw-Hill Book Co., Inc., 1927.

----: The oxidative removal of lactic acid. J. Physiol. 48:x-xi, Feb. 14, 1914. (Cambridge, Eng.)

----: Oxygen and violent exercise. Discovery 4:64-69, 1923.

----: The physiological basis of athletic records. Sci. Monthly 21:409-428, 1925. (Also in
Nature 116:544-548, Oct. 10, 1925.)

----, and Long, C. N. H.: Muscular exercise, lactic acid and the supply and utilization of oxygen.
Ergebn. Physiol. 24:43-51, 1925. (London)

----, ----, and ----: Muscular exercise, lactic acid, and the supply and utilisation of oxygen.
Parts I-III. Proc. Roy. Soc. 96B:438-475, Sept. 1, 1924. (London)

----, ----, and ----: Muscular exercise, lactic acid, and the supply and utilisation of oxygen. Parts
IV-VI. Proc. Roy. Soc. 97B:84-138, Nov. 1, 1924. (London)

----, ----, and ----: Muscular exercise, lactic acid, and the supply and utilization of oxygen.
Part VII. Proc. Roy. Soc. 97B:155-167, Dec. 1, 1924.

----, and Lupton, Hartley: Muscular exercise, lactic acid, and the supply and utilization of oxygen.
Quart. J. Med. 16:135-171, Jan., 1923. (Manchester, Eng.)

----, and ----: The oxygen consumption during running. J. Physiol. 56:xxxii-xxxiii, May 20, 1922,

----, and Meyerhoff, Otto: Über die Vorgänge bei der Muskelkontraktion. Ergebn. Physiol. 22:
299-327, 1923. (Manchester, Eng. and Kiel, Ger.)

Hill, Leonard: An address on the influence of muscular exercise and open air on the bodily
functions. Brit. Med. J. 2:599-606, Sept. 14, 1912. (London)

----: Oxygen and muscular exercise as a form of treatment. Brit. Med. J. 2:967-968, Oct. 3,
1908. (London)

----, and Flack, Martin: The effect of excess of carbon dioxide and of want of oxygen upon the
respiration and the circulation. J. Physiol. 37:77-111, 1908.

Hill, Leonard; and Flack, Martin: The influence of oxygen inhalations on muscular work. J. Physiol. 40:347-372, 1910.

---- and ----: The influence of oxygen on athletes. (Prel. comm.) J. Physiol. 38:xxviii-xxxvi, Jan. 23, 1909. (London)

----, ----, and Just, T. H.: The influence of oxygen inhalations on athletes. Brit. Med. J. 2:499-500, Aug. 22, 1908. (London)

----, and Mackenzie, J.: The effect of oxygen inhalation on muscular exertion. J. Physiol. 39:xxxiii-xxxv, Dec. 11, 1909. (London)

Hillestad, Leif K.: The peripheral blood flow in intermittent claudication. I. The significance of the postural tests. Acta Med. Scand. 172:301-305, Sept., 1962. (Oslo)

----: The peripheral blood flow in intermittent claudication. II. The significance of skin thermometry. Acta Med. Scand. 172:307-314, Sept., 1962. (Oslo)

----: The peripheral blood flow in intermittent claudication. III. The significance of oscillometry. Acta Med. Scand. 172:573-583, Nov., 1962. (Oslo)

----: The peripheral blood flow in intermittent claudication. IV. The significance of the claudication distance. Acta Med. Scand. 173:467-478, Apr., 1963. (Oslo)

----: The peripheral blood flow in intermittent claudication. V. Plethysmographic studies. The significance of the calf blood flow at rest and in response to timed arrest of the circulation. Acta Med. Scand. 174:23-41, July, 1963. (Oslo)

----: The peripheral blood flow in intermittent claudication. VI. Plethysmographic studies. The blood flow response to exercise with arrested and with free circulation. Acta Med. Scand. 174:671-685, Dec., 1963. (Oslo)

----: The peripheral blood flow in intermittent claudication. VII. The difference between the hyperemias following free and ischemic exercise and the effect of the included period of ischemia upon the latter. A comparison of the tests for evaluation of the blood flow and of various methods for gauging the hyperemia. A note on the use of plethysmography in clinical studies. Acta Med. Scand. 174:687-700, Dec., 1963. (Oslo)

Hillman, Robert W.; and Rosner, Martin C.: Effects of exercise on blood (plasma) concentrations of vitamin A, carotene and tocopherols. J. Nutr. 64:605-613, Apr. 10, 1958. (Brooklyn)

Hilpert, P.; Schlosser, D.; Barbey, K.; and Bartels, H.: Regulation von Atmung und Kreislauf durch den O_2-Druck im venösen Mischblut. Pflüger Arch. ges. Physiol. 279:1-16, Mar. 12, 1964. (Tübingen)

Himbert, J.; Scébat, L.; and Théard, A.: Influence de l'effort sur la circulation et les fonctions du rein chez les cardiaques. Sem. Hôp. Paris 32:415-423, Feb. 6, 1956.

Himwich, Harold E.; and Rose, Milton I.: The respiratory quotient of exercising muscle. Proc. Soc. Exp. Biol. Med. 24:169-170, Nov., 1926. (New Haven, Conn.)

Hippisley, John Cox: Remarks on the tread-wheel. London Med. & Phys. J. 50:273-274, Oct., 1823.

Hirsch Carl: Ueber die Beziehungen zwischen dem Herzmuskel und der Körpermusculatur und über sein Verhalten bei Herzhypertrophie. Deutsch. Arch. klin. Med. 64:597-634, 1899; 68:55-86, Aug. 16, 1900. (Leipzig)

Hirschberg, Gerald G.: Bard, Gregory, Ralston, H. J.; and Wilkie, Lorine R.: Energy cost of
stand-up exercises in normal and hemiplegic subjects. Amer. J. Phys. Med. 43:43-45,
Apr., 1964. (San Francisco)

Hislop, H. J.: Quantitative changes in human muscular strength during isometric exercise. J.
Amer. Phys. Ther. Ass. 43:21-38, Jan., 1963.

----: Response of immobilized muscle to isometric exercise. J. Amer. Phys. Ther. Ass. 44:339-347,
May, 1964.

Hoagland, Hudson: Adventures in biological engineering. Science 100:63-67, July 28, 1944.
(Worchester, Mass.)

Hobbs, Robert E.: March hemoglobinuria: a report of two cases. Amer. J. Clin. Path. 14:485-488,
Sept., 1944.

Hochrein, M.; Dill, D. B.; and Henderson, L. J.: Das physikalisch-chemische System des Blutes in
seiner Beziehung zu Atmung und Kreislauf. Naunyn Schmiedeberg Arch. exp. Path. 143:
129-146, 1929. (Boston)

----, ----, and ----: Das physikalisch-chemische System des Blutes in seiner Beziehung zu Atmung
und Kreislauf. IV. Mitteilung: Kohlensaureatmung und Hyperpnoe. Naunyn Schmiedeberg Arch.
exp. Path. 143:170-183, 1929. (Boston)

----, Talbott, J. H.; Dill, D. B.; and Henderson, L. J.: Das physikalisch-chemische System des Blutes
in seiner Beziehung zu Atmung und Kreislauf. II. Mitteilung: Die Bestimmung der Blutzirkulation in
Ruhe und Arbeit. Naunyn Schmiedeberg Arch. exp. Path. 143:147-160, 1929. (Boston)

Hock, Raymond J.: Effect of altitude on endurance running of Peromyscus maniculatus. J. Appl.
Physiol. 16:435-438, May, 1961. (Big Pine, Calif.)

Hockaday, T. D. R.; Downey, J. A.; and Mottram, R. F.: A case of McArdle's syndrome with a
positive family history. J. Neurol. Neurosurg. Psychiat. 27:186-197, June, 1964. (Oxford)

Hodgkins, Jean: Influence of unilateral endurance training on contralateral limb. J. Appl. Physiol.
16:991-993, Nov., 1961. (Santa Barbara, Calif.)

Hodgkinson, C. Paul: Effect of violent exercise on fibrinogen level. Henry Ford Hosp. Med. Bull.
6:48-54, Mar., 1958. (Detroit)

Hodgson, P.: Study of some relationships between performance tests and certain physiological
measures associated with maximal and submaximal work. Res. Quart. 17:208-224, Oct., 1946.

Højensgård, I. C.; and Sturup, H.: On the function of the venous pump and the venous return from the
lower limbs. Acta Dermvener. 32(Suppl. 29): 169-176, 1952. (Copenhagen)

----, and ----: Static and dynamic pressures in superficial and deep veins of the lower extremity in
man. Acta Physiol. Scand. 27:49-67, Dec. 20, 1952. (Copenhagen)

Hoff, Hebbel E.: Medical progress: Physiology. New Eng. J. Med. 229:543-550, Sept. 30, 1943.
(Montreal)

Hoffman, S. A.; Paschkis, K. E.; DeBias, D. A.; Cantarow, A.; and Williams, T. L.: The influence
of exercise on the growth of transplanted rat tumors. Cancer Res. 22:597-599, June, 1962.
(Philadelphia)

Hoffman, A.: Weitere Untersuchungen über den Einfluss des Trainings auf die Skeletmuskulatur.
Anat. Anz. 96:191-203, Dec. 15, 1947.

Holland, P. D. J.: March haemoglobinuria. Irish J. Med. Sci., 6th series:183-185, Apr.,
    1955. (Dublin)

Hollander, William; Madoff, Irving M.; and Chobanian, Aram V.: Local myocardial blood flow
    as indicated by the disappearance of NaI[131] from the heart muscle: studies at rest, during
    exercise and following nitrite administration. J. Pharmacol. Exp. Ther. 139:53-59, Jan.,
    1963. (Boston)

Hollmann, Werner: Der Arbeits - und Trainingseinfluss auf Kreislauf und Atmung; eine klinische
    und physiologische Betrachtung. Dormstadt, Steinkopf, 1959.

----: (Possible injury to heart and blood circulation by physical strain) (Ger). Aerztl. Wschr.
    14:605-609, Aug. 7, 1959.

Holloszy, John O.: The epidemiology of coronary heart disease: national differences and the role
    of physical activity. J. Amer. Geriat. Soc. 11:718-725, Aug., 1963. (Urbana, Ill.)

----, Skinner, James S.; Barry, Alan J.; and Cureton, Thomas K.: Effect of physical conditioning
    on cardiovascular function; a ballistocardiographic study. Amer. J. Cardiol. 14:761-770,
    Dec., 1964. (Urbana, Ill. and Washington, D.C.)

----, ----, Toro, Gelson; and Cureton, Thomas K.: Effects of a six month program of endurance
    exercise on the serum lipids of middle-aged men. Amer. J. Cardiol. 14:753-760, Dec.,
    1964. (Urbana, Ill. and Washington, D.C.)

Holmes, Richard; and Rasch, Philip J.: Effect of exercise on number of myofibrils per fiber in
    sartorius muscle of the rat. Amer. J. Physiol. 195:50-52, Oct., 1958. (Los Angeles)

Holmgren, Alf: Circulatory changes during muscular work in man; with special reference to
    arterial and central venous pressures in the systemic circulation. Scand. J. Clin. Lab.
    Invest. 8(Suppl. 24):1-97, 1956. (Stockholm)

----, Jonsson, Bengt; Levander, Maj; Linderholm, Håkan; Mossfeldt, Folke; Sjöstrand, Torgny; and
    Ström, Gunnar: Effect of physical training in vasoregulatory asthenia, in Da Costa's syndrome,
    and in neurosis without heart symptoms. Acta Med. Scand. 165:89-103, Oct. 16, 1959.
    (Stockholm and Nynäshamn)

----, ----, ----, ----, Sjöstrand, Torgny; and Ström, Gunnar: Low physical working capacity in
    suspected heart cases due to inadequate adjustment of peripheral blood flow (vasoregulatory
    asthenia). Acta Med. Scand. 158:413-436, Oct. 15, 1957. (Stockholm)

----, ----, and Sjöstrand, Torgny: Circulatory data in normal subjects at rest and during exercise
    in recumbent position, with special reference to the stroke volume at different work intensities.
    Acta Physiol. Scand. 49:343-363, Aug. 25, 1960. (Stockholm)

----, and Linderholm, Håkan: Oxygen and carbon dioxide tensions of arterial blood during heavy and
    exhaustive exercise. Acta Physiol. Scand. 44:203-215, Dec. 15, 1958. (Stockholm)

----, and McIlroy, Malcolm B.: Effect of temperature on arterial blood gas tensions and pH during
    exercise. J. Appl. Physiol. 19:243-245, Mar., 1964. (Stockholm)

Holmgren, Alf; Mossfeldt, F.; Sjöstrand, T.; and Ström, G.: Effect of training on work
    capacity, total hemoglobin, blood volume, heart volume and pulse rate in recumbent
    and upright positions. Acta Physiol. Scand. 50:72-83, Sept. 30, 1960. (Stockholm)

----, and Ovenfors, C. O.: Heart volume at rest and during muscular work in the supine and in the
    sitting positions. Acta Med. Scand. 167:267-277, July 15, 1960. (Stockholm)

----, and Pernow, B.: The reproducibility of cardiac output determination by the direct Fick
    method during muscular work. Scand. J. Clin. Lab. Invest. 12:224-227, 1960. (Stockholm)

----, and Strandell, Tore: On the use of chest-head leads for recording of electrocardiogram during
    exercise. Acta Med. Scand. 169:57-62, Jan., 1961. (Stockholm)

----, and ----: The relationship between heart volume, total hemoglobin and physical working
    capacity in former athletes. Acta Med. Scand. 163:149-160, Feb. 25, 1959. (Stockholm)

----, and Ström, Gunnar: Blood lactate concentration in relation to absolute and relative work load
    in normal men, and in mitral stenosis, atrial septal defect and vasoregulatory asthenia. Acta
    Med. Scand. 163:185-193, Mar. 4, 1959. (Stockholm)

Hon, Edward H.; and Wohlgemuth, Richard: The electronic evaluation of fetal heart rate. IV. The
    effect of maternal exercise. Amer. J. Obstet. Gynec. 81:361-371, Feb., 1961. (New Haven,
    Conn.)

Hooker, D. R.: The effect of exercise upon the venous blood pressure. Amer. J. Physiol. 28:235-248,
    Aug. 1, 1911. (Baltimore)

----, Wilson, D. W.; and Connett, Helene: The perfusion of the mammalian medulla: the effect
    of carbon dioxide and other substances on the respiratory and cardiovascular centers. Amer. J.
    Physiol. 43:351-361, May 1, 1917. (Baltimore)

Horiuchi, Kiyoshi: Über den Einfluss der Gehirndurchblutung auf die Ermüdung. Arbeitsphysiol.
    1:75-84, Feb. 1, 1928. (Berlin)

Hornbein, Thomas F.; and Roos, Albert: Effect of mild hypoxia on ventilation during exercise. J.
    Appl. Physiol. 17:239-242, Mar., 1962. (St. Louis, Mo.)

Horst, Kathryn; Mendel, Lafayette B.; and Benedict, Francis G.: The influence of previous exercise
    upon the metabolism, the rectal temperature, and the body composition of the rat. J. Nutr. 7:
    251-275, Mar., 1935. (Boston, Mass. and New Haven, Conn.)

Horwitt, M. K.; and Kreisler, O.: The determination of early thiamine-deficient states by estimation
    of blood lactic and pyruvic acids after glucose administration and exercise. J. Nutr. 37:411-427,
    Apr., 1949. (Elgin, Ill.)

Hough, Theodore: Certain aspects of influence of muscular exercise upon respiratory system. Trans.
    XV Int. Congr. Hyg. & Demog., Washington 2:651-659, 1913.

----: Ergographic studies in muscular soreness. Amer. J. Physiol. 7:76-92, Apr., 1902. (Boston)

----: The influence of muscular activity upon the alveolar tensions of oxygen and carbon dioxide.
    Amer. J. Physiol. 30:18-36, Apr., 1912. (Charlottesville)

Hough, Theodore: Physiological effects of moderate muscular activity and strain. Amer. Phys. Educat. Rev. 14:207-215, 1909.

Howell, M. L.: Effect of blood loss upon performance in the Balke-Ware treadmill test. Res. Quart. Amer. Ass. Health Phys. Educ. 35:156-165, May, 1964.

Howenstine, James A.: Exertion-induced myoglobinuria and hemoglobinuria; simultation of acute glomerulonephritis. J.A.M.A. 173:493-499, June 4, 1960. (Boston)

Huang, M. H.; Yu, K. J.; Chin, H. Y.; and Hou, H. F.: Ballistocardiographic changes in hypertension and hypertension associated with coronary heart disease. Chin. Med. J. 82:202-207, Apr., 1963.

Hubač, M.; Borsky, I.; Strelka, F.; et al: Körperliche Beanspruchung bei der Arbeit mit verchiedenen Typen von Motorsägen. Int. Zeits. angew. Physiol. 20:111-124, Oct. 16, 1963.

Huckabee, William E.: Relationships of pyruvate and lactate during anaerobic metabolism. I. Effects of infusion of pyruvate or glucose and of hyperventilation. J. Clin. Invest. 37:244-254, Feb., 1958. (Boston)

----: Relationships of pyruvate and lactate during anaerobic metabolism. II. Exercise and formation of O_2-debt. J. Clin. Invest. 37:255-263, Feb., 1958. (Boston)

----: Relationships of pyruvate and lactate during anaerobic metabolism. III. Effect of breathing low-oxygen gases. J. Clin. Invest. 37:264-271, Feb., 1958. (Boston)

----: The role of anaerobic metabolism in the performance of mild muscular work. II. The effect of asymptomatic heart disease. J. Clin. Invest. 37:1593-1602, Nov., 1958. (Boston)

----, and Judson, Walter E.: The role of anaerobic metabolism in the performance of mild muscular work. I. Relationship to oxygen consumption and cardiac output and the effect of congestive heart failure. J. Clin. Invest. 37:1577-1592, Nov., 1958. (Boston)

Hünnekens, H.; and Kiphard, E.: Motoskopische Untersuchungen beim Trampolinspringen. Acta Paedopsychiat. 30:324-341 (Concl.), Sept.-Oct., 1963. (Gütersloh)

Hugenholtz, Paul G.; and Nadas, Alexander S.: Exercise studies in patients with congenital heart disease. Pediatrics 32(Suppl.):769-775, Oct., 1963. (Boston)

Hughes, Frederick D.; and Sterner, James H.: The working cardiac. Med. Rec. Ann. 57:461-467, Aug., 1964. (Rochester, N.Y.)

Hughes, J. Rowland: Ischaemic necrosis of the anterior tibial muscles due to fatigue. J. Bone Joint Surg. 30B:581-594, Nov., 1948. (Liverpool)

Hugh-Jones, P.: A simple standard exercise test and its use for measuring exertion dyspnoea. Brit. Med. J. 1:65-71, Jan. 12, 1952. (Cardiff)

Huidobro, F.; Guzmán, D.; and Andía, M.: Variaciones del poder colinoesterárasico del suero sanguíneo durante el ejercicio muscular violento y en los estados de shock hipoglicémico. Rev. Med. Aliment. 6:38-40, Oct., 1943-Jan., 1944.

Hulth, Anders; and Olerud, Sven: Disuse of extremities. II. A microangiographic study in the rabbit. Acta Chir. Scand. 120:388-394, Jan., 1961. (Uppsala)

Humphreys, P. W.; and Lind, A. R.: Blood flow through active muscles of the forearm during sustained hand-grip contractions. J. Physiol. 163:18P-19P, Aug., 1962. (Oxford)

Humphreys, P. W.; and Lind, A. R.: The energy expenditure of coal-miners at work. Brit. J. Indust. Med. 19:264-275, Oct., 1962. (Oxford)

Hundt, Alan G.; and Premack, David: Running as both a positive and negative reinforcer. Science 142:1087-1088, Nov. 22, 1963. (Columbia)

Hurtel: Conséquences des exercices physiques sur la tenue, la discipline et les études; ce que devrait être le medecin de lycee. Vie Med. 2:1162-1164, 1921.

Hutchings, R. H.: Physiology of exercise. Nat. Hosp. San. Rec. 2:1-6, 1898-1899.

Hutchinson, Benj: Observations on the treadmill. London Med. & Phys. J. 50:112-118, Aug., 1823.

Huycke, E. J.; and Kruhøffer, P.: Effects of insulin and muscular exercise upon uptake of hexoses by muscle cells. Acta Physiol. Scand. 34:232-249, Oct. 27, 1955. (Copenhagen)

Hyde, I. H.; Root, C. B.; and Curl, H.: A comparison of the effects of breakfast, of no breakfast and of caffeine on work in an athlete and a non-athlete. Amer. J. Physiol. 43:371-394, June 1, 1917.

Hyman, Chester: The circulation of blood through skeletal muscle. Pediatrics 32(Suppl.):671-679, Oct., 1963. (Los Angeles)

----, Paldino, R. L.; and Zimmermann, Emery: Local regulation of effective blood flow in muscle. Circ. Res. 12:176-181, Feb., 1963. (Los Angeles)

Hyman, Richard M.; Soloman, Cyril; and Silberblatt, John: Further experience with exfoliative cytology of urinary tract; increase in exfoliation by exercise. Amer. J. Clin. Path. 26:381-383, Apr., 1956. (New York)

Iakovlev, N. N.; Leshkevich, L. G.; Rogozkin, V. A.; et al: Adaptatsiia lits srednego i starshego vozrasta k intensivnoi myshechnoi deiatel'nosti. (The adaptation of middle-aged and elderly persons to strenuous muscular activity) (Russ). Fiziol. Zh. SSSR Sechenov. 49:1067-1070, Sept., 1963.

Iampietro, P. F.; and Goldman, R. F.: Prediction of energy cost of treadmill work. U. S. Civil Aeromed. Res. Inst. 62-5:4P, Apr., 1962.

Iannacone, A.; Zazo, S.; and Cicchella, G.: (Variation of the plasma adrenalin and noradrenalin content induced in man by the maximum muscular effort of brief duration) (It). Arch. Fisiol. 60:339-348, Sept. 25, 1961.

Iaria, C. T.; Jalar, U. H.; and Kao, F. F.: The peripheral neural mechanism of exercise hyperpnoea. J. Physiol. 148:49P-50P, 1959.

Iatridis, Sotirios G.; and Ferguson, John H.: Effect of physical exercise on blood clotting and fibrinolysis. J. Appl. Physiol. 18:337-344, Mar., 1963. (Chapel Hill)

Idbohrn, Hans; and Wahren, John: The origin of blood withdrawn from deep forearm veins during rhythmic exercise. Acta Physiol. Scand. 61:301-313, Aug., 1964. (Stockholm)

Ikkala, E.: Lihastyön aiheuttamat hematologiset muutskset. (Hematological changes associated with muscular exercise) (Fin). Duodecim 80:115-117, 1964.

----, Myllylä, G.; and Sarajas, H. S. S.: Haemostatic changes associated with exercise. Nature 199: 459-461, Aug. 3, 1963. (Helsinki)

Ikkos, Danae; and Hanson, John S.: Response to exercise in congenital complete atrioventricular block. Circulation 22:583-590, Oct., 1960. (Stockholm)

Inouye, K.: Influence of bodily exercise upon capillaries of body surface. Acta Sch. Med. Univ. Imp. Kioto 14:271-275, 1932.

Isaacs, Raphael; and Gordon, Burgess: The effect of exercise on the distribution of corpuscles in the blood stream. Amer. J. Physiol. 71:106-111, Dec., 1924. (Boston)

Iseri, Lloyd T.; Evans, John R.; and Evans, Michael: Pathogenesis of congestive heart failure. Correlation between anaerobic metabolism and plasma volume changes following exercise. Ann. Intern. Med. 59:788-797, Dec., 1963. (Downey and Los Angeles)

Ismizaki, T.; Yasui, A.; Harafuji, S.; et al: (Changes in the physical capacities of the ground self-defense force personnel by training) (Jap). Nat. Def. Med. J. 11:63-65, Feb., 1964.

Israel, S.: Das Verhalten des arteriellen Blutdrucks an verschiedenen Messtellen bei körperlicher Belastung. Zeits. ges. inn. Med. 14:432-435, May 1, 1959.

Issekutz, B., Jr.; Birkhead, N. C.; and Rodahl, K.: Effect of diet on work metabolism. J. Nutr. 79:109-115, Jan., 1963.

----, ----, and ----: Use of respiratory quotients in assessment of aerobic work capacity. J. Appl. Physiol. 17:47-50, Jan., 1962. (Philadelphia)

Issekutz, B., Jr.; and Miller, Harvey: Plasma free fatty acids during exercise and the effect of
    lactic acid. Proc. Soc. Exp. Biol. Med. 110:237-239, June, 1962. (Philadelphia)

----, Miller, H. L.; and Rodahl, K.: Effect of exercise on FFA metabolism of pancreatectomized
    dogs. Amer. J. Physiol. 205:645-650, Oct., 1963. (Philadelphia)

----, ----, Paul, P.; and Rodahl, K.: Source of fat oxidation in exercising dogs. Amer. J.
    Physiol. 207:583-589, Sept., 1964. (Philadelphia)

----, and Rodahl, K.: Respiratory quotient during exercise. J. Appl. Physiol. 16:606-610, July, 1961.
    (Philadelphia)

Ivanhova, M. P.: Izmenenie electricheskoĭ aktivenosti v razlichnykh oblastiakh kory mosga vo vremia
    vypolneniia myshechnoĭ raboty. (Changes in the electrical activity in different sections of the
    cerebral cortex during the performance of muscular work) (Russ). Zh. Vyssh. Nerv. Deiat.
    Pavlov. 13:972-979, Nov.-Dec., 1963.

Jack, W. B.: Commando training and its medical problems. J. Roy. Nav. Med. Serv. 50:140-154, Autumn, 1964.

Jackson, D. C.; and Hammel, H. T.: Hypothalamic "set" temperature decreased in exercising dog. Life Sci. 8:554-563, Aug., 1963. (Philadelphia and New Haven)

----, ----: Reduced set point temperature in exercising dog. Techn. Docum. Rep. AMRL-TDR-63-93. U. S. Air Force 6570 Aerospace Med. Res. Lab. 1-16, Oct., 1963.

Jacob, J.; and Michaud, G.: Actions de divers agents pharmacologiques sur les temps d'épuisement et le comportement de souris nageant a 20° C. I. Description de la technique. - Actions de l'amphétamine, de la cocaïne, de la caféïne, de l'hexobarbital et du méprobamate. Arch. Int. Pharmacodyn. 133:101-115, Aug.-Sept., 1961. (Paris)

----, and ----: Actions de divers agents pharmacologiques sur les temps d'épuisement et le comportement de souris nageant a 20° C. II. Analgésiques (morphine, dextromoramide, méthadone, péthidine et 3570 CT). Influence de la répétition de l'épreuve. Arch. Int. Pharmacodyn. 135:462-471, Feb. 1, 1962. (Paris)

----, ----: (The effect of various pharmacological agents (amphetamine, cocaine, caffeine, hexobarbital, meprobamate, morphine, dextromoramide, 1-methadone, pethidine and CT 3570) on the time of exhaustion and behavior of animals swimming at 20° C.) (Fr). Med. Exp. 2:323-328, 1960.

Jacobson, Eugene D.; and Bass, David E.: Effects of sodium salicylate on physiological responses to work in heat. J. Appl. Physiol. 19:33-36, Jan., 1964. (Natick)

Jacobson, Gary; Seltzer, Carl C.; Bondy, Philip K.; and Mayer, Jean: Importance of body characteristics in the excretion of 17-ketosteroids and 17-ketogenic steroids in obesity. New Eng. J. Med. 271:651-656, Sept. 24, 1964. (Boston and New Haven)

Jacobsson, S.; and Kjellmer, I.: Accumulation of fluid in exercising skeletal muscle. Acta Physiol. Scand. 60:286-292, Mar., 1964. (Göteborg)

----, and ----: Flow and protein content of lymph in resting and exercising skeletal muscle. Acta Physiol. Scand. 60:278-285, Mar., 1964. (Göteborg)

Jacono, A.; and Juliani, G.: (Observations on a case of transitory flutter, atrial fibrillation and atrioventricular dissociation after exertion) (It). Riforma Med. 76:429-431, Apr. 21, 1962.

Jacquelin, A.; Gratay, A.; Chiron, J. P.; Olivo, H. T.; Schwartz, B.; and Schwartz, D.: L'asthme a dyspnée d'effort exclusive. Sem. Hôp. Paris 38:599-603, Feb. 20, 1962.

Jaeger, M. J.; and Otis, A. B.: Effects of compressibility of alveolar gas on dynamics and work of breathing. J. Appl. Physiol. 19:83-91, Jan., 1964.

Jakoubek, B.; Gutmann, E.; Hajek, I.; et al: Changes in protein metabolism of peripheral nerve during functional activity. Physioc. Bohemoslov. 12:553-561, 1963.

----, and Svorad, D.: Über die Veränderungen in der Konzentration des Gehirnglykogens bei körperlicher Belastung. Pflüger Arch. ges. Physiol. 268:444-448, Feb. 24, 1959. (Prague)

James, William H.; and Elgindi, Ibrahim M.: Effect of strenuous physical activity on blood
    vitamin A and carotene in young men. Science 118:629-630, Nov. 20, 1953. (Baton
    Rouge)

Janda, F.: Suitability of physical work with regard to the development of children and adolescents.
    Rev. Czech. Med. 9:82-93, 1963.

Jang, Evangeline; Taylor, Fletcher B., Jr.; and Bickford, Arthur F.: Effect of exercise on the time
    of clot lysis in normal subjects and patients with cirrhosis of the liver. Clin. Sci. 27:9-13, Aug.,
    1964. (San Francisco)

Janota-Lukaszewska, Janina; and Romanowski, Wieslaw: γ-Amino-butyric acid content in the brain
    after a single and prolonged physical effort. Acta Physiol. Pol. 15:187-191, 1964. (Warsaw)

Jansen, G.: Lärmewïrkung bei körperlicher Arbeit. Int. Zeits. angew. Physiol. 20:233-239, Feb.
    21, 1964.

Jarisch, A.; and Liljestrand, G.: Uber das Verhalten des Kreislaufes bei Muskelarbeit nach dem Essen
    und bei Flussigkeitszufuhr. Skand. Arch. Physiol. 51:235-248, May, 1927.

Jasinski, B.: Die klinische Bedeutung von Fahrradergometerversuchen zur Beurteilung der verminderten
    Leistungsfähigkeit, nebst Bemerkungen zu dem Verhalten der Milchsäure im Blute wahrend und
    nach der Arbeit bei verschiedenen Erkrankungen. Helv. Med. Acta 14:117-136, Apr., 1947.
    (Winterthur)

Jasmin, Gaétan; and Bois, Pierre: Effect of centrally acting drugs upon muscular exercise in rats.
    Canadian J. Biochem. Physiol. 37:417-423, Mar., 1959.

Jenkins, D. J.: Effect of B-sympathetic blockade on non-esterified-fatty-acid and carbohydrate
    metabolism at rest and during exercise. Lancet 2:1184-1185, Nov. 28, 1964. (Oxford)

Jeyasingham, K.: Some studies in ear oximetry. Ceylon Med. J. 7:23-31, Mar., 1962.

Jørgensen, G.: Experimental investigation of the venous pressure with special reference to the regulation
    of the circulation. Copenhagen, Danish Science Press, 1954.

Johansson, J. E.: Ueber die Einwirkung der Muskeltätigkeit auf die Athmung und die Herzthätigkeit.
    Skand. Arch. Physiol. 5:20-66, 1895. (Stockholm)

----, and Koraen, Gunnar: Untersuchungen über die Kohlensäureabgabe bei statischer und negativer
    Muskelthätigkeit. Skand. Arch. Physiol. 13:229-250, 1902. (Stockholm)

----, and ----: Wie wird Kohlensäureabgabe bei Muskelarbeit von Nahrungszufuhr beeinflusst?
    Skand. Arch. Physiol. 13:251-268, 1902. (Stockholm)

Johnson, B. L.; Jokl, E.; and Jokl, P.: The effect of exercise upon the duration of the triceps surae
    stretch reflex. J. Ass. Phys. Ment. Rehab. 17:172-176, Nov.-Dec., 1963.

Johnson, Mary Louise; Burke, Bertha S.; and Mayer, J.: Relative importance of inactivity and over-
    eating in the energy balance of obese high school girls. Amer. J. Clin. Nutr. 4:37-44, Jan.-
    Feb., 1956. (Boston)

Johnson, Robert E.: Caloric requirements under adverse environmental conditions. Fed. Proc. 22:1439-1446,
    Nov.-Dec., 1963. (Urbana)

Johnson, R. E.; and Edward, H. T.: Lactate and pyruvate in blood and urine after exercise. J. Biol. Chem. 118:427-432, Apr., 1937. (Boston)

----, and Passmore, R.: Interrelations among post-exercise ketosis (Courtice-Douglas effect), hydration, and metabolic state. Metabolism 9:443-451, May, 1960. (Edinburgh)

Johnson, Robert Lee, Jr.; Spicer, W. S.; Bishop, J. M.; and Forster, Robert E.: Pulmonary capillary blood volume, flow, and diffusing capacity during exercise. J. Appl. Physiol. 15:893-902, Sept., 1960. (Philadelphia)

Johnson, Thomas F.; and Wong, Harry Y. C.: Effects of training and competitive swimming on serum proteins. J. Appl. Physiol. 16:807-809, Sept., 1961. (Washington)

Jokl, Ernst: Blutuntersuchungen an Sportsleuten. Arbeitsphysiol. 4:379-389, 1931. (Breslau)

----: Beiträge zur Physiologie des Laufens und Hürdenlaufens. Arbeitsphysiol. 1:296-305, 1929. (Breslau)

----: Exercise and cardiac stroke force. J. Ass. Phys. Ment. Rehab. 18:148-163, Nov.-Dec., 1964.

----, and Suzman, M. M.: Mechanisms involved in acute fatal nontraumatic collapse associated with physical exertion. Amer. Heart J. 23:761-765, June, 1942. (Johannesburg)

----, and Wolffe, J. B.: Sudden non-traumatic death associated with physical exertion in identical twins. Acta Genet. Med. 3:245-246, May, 1954.

Jones, C. Handfield: The effect of brief exertion on the radial tracing. Lancet 1:810, June 3, 1876. (London)

Jones, Evelyn M.; Montoye, Henry J.; Johnson, Perry B.; Martin, Sister M. John Martin; Van Huss, Wayne D.; and Cederquist, Dena: Effects of exercise and food restriction on serum cholesterol and liver lipids. Amer. J. Physiol. 207:460-466, Aug., 1964. (East Lansing)

Jones, J.: Investigations on the effects of prolonged muscular exercise on the excretion of urea, uric acid, phosphoric acid, sulphuric acid and chloride of sodium. New Orleans Med. Surg. J. 5:853-867, 1877-1878.

Jones, Maxwell Shaw and Mellersh, Veronica: A comparison of exercise response in anxiety states and normal controls. Psychosom. Med. 8:180-187, May-June, 1946. (London)

----, and ----: A comparison of the exercise response in anxiety states in various groups of neurotic patients. Psychosom. Med. 8:192-194 May-June, 1946. (London)

----, and Scarisbrick, Ronald: Effect of exercise on soldiers with effort intolerance. Lancet 2:331-332, Sept. 11, 1943. (London)

----, and ----: The effect of exercise on soldiers with neurocirculatory asthenia. Psychosom. Med. 8:188-192, May-June, 1946. (London)

Jones, William B.; and Foster, Glenn L.: Determinants of duration of left ventricular ejection in normal young men. J. Appl. Physiol. 19:279-283, Mar., 1964.

Jonsell, Sonie; and Sjöstrand, Torgny: Herzgrösse und Vitalkapazität bei Schwankungen der Blutverteilung. Acta Physiol. Scand. 3:49-53, Nov. 15, 1941. (Stockholm)

Jonsson, B.; Linderholm, H.; and Pinardi, G.: Atrial septal defect: a study of physical working capacity and hemodynamics during exercise. Acta Med. Scand. 159:275-294, Dec. 12, 1957. (Stockholm)

----, and Lukianski, M.: Systemic arterial pressure during exercise in patients with pulmonary hypertension. Acta Med. Scand. 173:73-81, Jan., 1963. (Stockholm)

Jouve, A.; Rochu, P.; Monteix, R.; and Schlaefflin, G.: Les modifications électrocardiographiques après effort prolongé (courses de fond) chez des adolescents. Presse Méd. 65:1387-1389, Aug. 17, 1957. (Marseilles)

Judge, Richard D.; Wilson, William S.; and Siegel, John H.: Hemodynamic studies in patients with implanted cardiac pacemakers. New Eng. J. Med. 270:1391-1395, June 25, 1964. (Ann Arbor, Mich.)

Judson, Walter E.; Hollander, William; Hatcher, J. D.; and Halperin, Meyer H.: The effects of exercise on cardiovascular and renal function in cardiac patients with and without heart failure. J. Clin. Invest. 34:1546-1558, Oct., 1955. (Boston)

----, ----, and Wilkins, Robert W.: The effect of exercise in the supine position on cardiovascular and renal function in hypertensive patients before and during chronic oral hydralazine therapy. J. Lab. Clin. Med. 49:672-683, May, 1957. (Boston)

Julich, Horst: Das Verhalten von Sauerstoffdruck sowie Kohlensäuregehalt im Arterienblut bei Gesunden und Kranken nach körperlicher Belastung. Zeits. ges. inn. Med. 18:928-932, Oct., 1963.

----, and Eisfeld, Gunter: Der Einfluss von körperlicher Arbeit auf das Verhalten von Milchsäure, Brenztraubensäure und Citronensäure im Blut. Zeits. klin. Med. 156:222-235, Jan. 20, 1960. (Halle)

Jundell, I.; and Fries, K. A. E.: Die Anstrengungsalbuminurie. Nord. Med. Ark. 44; Afd. II:1-154, 1911.

Junkmann, K.; and Witzel, H.: Chemie und Pharmakologie der Corticoide. Zeits. Vitamin Hormon Fermentforsch. 13:49-128, 1963.

----, and ----: Chemie und Pharmakologie der Corticoide. Zeits. Vitamin Hormon Fermentforsch. 13: 129-208, 1963.

----, and ----: Chemie und Pharmakologie der Corticoide. Zeits. Vitamin Hormon Fermentforsch. 13: 209-304, 1963.

Juurup, A.; and Muido, L.: On acute effects of cigarette smoking on oxygen consumption, pulse rate, breathing rate, and blood pressure in working organisms. Acta Physiol. Scand. 11:48-60, 1946.

Kägi, Hans Rudolf: Der Einfluss von Muskelarbeit auf die Blutkonzentration der Nebennieren-
rindenhormone. Helv. Med. Acta 22:258-267, Aug., 1955. (Zürich)

Kahler, Richard L.; Gaffney, Thomas E.; and Braunwald, Eugene: The effects of autonomic nervous
system inhibition on the circulatory response to muscular exercise. J. Clin. Invest. 41:1981-1987,
Nov., 1962. (Bethesda)

----, Thompson, Ronald H.; Buskirk, Elsworth R.; Frye, Robert L.; and Braunwald, Eugene: Studies
on digitalis. VI. Reduction of the oxygen debt after exercise with digoxin in cardiac patients
without heart failure. Circulation 27:397-405, Mar., 1963. (Bethesda)

Kahn, Harold A.: The relationship of reported coronary heart disease mortality to physical activity of
work. Amer. J. Public Health 53:1058-1067, July, 1963. (Bethesda)

Kaindl, F.; and Pärtan, J.: Die periphere arteriovenöse Sauerstoffdifferenz bei Durchblutungsänderungen
durch Muskelarbeit und Vasodilatantien. Wien. Zeits. inn. Med. 38:413-417, Oct., 1957.

Kalk, H.; and Bonis, A.: Über den Ammoniakgehalt des Blutes nach Muskelarbeit. Zeits. klin. Med.
123:731-741, 1933. (Berlin)

Kalliomäki, J. L.; Pulkkinen, M.; and Savola, P.: Lactic acid response to muscular exercise in rheumatoid arthritis. Ann. Med. Exp. Fenn. 35:441-445, 1957.

Kaltenbach, M.; and Klepzig, H.: Das EKG während Belastung und seine Bedeutung für die Erkennung
der Koronarinsuffizienz. Zeits. Kreislaufforsch. 52:486-497, May, 1963. (Frankfurt and Taunusheim)

Kaltreider, Nolan L.; and Meneely, George R.: The effect of exercise on the volume of the blood.
J. Clin. Invest. 19:627-634, July, 1940. (Rochester, N.Y.)

Kanematsu, H.: (On sinus arrhythmia in children. 3. Changes in sinus arrhythmia with the injections
of adrenaline, noradrenaline, pilocarpine, and atropine and movement load) (Jap). Acta Paediat.
Jap. 68:101-106, Feb., 1964.

Kao, Frederick F.: Regulation of respiration during muscular activity. Amer. J. Physiol. 185:145-151,
Apr., 1956.

----, Michel, C. C.; and Mei, S. S.: Carbon dioxide and pulmonary ventilation in muscular exercise.
J. Appl. Physiol. 19:1075-1080, Nov., 1964. (Brooklyn)

----, ----, ----, and Li, W. K.: Somatic afferent influence on respiration. Ann. N. Y. Acad.
Sci. 109:696-711, June 24, 1963. (Brooklyn)

----, and Ray, Louise H.: Regulation of cardiac output in anesthetized dogs during induced muscular work.
Amer. J. Physiol. 179:255-260, Nov., 1954. (New York and Brooklyn)

----, and ----: Respiratory and circulatory responses of anesthetized dogs to induced muscular work.
Amer. J. Physiol. 179:249-254, Nov., 1954. (New York and Brooklyn)

----, Schlig, Barbara B.; and Brooks, Chandler McC.: Regulation of respiration during induced
muscular work in decerebrate dogs. J. Appl. Physiol. 7:379-386, Jan., 1955. (Brooklyn)

----, and Suckling, Eustace E.: A method for producing muscular exercise in anesthetized dogs and
its validity. J. Appl. Physiol. 18:194-196, Jan., 1963. (Brooklyn)

Kärki, N. T.: The urinary excretion of noradrenaline and adrenaline in different age groups, its diurnal variation and the effect of muscular work on it. Acta Physiol. Scand. 39(Suppl. 132): 1-96, 1956. (Turku)

----; and Vasama, R.: (Urinary excretion of noradrenaline and adrenaline during muscular exercise) (Fin). Sotilaslaak. Aikak. 34:59-69, 1959.

Karlan, Samuel C.; and Cohn, Clarence: Hypoglycemic fatigue. J.A.M.A. 130:553-555, Mar. 2, 1946.

Karpenko, L. I.: (Correlation of the indices of external respiratory function and blood circulation after physical stress during the 1st stage of cardiac insufficiency) (Russ). Ter. Arkh. 35:106-109, Mar., 1963.

Karpovich, Peter V.: Physiological and psychological dynamogenic factors in exercise. Arbeitsphysiol. 9:626-629, 1937.

----, and Hale, Creighton J.: Effect of warming-up upon physical performance. J.A.M.A. 162: 1117-1119, Nov. 17, 1956. (Springfield, Mass.)

Karvonen, Matti J.: Electromyographic and energy expenditure studies of rhythmic and paced lifting work. Ann. Acad. Sci. Fenn. (Med.) 106(Suppl. 19):1-11, 1964. (Helsinki)

----: Körperliche Tätigkeit, Cholesterinstoffwechsel und Arteriosklerose. Schweiz. Zeits. Sportmed. 9:90-100, 1961. (Helsinki)

Kasalický, J.; Widimský, J.; and Dejdar, R.: The effect of muscular exercise, oxygen inhalation, serpasil and priscol on the lesser circulation in silicosis. Cor Vasa 5:264-272, 1963.

Kasanen, A.; Kallio, V.; and Forsström, J.: The significance of psychic and socio-economic stress and other modes of life in the etiology of myocardial infarction. Ann. Med. Intern. Fenn. 52(Suppl. 43):1-40, 1963. (Turku)

Kattus, Albert A.; Sinclair-Smith, Bruce; Genest, Jacques; and Newman, Elliot V.: The effect of exercise on the renal mechanism of electrolyte excretion in normal subjects. Bull. Johns Hopkins Hosp. 84:344-368, Apr., 1949. (Baltimore)

Katz, Gerhard: Über den Adrenalingehalt des peripheren menschlichen Blutes bei Muskelarbeit. Zeits. klin. Med. 123:154-158, 1934. (Berlin)

Katzenstein, George: Ueber die Einwirkung der Muskelthätigkeit auf den Stoffverbranch des Menschen. Pflüger Arch. ges. Physiol. 49:330-404, 1891.

Kaufman, W. C.: Human tolerance limits for some thermal environments of aerospace. Aerospace Med. 34:889-896, Oct., 1963. (Wright-Patterson Air Force Base)

Kaufmann, G.: Über Kreislaufzeiten und Blutverteilung bei Arbeit. Cardiologia 30:102-114, 1957. (St. Gallen)

Kaufmann, W.; Nieth, H.; Heckermann, H.; et al: Exkretionsfunktion und Hämodynamik der Nieren bei körperlicher Belastung Herzkranker unter Thermoindifferenzbedingungen. Verh. deutsch. ges. Kreislaufforsch. 30:340-345, 1964.

Kaup, I.: Arbeit und Erholung als Atmungsfunktion des Blutes. Vorläufige Mitteilung. Arbeitsphysiol. 2:541-574, May 9, 1930. (Munich)

Kaup, J.; and Grosse, A.: Herzminutenvolumen in Ruhe und Arbeit nach der Jodäthyl und Stickoxydulmethode. Zeits. Kreislaufforsch. 21:44-48, Jan. 15, 1929.

----, and ----: Zur Bestimmung des Minutenvolumens mit Aethyljodid. Arbeitsphysiol. 1:357-376, Jan. 9, 1929. (Munich)

Kawamoto, K.: Effect of exercise on colloidal osmotic pressure of serum in rabbit. (Abstract) Far East Sci. Bull. 1:39, Sept., 1941.

Kayne, Herbert L.; and Alpert, Norman R.: Oxygen consumption following exercise in the anesthetized dog. Amer. J. Physiol. 206:51-56, Jan., 1964. (Chicago)

Kayser, Charles: Physiologie du travail et du sport. Paris, Hermann, 1947.

Keatinge, W. R.: The effect of work and clothing on the maintenance of the body temperature in water. Quart. J. Exp. Physiol. 46:69-82, Jan., 1961. (Cambridge, Eng.)

Keck, Ernst W. O.; Allwood, Michael J.; Marshall, Robert J.; and Shepherd, John T.: Effects of catecholamines and atropine on cardiovascular response to exercise in the dog. Circ. Res. 9: 566-570, May, 1961. (Rochester, Minn.)

Keener, H. A.; Canty, T. J.; and Prevost, J. V.: Thrombosis of axillary vein caused by strain or effort; report of a case occurring in a deep-sea diver; and a brief resumé of the subject. U. S. Naval Med. Bull. 40:687-692, July, 1942.

Keeney, Clifford E.: Effect of training on eosinophil response of exercised rats. J. Appl. Physiol. 15:1046-1048, Nov., 1960. (Springfield, Mass.)

----, and Laramie, David W.: Effect of exercise on blood coagulation. Circ. Res. 10:691-695, Apr., 1962. (Springfield, Mass.)

Keith, M. Helen; and Mitchell, H. H.: The effect of exercise on vitamin requirements. Amer. J. Physiol. 65:128-138, June, 1923. (Urbana)

Kekcheyev, Krikor: Expediting visual adaptation to darkness. Nature 151:617-618, May 29, 1943. (Moscow)

Kektscheew, K.; and Braitzewa, L.: Material zur physiologischen Untersuchung der statischen Arbeit. Arbeitsphysiol. 2:526-540, May 9, 1930. (Moscow)

Keller, W. D.; and Kopf, H.: (Differences in anthropological measurements in 4 groups of young men with different physical activity) (Ger). Int. Zeits. angew. Physiol. 19:110-119, 1961.

Kennaway, E. L.: The effects of muscular work upon the excretion of endogenous purines. J. Physiol. 38:1-27, Dec. 30, 1908. (London)

Kerimov, S. M.; Akopian, A. K.; Tagizade, Z. A.; et al: K izucheniiu ateroskleroza (Soderzhanie kholesterina krovi u lits fizicheskogo truda). (On the study of atherosclerosis (cholesterol content of the blood in persons engaged in physical labor)) (Russ). Azerbaidzh. Med. Zh. 2:42-48, Feb., 1964.

Kerkhof, Arthur C.; and Kolars, Charles P.: Deer hunting and the heart. (A preliminary report.) Minnesota Med. 46:1092; 1126; 1189, Nov., 1963. (Minneapolis)

Kern, R.: Über das Verhalten von Augendruck, Blutdruck und Körpergewicht bei extremer körperlicher Dauerleistung. Ophthalmologica 147:82-92, 1964.

Kesseler, Karlheinz; Egli, Hans; and Wachholder, Kurt: Über die Einwirkung körperlicher Arbeit auf die Blutgerinnung. Klin. Wschr. 35:1088-1089, Nov. 1, 1957. (Bonn)

Kettel, L. J.; Overbeck, H. W.; Daugherty, R. M.; Lillehei, J. P.; Coburn, R. F.; and Haddy, F. J.: Responses of the human upper extremity vascular bed to exercise, cold, levoarterenol, angiotensin, hypertension, heart failure, and respiratory tract infection with fever. J. Clin. Invest. 43:1561-1575, Aug., 1964. (Minneapolis, Chicago and Oklahoma City)

Keul, J.; Reindell, H.; and Roskamm, H.: Zur Belastbarkeit des jugendlichen Organismus. Herzvolumen und Leislungsfähigkeit bei Jugendlichen nach langjahriger Trainingsbelastung. Int. Zeits. angew. Physiol. 19:287-329, 1962.

Keys, Ancel: The recovery following brief severe exercise. J. Biol. Chem. 105:xlvi, May, 1934. (Boston)

----, Anderson, Joseph T.; Aresu, Mario; Biörck, Gunnar; Brock, John F.; Bronte-Stewart, B.; Fidanza, F.; Keys, Margaret H.; Malmros, Haquin; Poppi, Arrigo; Posteli, Teodoro; Swahn, Bengt; and Del Vecchio, Alfonso: Physical activity and the diet in populations differing in serum cholesterol. J. Clin. Invest. 35:1173-1181, Sept., 1956. (Minneapolis)

----, and Blackburn, Henry: Background of the patient with coronary heart disease. Progr. Cardiov. Dis. 6:14-44, July, 1963. (Minneapolis)

Kimeldorf, D. J.; and Baum, S. J.: Alterations in organ and body growth of rats following daily exhaustive exercise, x-irradiation, and post-irradiation exercise. Growth 18:79-96, June, 1954. (San Francisco)

----, and Jones, D. C.: The relationship of radiation dose to lethality among exercised animals exposed to roentgen rays. Amer. J. Physiol. 167:626-632, Dec., 1951. (San Francisco)

----, ----, and Castanera, T. J.: Effect of x-irradiation upon the performance of daily exhaustive exercise by the rat. Amer. J. Physiol. 174:331-335, Sept., 1953. (San Francisco)

----, ----, and Fishler, M. C.: The effect of exercise upon the lethality of roentgen rays for rats. Science 112:175-176, Aug. 11, 1950. (San Francisco)

Kimura, Eüichi; Ushiyama, S.; Kojima, Naohiko; et al: (Effectiveness of segontin in angina pectoris. Evaluation of O-2 deficiency and exercise load) (Jap). J. Ther. 46:162-165, Jan., 1964. (Tokyo)

----, Ushiyama, Kiyoji; Kojima, Naohiko; Hayakawa, Hirokazu; and Yoshida, Koichi: Exercise test and anoxia test in the diagnosis of angina pectoris. A comparative study. Jap. Heart J. 4:313-322, July, 1963. (Tokyo)

Kinnen, Edwin; Kubicek, William; and Patterson, R.: Thoracic cage impedance measurements. Impedance plethysmographic determination of cardiac output (a comparative study). Tech. Docum. Rep. No. SAM-TDR-64-15. U. S. Air Force Sch. Aerospace Med. 1-8, Mar., 1964. (Minneapolis)

Kinzius, H.; and Kötter, F.: Der Adrenalinogenspiegel des Blutes nach sportlichen Laufübungen. Arbeitsphysiol. 14:363-368, 1951.

Kinzlmeier, H.; Wolf, F.; and Henning, N.: Die Prüfung der Leberdurchblutung mit Radiobengalrot unter Muskelarbeit und lokalen thermischen Reizen. Gastroenterologia 91:303-314, 1959. (Erlangen)

Kirchhoff, H. W.; Reindell, H.; and Gebauer, A.: Untersuchungen über die Sauerstoffaufnahme, Kohlensäureabgabe, das Atemminutenvolumen, Atemäquivalent und den respiratorischen Quotienten wahrend koperlicher Belastung bei Normalpersonen und Hochleistungssportlern. Deutsch. Arch. klin. Med. 203:423-447, Nov. 7, 1956. (Freiburg)

Kirschner, Henryk: Analysis of "simple" and "complex" rhythm efficiency of muscular work. Acta Physiol. Pol. 14:182-195, 1963. (Warsaw)

Kjellberg, Sven Roland; Rudhe, Ulf; and Sjöstrand, Torgny: The amount of hemoglobin (blood volume) in relation to the pulse rate and heart volume during work. Acta Physiol. Scand. 19:152-169, Dec. 23, 1949. (Stockholm)

----, ----, and ----: Increase of the amount of hemoglobin and blood volume in connection with physical training. Acta Physiol. Scand. 19:146-151, Dec. 23, 1949. (Stockholm)

----, ----, and ----: The influence of the autonomic nervous system on the contraction of the human heart under normal circulatory conditions. Acta Physiol. Scand. 24:350-360, Feb. 12, 1952. (Stockholm)

Kjellmer, Ingemar: The effect of exercise on the vascular bed of skeletal muscle. Acta Physiol. Scand. 62:18-30, Sept.-Oct., 1964. (Göteborg)

----: An indirect method for estimating tissue pressure with special reference to tissue pressure during exercise. Acta Physiol. Scand. 62:31-40, Sept.-Oct., 1964. (Göteborg)

----: The role of potassium ions in exercise hyperaemia. Med. Exp. 5:56-60, 1961.

Kleinerman, Jerome; and Sancetta, Salvatore M.: Effect of mild steady state exercise on cerebral and general hemodynamics of normal untrained subjects. (Abstract) J. Clin. Invest. 34: 945-946, June, 1955.

Kleinschmidt, A.: Klinische Aspeckte der benignen Proteinurie. Deutsch. med. Wschr. 88:2283-2288, Nov. 22, 1963.

Klepping, J.; Truchot, R.; Didier, J. P.; Escousse, A.; and Eygonnet, J. P.: Etude de l'élimination urinaire de l'acide vanillylmandélique (VMA) pendant l'effort comme critére de la capacité de' d'adaptation a l'exercice musculaire. Comptes Rend. Soc. Biol. 158:2007-2009, 1964. (Dijon)

Klepzig, H.; Müller, D.; and Reindell, H.: Uber das EKG wahrend Belastung und seine klinische Bedeutung. Zeits. Kreislaufforsch. 45:741-750, Oct., 1956. (Freiburg)

Kliment, V.; Zachar, V.; Ditteová, V.; et al: Pokus o hodnotenie vplyvu nadmernej fyzickey námahy na estrus a maternicový sval krýs. (An attempt to evaluate the effect of extreme physical exertion on the estrus and myometrium in rats) (Cz). Cesk. Gynek. 28:501-503, Sept., 1963.

Klink, K.; and Bürkmann, I.: Das Verhalten der arteriellen O_2-Sättigung und des arteriellen O_2-Druckes in der Erholungszeit nach körperlicher Belastung von Gesunden und Lungenkranken. Zeits. ges. inn. Med. 19:188-192, Feb., 15, 1964.

Klug, Paul: Ueber Veranderung der Blutzusammensetzung bei körperlichen Anstrengungen. Würzburg, P. Scheiner, 1904.

Knipping, H. W.; and Valentin, H.: Das Herz des Schwerarbeiters und des Hochleistungssportlers. Munchen. med. Wschr. 103:11-15, Jan. 6, 1961. (Köln)

Knoll, Wilhelm: Kritisches zur Physiologie der Leibesübungen. Schweiz. med. Wschr. 58:1262-1264, Dec. 22, 1928.

----, and Arnold, Arno: Normale und pathologische Physiologie der Leibesübungen. Leipzig, J.A. Barth, 1933.

Knott, John: Physical overexertion and its effects on health. Amer. Med. 7:148-150, Jan. 23, 1904. (Dublin)

Knox, J. A. C.: The effect of the static and of the dynamic components of muscular effort on the heart rate. J. Physiol. 113:36-42, Mar. 19, 1951. (London)

----: The heart rate with exercise in patients with auricular fibrillation. Brit. Heart J. 11:119-125, Apr., 1949. (London)

Knudsen, E. O. Ernebo: See Ernebo-Knudsen, E. O.

Knuttgen, Howard G.: Oxygen debt, lactate, pyruvate, and excess lactate after muscular work. J. Appl. Physiol. 17:639-644, July, 1962. (Copenhagen)

----: Oxygen uptake and pulse rate while running with undetermined and determined stride lengths at different speeds. Acta Physiol. Scand. 52:366-371, July-Aug., 1961. (Copenhagen)

Kobayashi, I.: Cases of spontaneous tibia fracture caused by running. (Abstract) Far East. Sci. Bull. 3:18, June, 1943.

Kobernick, Sidney D.; and Hashimoto, Y.: Histochemistry of atherosclerosis. I. Induced lesions of the aorta of cholesterol-fed, exercised, and sedentary rabbits. Lab. Invest. 12:638-647, June, 1963. (Detroit)

----, and ----: Histochemistry of atherosclerosis. II. Spontaneous degenerative lesions of aorta of exercised and sedentary rabbits. Lab. Invest. 12:685-696, July, 1963. (Detroit)

----, and Niwayama, G.: Physical activity in experimental cholesterol atherosclerosis of rabbits. Amer. J. Path. 36:393-409, Apr., 1960. (Detroit)

----, ----, and Zuchlewski, Alexander C.: Effect of physical activity on cholesterol atherosclerosis in rabbits. Proc. Soc. Exp. Biol. Med. 96:623-628, Dec., 1957. (Detroit)

König, Erwin; and Zöllner, Nepomuk: Über das Verhalten des peripheren Venendruckes während und nach körperlicher Arbeit. Deutsch. Arch. klin. Med. 204:107-122, Aug. 5, 1957. (Munich)

Koessling, F. K.: Comparative studies on the regulation of performance-heartbeat frequency in trained and untrained persons with the method of pulse time registration) (Ger). Med. Welt 31:1567-1572, July 30, 1960.

Kohlrausch, W.: Der Atemtypus bei verschiedenen sportlichen Uebungen. München. med. Wschr. 68:1515, Nov. 25, 1921.

Kohlrausch, W.: Die Wirkungsweise der Leibesübungen auf Kräftige und Schwächliche nach den Erfahrungen an Berliner Studenten. Med. Welt 8:909-911, June 30, 1934.

----: Zur Kenntnis des Trainingszustandes. Arbeitsphysiol. 2:46-50, 1930. (Berlin)

Kokas, E.; and Kurucz, J.: Die Wirkung der Hypothalamusverletzung aud die Nebenniere und auf die Arbeitsleistung. Schweiz. med. Wschr. 86:1067-1070, Sept. 15, 1956. (Budapest)

----, and Miczbán, I.: Die Wirkung von Guanylnucleotiden auf die Arbeitsfähigkeit sowie auf die Hypertrophie von Herz und Nebennieren bei der Ratte. Zeits. Vitamin Hormon Fermentforsch. 11:310-319, Feb. 20, 1961. (Budapest)

Kommerell, Burkhard: Über den Einfluss des Schilddrüsenhormons auf den Arbeitsstoffwechsel des Hundes. Arbeitsphysiol. 1:586-594, 1929. (Berlin)

Konishi, F.: The effect of exercise on calcium and phosphorus balance in young adult men. Army Med. Nutrition Lab. Report 211, pages 1-17, Sept. 6, 1957.

Konttinen, Aarne: Lihastyön biokemiallinen perusta. (Biochemical basis of muscular work) (Fin). Duodecim 80:110-114, 1964.

----, Sarajas, H. S.; Frick, M. H.; and Rajasalmi, M.: Arteriovenous relationship of non-esterified fatty acids, triglycerides, cholesterol and phospholipids in exercise. Ann. Med. Exp. Fenn. 40: 250-256, 1962.

----, and Somer Timo: Effect of muscular exercise on plasma viscosity in correlation with postprandial triglyceridemia. J. Appl. Physiol. 18:991-993, Sept., 1963. (Helsinki)

Kontos, Hermes A.; Harley, Eugene L.; Wasserman, Albert J.; Kelly, John J., III; and Magee, Joseph H.: Exertional idiopathic paroxysmal myoglobinuria. Evidence of a defect in skeletal muscle metabolism. Amer. J. Med. 35:283-292, Aug., 1963. (Richmond)

----, Shapiro, William; and Patterson, John L., Jr.: Observations on dyspnea induced by combinations of respiratory stimuli. Amer. J. Med. 37:374-385, Sept., 1964. (Richmond)

Koriakina, A. F.; Kossowskaja, E. B.; and Krestownikoff, A. N.: Ueber die Schwankungen des Chloridgehaltes im Blut, Harn und Schweiss bei Muskeltätigkeit. Arbeitsphysiol. 2:461-473, Mar. 25, 1930. (Leningrad)

----, and Krestownikoff, A. N.: Ueber die quantitativen verhältnisse von Milchsäure in Schweiss und von Eiweiss im Harn bei Muskelarbeit. Arbeitsphysiol. 2:421-426, Jan. 25, 1930.

Korner, P. I.: The normal human blood pressure during and after exercise, with some related observations on changes in heart rate and the blood flow in the limbs. Aust. J. Exp. Biol. Med. Sci. 30:375-384, Oct., 1952. (Sydney)

----: Reflex regulation of post-exercise blood pressure. Aust. J. Exp. Biol. Med. Sci. 30: 385-394, Oct., 1952. (Sydney)

Korotkoff, E.: Le travail, facteur d'équilibre humain. Concours Med. 85:5951-5954, Nov. 2, 1963.

Kosilov, S. A.: Fiziologicheskie osnovy rezhima truda i otdykha i povysheniia rabotosposobnosti. (Physiological principles of work and rest and of the increase of working capacity) (Russ). Nerv. Sist. 4:173-175, 1963.

Kosilov, S. A.: (On the relationship between the 1st and 2nd signal systems during work) (Russ). Zh. Vyss. Nerv. Deiat. Pavlov. 10:481-487, July-Aug., 1960.

----: (Physiological factors determining the rate of working movements) (Russ). Fiziol. Zh. SSSR Sechenov. 49:141-148, Feb., 1963.

Koster, L.; Alers, C. J.; Van Ham, E. H.; and Van Westreenen, E. Reactions to heavy physical exertion and Thorn tests in the analysis of physical insufficiency syndromes. Acta Med. Scand. 150:63-79, Sept. 11, 1954. (Utrecht)

Kotilainen, Martii; and Kotilainen, Anja: The effect of weight reduction on pulse rate, blood pressure, ventilation and oxygen consumption during rest and in connection with muscular exercise. Acta Med. Scand. 171:569-573, May, 1962. (Helsinki)

Kottmeyer, Günther: Die Wirkung der Crataegussäuren auf den venösen Blutmilchsäurespiegel des Menschen während und nach dosierter Arbeit am Ergometer. Klin. Wschr. 33:867-869, Sept. 15, 1955. (Giessen)

Kouwenhoven, W. B.; Starzl, T. E.; and Baker, B.: A low cost treadmill for experimental animals. J. Appl. Physiol. 7:347-348, Nov., 1954. (Baltimore)

Kozawa, S.: The mechanical regulation of the heart beat in the tortoise. J. Physiol. 49:233-245, May 12, 1915. (London)

Kozlowski, Stanislaw; and Saltin, Bengt: Effect of sweat loss on body fluids. J. Appl. Physiol. 19: 1119-1124, Nov., 1964. (Stockholm)

Kral, J.: Les phénomènes anaphylactiques après l'effort. Bruxelles Méd. 28:571-583, Mar. 14, 1948.

----, Schmid, L.; Zenisek, A.; and Stolz, I.: (An attempt at explanation of the activity of heteroauxin in the urine after athletic exertion) (Ger). Med. Welt 31:1595-1598, July 30, 1960.

----, Zenisek, A.; and Hais, I. M.: Sweat and exercise. J. Sport Med. 3:105-113, June-Sept., 1963.

Kramer, John D.; and Lurie, Paul R.: Maximal exercise tests in children; evaluation of maximal exercise tests as an index of cardiovascular fitness in children with special consideration of the recovery pulse curve. Amer. J. Dis. Child. 108:283-297, Sept., 1964. (Indianapolis)

Kramer, K.; and Gauer, Otto: Ueber die Regelung der Atmung bei Muskelarbeit. Pfluger Arch. ges. Physiol. 244:659-686, 1941.

----, and Quensel, W.: Untersuchungen über den Muskelstoffwechsel des Warmblüters. I. Mitteilung. Der Verlauf der Muskeldurchblutung während der tetanischen Kontraktion. Pflüger Arch. ges. Physiol. 239:620-743, 1937. (Heidelberg)

Krasno, Louis R.; and Kidera, George J.: Continuous electrocardiographic recording during exercise: its use in evaluating the effect of pentaerythritol tetranitrate. Angiology 14:417-425, Aug., 1963. (San Francisco)

Krasnova, A. F. (Krasnov): Sarkoplazmaticheskie belke myshts i belki synorotke krovi pri delitel'noi myshechnoi deiatel'nosti i otdykhe. (Sarcoplasmic muscle proteins following a prolonged muscular activity and at rest) (Russ). Ukr. Biokhim. Zh. 36:209-214, 1964.

Krasnova, A. F.: Vliianie fizicheskikh uprazhneniĭ na belkovye fraktsii syvorotki krovi u lits starshego vozrasta. (The influence of physical exercise on the blood serum protein fractions in elderly persons) (Russ). Fiziol. Zh. SSSR Sechenov. 50:756-761, June, 1964.

Krebs, Sir Hans: The Croonian Lecture, 1963. Gluconeogenesis. Proc. Roy. Soc. 159:545-564, Mar. 17, 1964. (Oxford)

----, and Yoshida, T.: Muscular exercise and gluconeogenesis. Biochem. Zeits. 338:241-244, 1963. (Oxford)

Kreisle, James E.; Queen, Dan M.; and Bowman, Barbara H.: Myoglobinuria following exhaustive muscular effort. Report of a case with determination of serum enzyme activities. Texas J. Med. 56:421-425, June, 1960. (Austin)

Kriz, K.: (Paroxysmal headache from exertion) (Cz). Cas. Lek. Cesk. 102:137-142, Feb. 8, 1963.

Kroeker, Edwin J.; and Wood, Earl H.: Comparison of simultaneously recorded central and peripheral arterial pressure pulses during rest, exercise, and tilted position in man. Circ. Res. 3:623-632, Nov., 1955. (Rochester, Minn.)

Krogh, August: The number and distribution of capillaries in muscles with calculations of the oxygen pressure head necessary for supplying the tissue. J. Physiol. 52:409-415, May 20, 1919. (Copenhagen)

----: On the influence of the venous supply upon the output of the heart. Scand. Arch. Physiol. 27:126-140, 1912. (Copenhagen)

----: The regulation of the supply of blood to the right heart. (With a description of a new circulation model.) Scand. Arch. Physiol. 27:227-248, 1912. (Copenhagen)

----: The respiratory exchange of animals and man. London; Longmans, Green and Co.; 1916.

----: The supply of oxygen to the tissues and the regulation of the capillary circulation. J. Physiol. 52:457-474, May 20, 1919. (Copenhagen)

----, and Lindhard, Johannes: The changes in respiration at the transition from work to rest. J. Physiol. 53:431-439, May 18, 1920. (Copenhagen)

----, and ----: A comparison between voluntary and electrically induced muscular work in man. J. Physiol. 51:182-201, July 3, 1917. (Copenhagen)

----, and ----: Measurements of the blood flow through the lungs of man. Scand. Arch. Physiol. 27:100-125, 1912. (Copenhagen)

----, and ----: The regulation of respiration and circulation during the initial stages of muscular work. J. Physiol. 47:112-136, Oct. 17, 1913.

----, and ----: The relative value of fat and carbohydrate as sources of muscular energy; with appendices on the correlation between standard metabolism and the respiration quotient during rest and work. Biochem. J. 14:290-363, July, 1920. (Copenhagen)

Krogh, Marie: The diffusion of gases through the lungs of man. J. Physiol. 49:271-300, May 12, 1915. (Copenhagen)

Kronfeld, D. S.; MacFarlane, W. V.; Harvey, Nancy; Howard, Beth; and Robinson, Kathleen W.: Strenuous exercise in a hot environment. J. Appl. Physiol. 13:425-429, Nov., 1958. (Brisbane, Australia)

Krumholz, Richard A.; Chevalier, Robert B.; and Ross, Joseph C.: Cardiopulmonary function in young smokers. A comparison of pulmonary function measurements and some cardiopulmonary responses to exercise between a group of young smokers and a comparable group of nonsmokers. Ann. Intern. Med. 60:603-610, Apr., 1964. (Indianapolis)

----, King, Leroy H., Jr.; and Ross, Joseph C.: Effect of pulmonary vascular engorgement on D_L during and immediately after exercise. J. Appl. Physiol. 18:1180-1182, Nov., 1963. (Indianapolis)

----, and Ross, Joseph C.: Effect of atropine and reserpine on pulmonary diffusing capacity during exercise in man. J. Appl. Physiol. 19:465-468, May, 1964. (Indianapolis)

Kruse, Robert D.; and Mathews, Donald K.: Bilateral effects of unilateral exercise: experimental study based on 120 subjects. Arch. Phys. Med. 39:371-376, June, 1958. (Cleveland, Ohio and Pullman, Wash.)

Kubicek, F.; and Scherrer, M.: Einfluss des Hämoglobingehalts auf Säure-Basen-Haushalt, Ventilation und O_2-Diffusion beim Gesunden während schwerer Arbeit. Schweiz. med. Wschr. 92:415-420, Apr. 7, 1962. (Vienna and Bern)

Kudrjawzew, Nikolaus: Über die Beeinflussung der muskulären Leistungsfähigkeit durch Ermudüngsstoffe. Arbeitsphysiol. 1:203-212, 1929. (Berlin)

Külbs: Ueber den einfluss der Bewegung auf den wachsenden und erwachsenen Organismus. Deutsch. med. Wschr. 38:1916-1920, Oct. 10, 1912. (Berlin)

Kuhn, W.: The production of mechanical energy on the principle of animal muscular action. Triangle 5:37-44, Apr., 1961. (Basel)

Kulczycki, A.: L'action sur le myocarde d'un effort épuisant. Bull. Int. Acad. Polon. Sci. Lett. Classe Méd.: 39-60, Jan.-Dec., 1952.

Kulenkampff, H.: Das Verhalten der Neuroglia in den Vorderhornern des Rückenmarks der weissen Maus unter dem Reiz physiologischer Tätigkeit. Zeits. Anat. Entwicklungsgesch. 116:304-312, 1952.

----: Das Verhalten der Vorderwurzelzellen der weissen Maus unter dem Reiz physiologischer Tätigkeit. Eine quantitativmorphologische Untersuchung. Zeits. Anat. Entwicklungsgesch. 116:143-156, 1951.

----: Mitosen im Spinalependym und die Beeinflussbarkeit ihres Auftretens durch körperliche Arbeit. Verh. Anat. Ges. 57:230-235, 1963.

Kumar, S.: Respiratory minute volume during moderate exercise. Indian J. Physiol. Pharmacol. 8:104-111, Jan., 1964.

Kurz, Edward R. H.: March hemoglobinuria. Brooklyn Hosp. J. 6:91-94, Apr., 1948. (Brooklyn)

Kusch, T.: Glutaminsaure-Brenztraubensäure-und-Glutaminsäure-Oxalessigsäure-transaminase unter dem Einfluss von Chlorpromazin, Reserpin, Serotonin und körperlicher Belastung. Acta Biol. Med. 11:485-493, 1963.

Lacroix, E.: Influence de l'exercice musculaire sur le débit splanchnique chez le chien. Arch. Int. Physiol. 71:108-111, Jan., 1913.

Lagerlöf, H.; Eliasch, H.; Werkö, L.; and Berglund, E.: Orthostatic changes of the pulmonary and peripheral circulation in man. Scand. J. Clin. Lab. Invest. 3:85-91, 1951. (Stockholm)

Lagrange, Fernand: Physiologie des exercices du corps. Paris; F. Alcan, 1888.

----: Physiology of bodily exercise. London, Keegan Paul, Trench and Co., 1889.

Lahiri, S.: Pulmonary ventilation of man at altitude. Indian J. Physiol. Pharmacol. 8:31-39, April, 1964.

Laird, D. A.: The effects of sugar in recovering mental and motor control after brief periods of exercises; preliminary investigation. Med. Rev. of Rev. 36:383-386, June, 1930.

Lamb, Lawrence E.; and Hiss, Roland G.: Influence of exercise on premature contractions. Amer. J. Cardiol. 10:209-216, Aug., 1962. (Brooks Air Force Base, Texas)

Lambertsen, Christian J.; Owen, S. G.; Wendel, Herbert; Stroud, Morris W.; Lurie, Abraham A.; Lochner, Wilhelm; and Clark, Gordon F.: Respiratory and cerebral circulatory control during exercise at .21 and 2.0 atmospheres inspired pO_2. J. Appl. Physiol. 14:966-982, Nov., 1959. (Philadelphia)

Lammers, B.: Arbeidstijd en rusttijd. Bedrijfsgeneeskundige aspecten. (Work time and rest time. Industrial medical aspects) (Dut). T. Soc. Geneesk. 41:631-633, Oct. 11, 1963.

----: Arbeidstijk en rusttijd. Probleemstelling. T. Soc. Geneesk. 41:625-626, Oct. 11, 1963.

Lamperi, S.; and Bianchini, E.: Studio elettroforetico delle proteine urinaire in soggetti normali e nefropatica sottoposti a lavoro muscolare. Minerva Nefrol. 4:17-21, Jan.-Mar., 1957.

Lampert, H.: Die Wirkung von Muskelanstrengung und nachfolgender Massage beim Gesunden; die Wirkung auf das Blut. Zeits. ges. phys. Ther. 39:238-253, Oct. 14, 1930.

Lancet Commission on Athletics. Lancet 1:999-1001, June 26; 2:218-219, Aug. 7, 1880.

Landen, H. C.: Über die Bedeutung des Trainingsfactors in der Gesamtkreislaufleistung alter Personen. Deutsch. med. Wschr. 68:168, Feb. 13, 1942.

Landis, Eugene M.; and Barger, A. Clifford: Experimental cardiac failure in dogs; effects of exhausting exercise. Trans. Ass. Amer. Physicians 65:64-74, 1952. (Boston)

----, Brown, E.; Fauteux, M.; and Wise, C.: Central venous pressure in relation to cardiac "competence", blood volume and exercise. J. Clin. Invest. 25:237-255, Mar., 1946. (Boston)

Láng, S.: A munka elötti vörös vérsejtszaporodás feltételes reflexe. (Conditioned reflex of increased erythrocytes before exertion) (Hun). Kiserl. Orvostud. 15:375-380, Aug., 1963.

Lange, Andersen K.   see Andersen, K. Lange

Langlois, J.-P.: Second souffle des coureurs. Médecine 2:915-917, Sept., 1921.

Larmi, Teuro K. I.: Regulation of tidal air in relation to ventilatory equivalent and oxygen removal
    in pulmonary insufficiency during exercise. Ann. Med. Exp. Fenn. 32:240-247, 1954.
    (Helsinki)

----: Spirometric and gas analytic studies in pulmonary insufficiency at rest and during graduated
    exercise. Scand. J. Clin. Lab. Invest. (suppl. 12) 6:1-144, 1954. (Helsinki)

Larrabee, Martin G.; Klingman, Jack D.; and Leicht, William S.: Effects of temperature, calcium
    and activity on phospholipid metabolism in a sympathetic ganglion. J. Neurochem. 10:549-570,
    Aug., 1963. (Baltimore)

Larrabee, R. C.: The effects of exercise on the heart and circulation. Boston Med. & Surg. J. 147:
    318-323; 328-330, Sept. 18, 1902. (Boston)

Larsson, Yngve; Persson, Bengt; Sterky, Göran; and Thoren, Claes: Effect of exercise on blood-lipids
    in juvenile diabetes. Lancet 1:350-355, Feb. 15, 1964.

----, ----, ----, and ----: Functional adaptation to vigorous training and exercise in diabetic and
    non-diabetic adolescents. J. Appl. Physiol. 19:629-635, July, 1964. (Stockholm)

Lashof, Joyce Cohen; Bondy, Philip K.; Sterling, Kenneth; and Man, Evelyn B.: Effect of muscular
    exercise on circulatory thyroid hormone. Proc. Soc. Exp. Biol. Med. 86:233-235, June, 1954.
    (New Haven, Conn.)

Lasser, Richard P.; and Amram, Salomao, S.: Distensibility of the pulmonary arterial vessels at rest
    and during exercise in patients with mitral stenosis. Amer. Heart J. 51:749-760, May, 1956.
    (New York)

Laudonnière-Augry, Marc Jules: Sur l'exercice, et son influence sur l'économie animale. Paris,
    Thèse numéro 106, vol. 147, 1819.

Laulanié, F.: De la marche du quotient respiratoire en fonction du travail musculaire et du repos
    consécutif. Arch. Physiol. Norm. Path. 5e série 8:572-586, 1896.

Laval, E.: De l'influence des exercices physiques sur l'excretion de l'acide urique. Rev. Méd. 16:
    384-392, 1896.

Laville, A.; Bouisset, S.; and Monod, H.: Etude d'un travail musculaire léger. II. Zone de moindre dépense
    énergétique (activité bimanuelle). Arch. Int. Physiol. 71:431-440, May, 1963.

Lavoisier, Antoine: Expérience sur la respiration des animaux, et sur les changements qui arrivent à
    l'air en passant par les poumons. Hist. Acad. Sci. pages 185-194, 1776. (Paris)

----, and Laplace, P. S. de: Mémoire sur la chaleur. Hist. Acad. Roy. Sci. 1780:355-408,
    (June 18, 1783) 1784.

----, and Seguin, Armand: Second mémoire sur la respiration des animaux. Ann. Chim. 91:318-334,
    1814. (Paris)

Lawaczeck, Heinz: Über den Mechanismus der Beeinflussung des Lactacidogengehalts von Froschmuskeln durch
    wechselnde Aussentemperatur. Hoppe-Seyler Zeits. physiol. Chem. 113:301-312, Apr. 5, 1921.
    (Frankfurt)

Lawrence, L. Theodore: Exercise and the heart. Delaware Med. J. 36:54-57, Mar., 1964.

Lawrie, R. A.: Effect of enforced exercise on myoglobin concentration in muscle. Nature 171: 1069-1070, June 13, 1953. (Cambridge, England)

Lazarev, N. V.; and Rusin, V. ia.: Novye materialy k kharakteristike sostoianiia nespetsificheski povyshennoĭ soprotivliamosti. (New data on the status of non-specific increased resistance) (Russ). Nerv. Sist. 4:149-152, 1963.

Lazzari, A.: Comportamento della frequenza cardiaca dopo sforzo in soggetti allenati e non allenati sottoposti alla prova dell'ipossia al 7 per cento. Gazz. Int. Med. Chir. 69:602-606, Mar. 31, 1964.

----: Comportamento della velocità di sedimentazione delle emazie in soggetti allenati e non allenati prima e dopo sforzo fisico. Gazz. Int. Med. Chir. 68:2887-2891, Dec. 31, 1963.

----: Durata della prova del massimo rendimento in soggetti allenati e non allenati sottoposti alla prova dell'ipossiema. Gazz. Int. Med. Chir. 69:179-184, Jan. 31, 1964.

----: Influenza dell'ATP sul reperto eritroleucocitario dopo sforzo in soggetti non allenati. Gazz. Int. Med. Chir. 69(Suppl.):3726-3731, Dec. 31, 1963.

----: Influenza della prova dell'ipossia sulla funzionalità renale di soggetti non allenati sottoposti alla prova del massimo rendimento. Gazz. Int. Med. Chir. 68:2883-2886, Dec. 31, 1963.

----: Il metabolismo intermedio nello sforzo fisico. II. Il metabolismo lipidico. Gazz. Int. Med. Chir. 69:1225-1229, July 15, 1964.

----: Le modificazioni del circolo cerebrale in seguite ad attività fisica. Gazz. Int. Med. Chir. 69:1340-1345, July 31, 1964.

----: Modificazioni del reperto eritroleucocitario in soggetti allenati a non allenati prima e dopo sforzo. Gazz. Int. Med. Chir. 68:2527-2531, Dec. 15, 1963.

----: Sui rapporti tra allenamento e metabolismo lipidico. I. Ricerche sperimentali in ratti sottoposti a dieta ipocolesterolemica carente in ac. pantotenico. Gazz. Int. Med. Chir. 69:1151-1154, June 30, 1964.

----: Il tempo di ripristino respiratorio in soggetti allenati previa somministrazione di ATP. Gazz. Int. Med. Chir. 69:674-678, Apr. 15, 1964.

----: Il tempo di ripristino della tensione arteriosa nella prova del massimo rendimento eseguita in ipossia. I. Ricerche eseguite in soggetti allenati. Gazz. Int. Med. Chir. 69:304-308, Feb. 15, 1964.

Leach, Robert E.; Zohn, David A. and Stryker, William S.: Anterior tibial compartment syndrome due to strenuous exercise. Milit. Med. 129:610-613, July, 1964. (San Diego and Washington)

----, ----, and ----: Anterior tibial compartment syndrome. Clinical and electromyographic aspects. Arch. Surg. 88:187-192, Feb., 1964. (San Diego)

Leake, Chauncey D.: Exercise and physiological aging. Geriatrics 19:227, Apr., 1964.

Lee, F. S.: Physical exercise from standpoint of physiology. Amer. Phys. Educat. Rev. 14:
216-223, 1910.

Lefebvre-des-Nottes, R.; and Girard, F.: La distribution dans les temps de la puissance développée
est-elle susceptible de modifier le rendement du travail musculaire? Comptes Rend. Soc. Biol. 151:
26-29, 1957.

Lefrançois, R.; and Dejours, P.: Etude des relations entre stimulus ventilatoire gaz carbonique et stimulus
ventilatoires neurogéniques de l'exercice musculaire chez l'homme. Rev. Franc. Etud. Clin.
Biol. 9:498-505, May, 1964.

Lehmann, G.: (Physiological bases of human work in high temperatures) (Fr). Concours Méd. 82:
2383-2388, May 7, 1960.

Lehmann, Gunther: Nochmals Aethyljodid und Schlagvolumen. Arbeitsphysiol. 1:595-599, June
28, 1929. (Dortmund)

----: Zur Bestimmung des Herzschlagvolumens mit Aethyljodid. Arbeitsphysiol. 1:114-129, May 21,
1928. (Berlin)

----, and Szakáll, L.: Weitere Untersuchungen über den Chlorumsatz bei Hitzearbeit. Arbeitsphysiol.
10:608-646, 1939. (Dortmund)

Lehmann, L.: Welchen Einfluss übt unter verschiedenen Verhältnissen die körperliche Bewegung, bis
zur ermüdenden Anstrengung gesteigert, auf den menschlichen Organismus, insonderheit auf den
Stoffwechsel aus? Arch. Ver. gemeinsch. Arb. Förd. Wissensch. Heilk. 4:484-520, 1860.

Lehoczky, T.; Halasy, M.; Simon, G.; Harmos, G.; et al: Myopathia glycogenica ikertestvérpárnál.
(Glycogenic myopathy in twins) (Hun). Ideggyogy Szemle 17:65-79, Mar., 1964.

----, ----, ----, and ----: Skeletal muscle glycogenosis in identical twins. Brit. Med. J. 2:802,
Sept. 26, 1964. (Budapest)

Leitão, J. A.; Lima, T.; Barreiros, M.; et al: Influência do exercício físico na fadiga intelectual.
(The influence of physical exercise on mental fatigue) (Por). J. Soc. Cienc. Med. Lisboa
127:651-730, Nov., 1963.

Lemarchands, H.: (The respiratory and circulatory adaptations of muscular exercise) (Fr). Gaz. Méd.
France 67:1093-1104, May 10, 1960.

Lepeschkin, E.; and Surawicz, B.: Characteristics of true-positive and false-positive results of
electrocardiographic Master two-step exercise tests. New Eng. J. Med. 258:511-520, Mar. 13,
1958. (Burlington, Vt.)

Leriche, R.: Le syndrome de la thrombose isolée de l'artère tibiale anterieure et son traitement.
Presse Méd. 58:1285, Nov. 18, 1950.

Leshkevich, L. G.: Vliianie myshechnoĭ deiatel'nosti i eksperimental'noĭ trenirovki na soderzhanie
i iodnoe chislo lipidor v tkaniakh krys. (Effect of muscular activity and experimental training
on the content of lipids and iodine level in rat tissues) (Uk). Ukr. Biokhim. Zh. 36:726-734,
1964.

Leusen, I. R.; (Blood circulation in muscular work) (Dut). Belg. T. Geneesk. 15:930-939, Sept. 1, 1959.

----: Chemosensitivity of the respiratory center. Influence of CO_2 in the cerebral ventricles on respiration. Amer. J. Physiol. 176:39-44, Jan. 1954. (Ghent)

----: Chemosensitivity of the respiratory center. Influence of changes in the H^+ and total buffer concentrations in the cerebral ventricles on respiration. Amer. J. Physiol. 176:45-51, Jan., 1954. (Ghent)

----: Influence du pH du liquide céphalorachidien sur la respiration. Experientia 6:272, July 15, 1950. (Ghent)

----, Demeester, G.; Bouckaert, J. J.: Chémo- et presso-récepteurs artériels et respiration au cours de l'exercice musculaire. Acta Physiol. Pharmacol. Neerl. 6:43-52, Oct., 1957.

----, ----, and ----: Influence du travail musculaire sur la circulation et la respiration chez le chien. Acta Cardiol. 13:153-172, 1958.

----, ----, and ----: Presso-récepteurs artériels et débit cardiaque au cours de l'exercice musculaire. Arch. Int. Physiol. 64:564-570, Nov., 1956.

----, and Lacroix, E.: Cardiac output during muscular exercise, role of the arterial pressoreceptors. Arch. Int. Pharmacodyn. 130:470-472, Mar. 1, 1961. (Ghent)

----, ----, and Demeester, G.: L'équilibre acide-base dans le sang et le liquide céphalo-rachidien pendant l'exercice musculaire. J. Physiologie 52:151-152, Jan.-Feb., 1960. (Ghent)

Levenson, Robert M.: Exercise tolerance of cardiac patients. Northwest Med. 55:288-290, Mar., 1956. (Seattle)

Levine, Herbert J.; Messer, Joseph V.; Neill, William A.; and Gorlin, Richard: The effect of exercise on cardiac performance in human subjects with congestive heart failure. Amer. Heart J. 66: 731-740, Dec., 1963. (Boston)

----, Neill, William A.; Wagman, Richard J.; Krasnow, Norman; and Gorlin, Richard: The effect of exercise on mean left ventricular ejection rate in man. J. Clin. Invest. 41:1050-1058, May, 1962. (Boston)

Levy, Arthur M.; Tabakin, Burton S.; and Hanson, John S.: Cardiac output in normal men during steady-state exercise utilizing dye-dilution technique. Brit. Heart J. 23:425-432, July, 1961. (Burlington, Vt.)

Lewalski, B.: Ocena wysilku fizycanego dokerów zatrudnionych przy malo zmechanizowanej pracy przeladunkowej. (Evaluation of the physical effort of longshoremen employed in a loading operation with minimum mechanization) (Pol). Bull. Inst. Mar. Med. Gdansk 14:191-197, 1963.

----: Poziom uropepsyny w moczu dokerów ciężko przy pracach malo zmechanizowanych. (The urinary uropepsin level in longshoremen under a heavy work load in areas with minimum mechanization) (Pol). Bull. Inst. Mar. Med. Gdansk 14:199-208, 1963.

Lewis, Benjamin M.; Lin, Tai-Hon; Noe, Frances E.; and Komisaruk, Richard: The measurement of pulmonary capillary blood volume and pulmonary membrane diffusing capacity in normal subjects; the effects of exercise and position. J. Clin. Invest. 37:1061-1070, July, 1958. (Detroit)

Lewis, Benjamin M.; and Morton, James W.: Effects of inhalation of CO_2, muscular exercise and epinephrine on maximal breathing capacity. J. Appl. Physiol. 7:309-312, Nov., 1954. (Philadelphia)

Lewis, C. M.: Studies in exercise tolerance as an aid to cardiological diagnosis and assessment. S. Afr. Med. J. 38:2-9, Jan. 4, 1964.

Lewis, John M.; Montero, Alfredo C.; Kinard, Sama, Jr.; Dennis, Edward W.; and Alexander, James K.: Hemodynamic response to exercise in isolated pulmonic stenosis. Circulation 29: 854-861, June, 1964. (Houston)

Lewis, Lena A.; Page, Irvine H.; and Brown, Helen B.: Effect of exercise on serum and hepatic lipids in rats fed high fat diets. Amer. J. Physiol. 201:4-8, July, 1961. (Cleveland)

Lewis, Sir Thomas: The soldier's heart and the effort syndrome. New York, P. B. Hoeber, 1919.

Liddell, F. D. K.: Estimation of energy expenditure from expired air. J. Appl. Physiol. 18: 25-29, Jan., 1963. (London)

Light, Arthur B.; and Warren, Clark R.: Urea clearance and proteinuria during exercise. Amer. J. Physiol. 117:658-661, Dec., 1936. (Lawrenceville, N. J.)

Lilienthal, J. L., Jr.; Railey, R. L.; and Proemmel, D. D.: Arterial oxyhemoglobin saturations at critical pressure-altitudes breathing various mixtures of oxygen and nitrogen: with a note on the effect of exercise. Amer. J. Physiol. 145:427-431, Jan., 1946. (Pensacola)

----, ----, ----, and Franke, R. E.: An experimental analysis in man of oxygen pressure gradient from alveolar air to arterial blood during rest and exercise at sea level and at altitude. Amer. J. Physiol. 147:199-216, Sept., 1946. (Pensacola)

Liljestrand, Åke: Respiratory reactions elicited from medulla oblongata of the cat. Acta Physiol. Scand. 29(Suppl. 106):321-393, 1953. (Stockholm)

Liljestrand, S. H.; and Wilson, D. Wright: The excretion of lactic acid in the urine after muscular exercise. J. Biol. Chem. 65:773-782, Oct., 1925. (Philadelphia)

----, and ----: The excretion of lactic acid in the urine after muscular exercise. Proc. Soc. Exp. Biol. Med. 21:426, May, 1924. (Philadelphia)

Lind, A. R.: A physiological criterion for setting thermal environmental limits for everyday work. J. Appl. Physiol. 18:51-56, Jan., 1963. (Oxford)

----: Physiological effects of continuous or intermittent work in the heat. J. Appl. Physiol. 18: 57-60, Jan., 1963. (Natick)

----: Practical assessment of intolerably hot conditions. Fed. Proc. 22:89-92, May-June, 1963. (Oxford)

----, and Bass, David E.: Optimal exposure time for development of acclimatization to heat. Fed. Proc. 22:704-708, May-June, 1963. (Natick)

Lindahl, Wallace W.; and Fatter, Mervin E.: March hemoglobinuria; a report of two cases. J. Urol. 53:805-807, June, 1945.

Linde, Leonard M.: An appraisal of exercise fitness tests. Pediatrics 32(Suppl.):656-659, Oct., 1963. (Los Angeles)

Lindell, S. E.; Svanborg, A.; Söderholm, B.; and Westling, H.: Haemodynamic changes in chronic constrictive pericarditis during exercise and histamine infusion. Brit. Heart J. 25:35-41, Jan., 1963. (Göteborg)

Lindhard, J.: Effect of posture on the output of the heart. Skand. Arch. Physiol. 30:395-408, 1913. (Copenhagen)

----: Über das minutenvolum des Herzens bei Ruhe und bei Muskelarbeit. Pflüger Arch. ges. Physiol. 161:233-383, June 1, 1915. (Copenhagen)

----: Über die Erregbarkeit des Atemzentrums bei Muskelarbeit. Arbeitsphysiol. 7:72-82, 1934.

Lipková, V.; and Rolný, D.: Spirometrické vyšetrenie ako podklad pre hodnotenic vplyva vyrobnej práce na organizmus chlapcov a dievčat. (Spirometric examinations as a basis of evaluating the influence of physical work on the organism of boys and girls) (Cz). Cesk. Hyg. 8:225-231, May, 1963.

Lipovetz, F. J.: Applied physiology of exercise. Minneapolis, Burgess Publishing Co., 1938.

Liska, S.; Hubač, M.; and Hajzoková, M.: Vplyv práce v hroúcom prostredí na aktivity krvných cholinesteráz. (Effect of work in a hot environment on blood cholinesterase activity) (Cz). Prac. Lek. 15:291-293, Sept., 1963.

Little, G. M.: The ventilatory cost of certain activities performed by patients. Tubercle 37:25-31, Jan.-Feb., 1956. (Godalming)

Litwak, Robert S.; Samet, Philip; Bernstein, William H.; Turkewitz, H.; and Lesser, Milton E.: The effect of exercise upon the mean diastolic left atrial - left ventricular gradient in mitral stenosis. J. Thorac. Surg. 34:449-468, Oct., 1957. (Miami)

Livingstone, Ronald A.: Blood flow in the calf of the leg after running. Amer. Heart J. 61:219-224, Feb., 1961. (Belfast)

Lloyd, Brian B.; Jukes, M. G. M., and Cunningham, John G. C.: The relation between alveolar oxygen pressure and the respiratory response to carbon dioxide in man. Quart. J. Exp. Physiol. 43:214-227, Apr., 1958. (Oxford)

Lloyd-Thomas, H. G.: The effect of exercise on the electrocardiogram in healthy subjects. Brit. Heart J. 23:260-270, May, 1961. (London)

Lob, M.; Miéville, C.; and Jéquier-Doge E.: Le contrôle continu de la saturation en oxygène du sang artériel (oxymétrie) pendant la spirométrie au repos et à l'effort. Helv. Med. Acta 17: 511-515, Oct., 1950. (Lausanne)

Lobyntsev, K. S.: O perestroike somaticheskoi myshechnoi tkani pod vliianiem reguliarnykh fizicheskikh nagruzok. (On the reconstruction of somatic muscle tissue under the influence of regular physical loads) (Russ). Arkh. Anat. 45:44-50, Oct., 1963.

Lochner, W.; and Nasseri, M.: Über den venösen Sauerstoffdruck, die Einstellung der Coronardurchblutung und den Kohlenhydratstoffwechsel des Herzens bei Muskelarbeit. Pflüger Arch. ges. Physiol. 269:407-416, Oct. 29, 1959. (Göttingen)

Loeschcke, Hans H.: Beziehung zwischen CO_2 und Atmung. Anaesthesist 9:38-46, Feb., 1960.

----: Homoiostase des arteriellen CO_2-Drucks und Anpassung der Lungenventilation an den Stoffwechsel als Leistung eines Regelsystems. Klin. Wschr. 38:366-376, Apr. 15, 1960. (Gottingen)

----, Koepchen, H. P.; and Gertz, K. H.: Über den Einfluss von Wasserstoffionenkonzentration und CO_2-Druck im Liquor cerebrospinalis auf die Atmung. Pflüger Arch. ges. Physiol. 266:569-585, May 14, 1958. (Göttingen)

----, Mitchell, R. A.; Katsaros, B.; Perkins, J. F.; and Konig, A.: Interaction of intracranial chemosensitivity with peripheral afferents to the respiratory centers. Ann. N. Y. Acad. Sci. 109:651-660, June 24, 1963. (San Francisco)

Loewy, A.; and Lewandowsky, M.: Untersuchungen über die Blutzirkulation gesunder und herzleidender Menschen bei Ruhe und Muskelarbeit. Zeits. ges. exp. Med. 5:321-348, 1917.

----, and Schrötter, H. von: Untersuchungen über die Blutcirculation beim Menschen. Zeits. exp. Path. Ther. 1:197-310, 1905.

Lofgren, Karl A.: Measurement of ambulatory venous pressure in the lower extremity. Surg. Forum 5: 163-168, (1954) 1955. (Rochester, Minn.)

Lofstedt, B.; and Wilson, O.: Försök över köldacklimatisering och fysisk träning på Hardangervidda 1963. (Study on cold acclimatization and physical training at Hardangervidda in 1963) (Sw). Nord. ·Hyg. T. 45:14-16, 1964.

Lokatkin, M. N.: Nekotorye osobennosti utilizatsii endogennogo zhira pri chastichnom golodanii i fizicheshoi nagryzke. (Some features of the utilization of endogenous fat during partial fasting and physical stress) (Russ). Vop. Pitan. 22:27-34, Sept.-Oct., 1963.

----: Utilization of endogenous fat in partial starvation and physical exertion. Fed. Proc. (Trans. Suppl.) 23:945-948, Sept.-Oct., 1964.

Loll, H.; and Hilscher, A.: Änderung der Substratkonzentration und der Enzymaktivität im Serum durch körperliche Belastung. Aerztl. Forsch. 12:85-86, Oct. 10, 1958.

Lombardo, Thomas A.; Rose, Leonard; Taeschler, Max; Tully, S.; and Bing, R. J.: The effect of exercise on coronary blood flow, myocardial oxygen consumption and cardiac efficiency in man. Circulation 7:71-78, Jan., 1953. (Birmingham, Ala., Baltimore, and Perry Poing)

Londe, Charles: De l'influence de l'exercice sur nos organes, et sur leurs fonctions dans l'état de santé. Paris, Thèse numéro 55, vol. 145, 1819.

Long, C. N. H.: The lactic acid in the blood of a resting man. J. Physiol. 58:455-460, May 23, 1924. (London)

----: Muscular exercise, lactic acid and the supply and utilization of oxygen. Part XIV. The relation in man between the oxygen intake during exercise and the lactic acid content of the muscle. Proc. Roy. Soc. 99B:167-172, Jan. 1, 1926.

Long, C. N. H.; and Grant, Rhoda: The recovery process after exercise in the mammal. I. Glycogen resynthesis in the fasted rat. J. Biol. Chem. 89:553-565, Dec., 1930. (Montreal)

----, and Lupton, H.: The removal of lactic acid during recovery from muscular exercise in man. J. Physiol. 57:lxvii-lxviii, May 19, 1923.

----, ----, and Hill, Archibald Vivian: The effect of fatigue on the relation between work and speed, in the contraction of human arm muscles. J. Physiol. 58:334-337, Mar. 14, 1924. (London)

Loosen, H.; Heinen, W.; and Creischer, M.: Blutgerinnung bei Belastung und peripherer Stauung als Beitrag zum Trainingsproblem. Zeits. ges. inn. Med. 7:520-523, June 1, 1952.

Lorentzen, F. Vogt: Lactic acid in blood after various combinations of exercise and hypoxia. J. Appl. Physiol. 17:661-664, July, 1962. (Oslo)

----: Non-esterified fatty acids in venous blood under different experimental conditions. Aerospace Med. 35:649-652, July, 1964.

Lorin, Alphonse: Sur l'influence de l'exercise sur l'économie animale dans l'état de santé et de maladie. Paris, Thèse numéro 160, vol. 158, 1820.

Lott, Bernice E.: Secondary reinforcement and effort: comment on Aronson's "The Effect of Effort on the Attractiveness of Rewarded and Unrewarded Stimuli". J. Abnorm. Soc. Psychol. 67: 520-522, Nov., 1963.

Loutsides, E.; Spanolios, G.; and Galankes, P.: (Comparative clinical, electrocardiographic, and biochemical observations of athletes before and after intensive exertion) (Fr). Rev. Méd. Moyen Orient 19:433-437, May-June, 1962.

Love, A. H. G.: The rate of blood flow and the oxygen saturation of the effluent blood following contraction of the muscles of the human forearm. Clin. Sci. 14:275-283, May, 1955.

Lowbury, E. J. L.; and Blakely, A. P. L.: Exertion haemoglobinuria: report of a case. Brit. Med. J. 1:12-13, Jan. 3, 1948.

Lowe, Harry, J.: Ventilation and acid-base balance. Bull. Millard Fillmore Hosp. 10:11-12, 1963. (Buffalo)

Lowenstein, Otto; and Loewenfeld, Irene E.: Disintegration of central autonomic regulation during fatigue and its reintegration by psychosensory controlling mechanisms. I. Disintegration. Pupillographic studies. J. Nerv. Ment. Dis. 115:1-21, Jan., 1952. (New York)

----, and ----: Disintegration of central autonomic regulation during fatigue and its reintegration by psychosensory controlling mechanisms. II. Reintegration. Pupillographic studies. J. Nerv. Ment. Dis. 115:121-145, Feb., 1952. (New York)

Lowenthal, Milton; Harpuder, Karl; and Blatt, Stanley D.: Peripheral and visceral vascular effects of exercise and postprandial state in supine position. J. Appl. Physiol. 4:689-694, Feb., 1952. (New York)

----, Tobis, Jerome S.; and Harpuder, Karl: Cardiovascular effects of exercise in the normal and cardiac. Brit. J. Phys. Med. 17:13-15, Jan., 1954. (New York)

Lowsley, Oswald S.: The effects of various forms of exercise on systolic, diastolic, and pulse pressures and pulse rate. Amer. J. Physiol. 27:446-466, Mar. 1, 1911. (Baltimore)

Lozada, B.; and Tempone, N. D.: Au sujet de l'électrocardiographie dans l'exercice. Acta Cardiol. 13:464-485, 1958.

Lubanska-Tomaszewska, L.: Wptyw treningu fizycznego na zawartość kwasów rybonukleinowych w narzadach o różnym metabliźmie biatkowym. (Effect of physical training on the content of ribonucleic acid in various organs with different forms of protein metabolism) (Pol). Acta Physiol. Pol. 15:819-829, Nov.-Dec., 1964.

Luck, James Murray; Thacker, Gilbert; and Marrack, John: Ammonia in the blood of epileptics. Brit. J. Exp. Path. 6:276-279, Dec., 1925. (London)

Lüthy, E.; Jeker, K.; and Stucky, P.: Kreislaufuntersuchungen bei Hyperventilation. Cardiologia 30: 139-144, 1957. (Bern)

Lukash, W. M.; and Frank, P. F.: The effects of physical activity and site on injection on penicillinemia following administration of 1.2 million units of benzathine penicillin G. Amer. J. Med. Sci. 246: 429-438, Oct. 1963. (Great Lakes, Ill.)

Lukiański, M.; Góralczyk, J.; and Jaroslawski, M.: Pomiary ciśnień krwi w sercu prawym a wyniki badan spirometrycynych. (Blood pressure measurement in the right heart and results of spirometric studies) (Pol). Gruzlica 31:907-912, Aug., 1963.

Lukin, L.: Instability of the "steady state" during exercise. Int. Zeits. angew. Physiol. 20:45-49, 1963.

----, and Ralston, H. J.: Oxygen deficit and repayment in exercise. Int. Zeits. angew. Physiol. 19: 183-193, 1962.

Lumia, V.; and Giamieri, D.: (Physical activity and blood cholesterol) (Ital). Gior. Geront. 8:615-618, Aug., 1960.

Lundberg, U.; and Gramvall, S.: Variations in pulse rate at a cycle ergometer test on Swedish Air Force pilots. Medd. Flyg. Navalmed. Namnd. 12:4-5, 1963.

Lundgren, Nils P. V.: The physiological effects of time schedule work on lumber-workers. Acta Physiol. Scand. 13(Suppl. 41):1-137, 1946. (Stockholm)

Lundin, Gunnar; and Strom, Gunnar: The concentration of blood lactic acid in man during muscular work in relation to the partial pressure of oxygen of the inspired air. Acta Physiol. Scand. 13: 253-266, Apr. 25, 1947. (Lund and Copenhagen)

Lundsgaard, Christen: Studies of oxygen in the venous blood. V. Determinations on patients with anemia. J. Exp. Med. 30:147-158, Aug. 1, 1919. (Copenhagen)

----: Untersuchungen über das Minutenvolumen des Herzens bei Menschen. III. Messungen an zwei Patienten mit totalem Herzblock. Deutsch. Arch. klin. Med. 120:481-496, Oct. 10, 1916. (Copenhagen)

----, and Moller, Eggert: Investigations on the immediate effect of heavy exercise (stair-running) on some phases of circulation and respiration in normal individuals. I. Oxygen and carbon dioxide content of blood drawn from the cubital vein before and after exercise. J. Biol. Chem. 55: 315-321, Feb., 1923. (Copenhagen)

Lundsgaard, Christen; and Moller, Eggert: Investigations on the immediate effect of heavy exercise (stair-running) on some phases of circulation and respiration in normal individuals. II. Oxygen and carbon dioxide content of blood drawn from a cubital vein at different intervals after exercise. J. Biol. Chem. 55:477-485, Mar., 1923. (Copenhagen)

----, and ----: Investigations on the immediate effect of heavy exercise (stair-running) on some phases of circulation and respiration in normal individuals. III. Effect of varying the amount and kind of exercise. J. Biol. Chem. 55:599-603, Apr., 1923. (Copenhagen)

Luongo, Edward P.: Work physiology in health and disease. J.A.M.A. 188:27-32, Apr. 6, 1964.

Lupton, Hartley: An analysis of the effects of speed on the mechanical efficiency of human muscular movement. With an appendix by A. V. Hill. J. Physiol. 57:337-353, Aug. 16, 1923. (Manchester)

----: The relation between the external work produced and the time occupied in a single muscular contraction in man. J. Physiol. 57:68-75, Dec. 22, 1922. (Manchester)

Lurie, Paul R.: Conversion of treadmill to cycle ergometer. J. Appl. Physiol. 19:152-153, Jan., 1964. (Indianapolis)

Lusk, Graham: The fundamental requirements of energy for proper nutrition. J.A.M.A. 70:821-824, Mar. 23, 1918. (New York)

Lyding, Georg: Untersuchungen über den Lactacidogenphosphorsäure- und Restphosphorsäuregehalt von Hühner- und Taubenmuskeln. Hoppe-Seyler Zeits. physiol. Chem. 113:223-244, Apr. 5, 1921. (Franfurt)

Lythgoe, R. J.; and Pereira, J. R.: Muscular exercise, lactic acid and the supply and utilization of oxygen. Part XI. Pulse rate and oxygen intake during the early stages of recovery from severe exercise. Proc. Roy. Soc., 98B:468-479, Oct. 1, 1925.

McAllister, Ferdinand F.; Bertsch, Robert; Jacobson, Julius, II; and D'Alessio, Gerald: The accelerating effect of muscular exercise on experimental atherosclerosis. Arch. Surg. 80: 54-60, Jan., 1960. (New York)

McArdle, B.; and Verel, D.: Responses to ischaemic work in the human forearm. Clin. Sci. 15: 305-318, May, 1956. (London)

MacCagno, A. L.; and Pellegrino, R.: Variazioni delgi elementi del sangue dopo sforzo e valutazione della funzionalità respiratoria. Lotta Tuberc. 24:930-938, Oct.-Nov., 1954.

Macchi, V.; and Corti, M.: (Muscular work and pathogenesis of congestive heart failure) (It). Minerva Med. 50:4127-4133, Dec. 15, 1959.

McCloy, C. H.: Venous pressure after exercise. Phys. Training 14:300-309, May, 1917. (Shanghai)

McConahay, T. P.; Robinson, S.; and Newton, J. L.: d-Aldosterone and sweat electrolytes. J. Appl. Physiol. 19:575-579, July, 1964. (Bloomington)

McCrea, F. D.; Eyster, J. A. E.; and Meek, W. J.: The effect of exercise upon diastolic heart size. Amer. J. Physiol. 83:678-689, Jan., 1928. (Madison)

McCurdy, J. H.: Physiology of exercise. Philadelphia, Lea and Febiger, 1924.

----: Physiology of exercise. Second edition. Philadelphia, Lea and Febiger, 1928.

McDonald, Ian: Statistical studies of recorded energy expenditure of man. Part II: Expenditure on walking related to weight, sex, age, height, speed and gradient. Nutr. Abstr. Rev. 31:739-762, July, 1961. (Aberdeen)

McDonald, Robert D.; Yagi, Kan; and Stockton, Eugene: Human-eosinophil response to acute physical exertion. Psychosom. Med. 23:63-66, Jan.-Feb., 1961. (Washington)

McDowall, R. J. A.: The function of the carotid sinus. Arch. Int. Pharmacodynam. 140:168-172, Nov. 1, 1962. (London)

----: The physiology of industrial hygiene: II. The physiologic effects of exercise and mental effort on the circulation, and their relation to industry. J. Industr. Hyg. 10:94-100, Mar., 1928. (London)

McGregor, Maurice; Adam, William; and Sekelj, Paul: Influence of posture on cardiac output and minute ventilation during exercise. Circ. Res. 9:1089-1092, Sept., 1961. (Montreal)

McIlroy, Malcolm B.: The respiratory response to exercise. Pediatrics 32(Suppl.):680-682, Oct., 1963. (San Francisco)

----, and Naimark, Arnold: Assessment of cardiovascular function. Biochem. Clin. 1:161-168, 1963. (San Francisco)

McKee, Wallace P.; and Bolinger, Robert E.: Caloric expenditure of normal and obese subjects during standard work test. J. Appl. Physiol. 15:197-200, Mar., 1960. (Kansas City, Kan.)

MacKenzie, Cosmo G.; and Riesen, Austin H.: The production by moderate exercise of a high incidence of bends at altitudes of 26,000 to 28,000 feet. J.A.M.A., 124:499-501, Feb. 19, 1944. (Greenville, S.C.)

McKenzie, R. Tait: The influence of exercise on the heart. Amer. J. Med. Sci. 145:69-74, Jan., 1913. (Philadelphia)

MacLaren, Archibald: Training in theory and practice, with appendix. London, Macmillan and Co., 1866.

McMichael, John; and Sharpey-Schafer, E. P.: Cardiac output in man by a direct Fick method. Effects of posture, venous pressure change, atropine, and adrenaline. Brit. Heart J. 6:33-40, Jan., 1944.

McMorris, Rex O.; and Elkins, Earl C.: A study of production and evaluation of muscular hypertrophy. Arch. Phys. Med. 35:420-426, July, 1954. (Columbus, Ohio and Rochester, Minn.)

McNelly, Walter C.: Some effects of training on the respiratory response to exercise. Amer. J. Physiol. 116:100-101, June, 1936.

MacPhail, J. M.: The effect of exercise on the circulation Brit. Med. J. 2:637-638, Oct. 30, 1915. (Edinburgh)

Maegraith, B. G.; Brown, G. M.; Rossiter, R. J.; Irvine, K. N.; Lees, J. C.; Parsons, D. S.; Partington, C. N.; Rennie, J. L.; and Havard, R. E.: The effect of muscular exercise in a hot moist invironment on the mepacrine concentrations of blood, plasma, and urine. Army Medical Research Unit, Oxford. Ann. Trop. Med. Parasit. 40:368-371, Dec., 1946. (Oxford)

Maestrini, D.: Sulla importanza dell'alterato ricambio organico (fatica), della struttura e dello stato colloidale della fibra, per la genesi delle cosi dette "contrazioni piccole insufficienti del cuore in scompenso" (casi clinici e sperimentali). Policlinico(Sez. prat.) 58:933-945, July 23, 1951.

Mager, M.; Iampietro, P. F.; and Goldman, Ralph F.: The effect of supplementary feeding on plasma free fatty acids during work. Metabolism 13:823-830, Sept., 1964. (Oklahoma City)

Maggio, M.; Stancari, V.; and Amorati, A.: Il test di Harward, lo LIP (Leistungs-Puls-Indez) di E. A. Mueller ed il massimo consumo di O_2 indiretto secondo Astrand in Giovani apprendisti (risultati preliminari). Rass. Med. Industr. 32:362-363, May-Aug., 1963.

Magnus, G.: Sur les gaz que contient le sang: oxygène, azote et acide carbonique. Ann. Chim. Phys. Série 2. 65:169-192, 1837.

Magri, G.; Dughera, L.; and Gamna, G.: Il fonocardiogramma da sforza nella volutazione del grado di stenosi mitralica. Minerva Med. 49:1258-1263, Apr. 4, 1958.

Mahomed, F. A.: The effect of prolonged muscular exertion on the circulatory system. Brit. Med. J. 1:359-361, Mar. 18, 1876. (London)

----: Observations on the circulation made on Mr. Weston during his late 500-mile walk. Lancet 1:432, Mar. 18, 1876. (London)

Mair, George B.: Frequency of micturition and albuminuria in service patients. Lancet 1:427-428, Apr. 3, 1943. (Aberdeen)

Maison, G. L.; Orth, O. S.; and Lemmer, K. E.: pH changes in rabbit and human striated muscles after contraction. Amer. J. Physiol. 121:311-324, Feb., 1938. (Madison)

Makin, Myer: A case of march haemoglobinuria. Brit. Med. J. 1:844, June 24, 1944.

Makinson, Donald H.: Changes in the ballistocardiogram after exercise in normal and abnormal subjects. Circulation 2:186-196, Aug., 1950. (Philadelphia)

Malhotra, M. S.; Ramaswamy, S. S.; and Ray, S. N.: Influence of body weight on energy expenditure. J. Appl. Physiol. 17:433-435, May, 1962. (Delhi)

----, Sen Gupta, J.; and Rai, R. M.: Pulse count as a measure of energy expenditure. J. Appl. Physiol. 18:994-996, Sept., 1963. (Delhi)

Malmcrona, Raoul: Haemodynamics in myocardial infarction. Acta Med. Scand. 176(Suppl. 417): 1-54, 1964. (Goteborg)

----, and Varnauskas, Ed: Haemodynamics during rest and exercise at the end of convalescence from myocardial infarction. Comparison with earlier and later stages of the disease. Acta Med. Scand. 175:19-30, Jan., 1964. (Goteborg)

Mandel, Morris J.; Robinson, Farrell R.; and Luce, Edward A.: SGOT levels in man and the monkey following physical and emotional exertion. Aerospace Med. 33:1216-1223, Oct., 1962. (Wright Air Force Base, Ohio)

Mangili, F.; Aghemo, P.; and Margaria, R.: Influence of high altitude on the pulse rate at work. Helv. Physiol. Pharmacol. Acta 22:66-69, 1964. (Milan)

Mankin, Harold T.; and Swan, H. J. C.: Arterial dilution curves of T-1824 during rest and exercise. Fed. Proc. 12:93, Mar., 1953. (Abstract) (Rochester, Minn.)

Mann, George V.: Diet, exercise, and coronary disease. Illinois Med. J. 116:20-21, July, 1959. (Nashville)

Mann, Richard H.; and Burchell, Howard B.: Premature ventricular contractions and exercise. Proc. Staff Meet. Mayo Clin. 27:383-389, Sept. 23, 1952. (Rochester, Minn.)

Mansfeld, G.: Die Ursache der motorischen Acceleration des Herzens. Pflüger Arch. ges. Physiol. 134:598-626, Oct. 8, 1910. (Budapest)

Marey: Modifications des mouvements respiratoires par l'exercice musculaire. Rev. Mil. Méd. Chir. 1:247-249, 1881.

Margaria, Rodolfo: Die Arbeitsfähigkeit des Menschen bei vermindertem Luftdruck. Arbeitsphysiol. 2:261-272, Oct. 21, 1929. (Turin)

----: Biochemistry of muscular contraction and recovery. J. Sport Med. 3:145-156, June-Sept., 1963. (Milan)

----: Cavagna, G. A.; and Saibene, F. P.: Possibilità di sfruttamento dell'elasticità del muscolo contratto durante l'esercizio muscolare. Boll. Soc. Ital. Biol. Sper. 39:1815-1817, Dec. 31, 1963. (Milan)

----, Cerretelli, P.; Aghemo, P.; and Sassi, G.: Energy cost of running. J. Appl. Physiol. 18: 367-370, Mar., 1963. (Milan)

Margaria, Rodolfo; Cerretelli, P.; and Chiumello, G.: (Effect of protracted muscular exercise on maximum oxygen consumption) (It). Boll. Soc. Ital. Biol. Sper. 37:1667-1669, Dec. 31, 1961. (Milan)

----, ----, DiPrampero, P. E.; Massari, C.; and Torelli, G.: Kinetics and mechanism of oxygen debt contraction in man. J. Appl. Physiol. 18:371-377, Mar., 1963. (Milan)

----, ----, and Mangili, F.: Balance and kinetics of anerobic energy release during strenuous exercise in man. J. Appl. Physiol. 19:623-628, July, 1964. (Milan)

----, ----, and ----: Le fonti energetiche nel lavoro muscolare strenuo di brevissima duranta. Boll. Soc. Ital. Biol. Sper. 39:1817-1819, Dec. 31, 1963. (Milan)

----, ----, Marchi, Spartaco; and Rossi, Luigi: Maximum exercise in oxygen. Int. Zeits. angew. Physiol. 18:465-467, 1961. (Milan)

----, Edwards, H. T.; and Dill, D. B.: The possible mechanisms of contracting and paying the oxygen debt and the role of lactic acid in muscular contraction. Amer. J. Physiol. 106:689-715, Dec., 1933. (Boston)

----, Milic-Emili, G.; Petit, J. M.; and Cavagna, G.: Mechanical work of breathing during muscular exercise. J. Appl. Physiol. 15:354-358, May, 1960. (Milan and Liege)

Marimpietri-Fabj, C.; Granata, A.; and Cricenti, F.: Alcuni dati sulla funzionalità ventilatoria prima e dopo attività lavoratira. Studio spirografico su un gruppo di saldatori e di sbavatori in un complesso metallurgico. Rass. Med. Industr. 32:584-592, Nov.-Dec., 1963.

Marino, A.: Physical stress and emetine cardiotoxicity. Experienta 17:116-117, Mar. 15, 1961. (Naples)

----, and Russo, E.: (Emetine cardiotoxicity and exertion) (It). Boll. Soc. Ital. Biol. Sper. 35:1244-1247, Oct. 15, 1959.

Maritz, J. S.; Morrison, J. F.; Peter, J.: Strydom, N. B.; and Wyndham, C. H.: A practical method of estimating an individual's maximal oxygen intake. Ergonomics 4:97-122, 1961.

Mark, Robert E.: Die Nachwirkung kurzdauernder schwerer körperlicher Arbeit. Arbeitsphysiol. 2:129-137, 1930. (Würzburg)

----, and Neumann, H.: Einfluss passiver Änderung der Körperlage auf Atmung und Pulsfrequenz beim Menschen. Zeits. ges. exp. Med. 80:150-163, 1931.

Marschak, M.: Die Blutverschiebungen beim Menschen bei hoher Umgebungstemperatur; das Minutenvolumen bei korperlicher Arbeit bei hoher Umgebungstemperatur. Zeits. ges. exp. Med. 77:133-143, 1931.

----: Eine Untersuchung uber den Gaswechsel und uber die Milchsaure und Alkalireserve im Blut bei statischer Arbeit. Arbeitsphysiol. 4:1-19, Feb. 18, 1931. (Moscow)

Marshall, Robert J.; and Shepherd, John T.: Effects of epinephrine on cardiovascular and metabolic responses to leg exercise in man. J. Appl. Physiol. 18:1118-1122, Nov., 1963. (Rochester, Minn.)

----, and ----: Exercise and the circulation. Circulation 27:323-327, Mar., 1963. (Rochester, Minn.)

----, and ----: Interpretation of changes in "central" blood volume and slope volume during exercise in man. J. Clin. Invest. 40:375-385, Feb., 1961. (Rochester, Minn.)

Martin, E. G.; Field, J., II; and Hall, V. E.: Tissue lactates and blood lactates as affected by muscular exercise. Proc. Soc. Exp. Biol. Med. 26:292-293, Jan., 1929. (Palo Alto)

----, and Gruber, C. M.: On the influence of muscular exercise on activity of bulbar centres. Amer. J. Physiol. 32:315-328, Oct., 1913. (Boston)

----, ----, and Lanham, T. H.: Body temperature and pulse rate after muscular exercise. Amer. J. Physiol. 35:211-223, 1914.

Martin, L.: Etude statistique de trois épreuves fonctionnelles d'aptitude à l'effort. Acta Belg. Arte Med. Pharm. Milit. 110:669-678, Dec., 1957.

Martin du Pan, R.: La glycémie pendant et après l'effort. Helv. Med. Acta 9:508-528, July, 1942. (Geneva)

Martynov, I. F.: (Evaluation of external respiratory function and blood circulation by means of physical exercise in patients with mitral stenosis in various stages of disease) (Russ). Ter. Arkh. 36:97-105, Mar., 1964.

Mascaretti, L.; and Morbelli, E.: Studio analitico delle curve di diluzione degli indicatori registrate durante lavori di intensita crecente nell'uomo sano. I. Le componenti temporali e di concentrazione. Folia Cardiol. 23:137-163, Mar.-Apr., 1964. (Milan)

----, ----, and Castelfranco, M.: (Adaptation of cardiac dynamics to work of increasing intensity) (It). Atti Soc. Ital. Cardiol. 22:325-326, 1962.

----, ----, and Regalia, F.: Gettata sistolica e frequenza cardiaca durante l'esercizio muscolare nell'individuo sano e in vari tipi di cardiopatie. Folia Cardiol. 23:491-506, Nov.-Dec., 1964. (Milan)

----, ----, and ----: Studio analitico delle curve di diluizione degli indicatori registrate durante lavori di intensità crescente nell'uomo sano. III. Rapporti tra le componenti di tempo, di concentrazione e di volume. Folia Cardiol. 23:395-422, Sept.-Oct., 1964. (Milan)

Mason, Gene W.: Medical and physiologic notes on mountain climbing. Anesth. Analg. 43:125-132, Mar.-Apr., 1964. (Everett, Wash.)

Mason, Robert E.: The Master test in patients with coronary artery disease and in normal subjects. Heart Bull. 8:67-69, July-Aug., 1959. (Baltimore)

Masoni, A.; Antonioli, G.; and Tomasi, A. M.: (The importance of effort in the development of myocardial infarct) (It). Arch. Pat. Clin. Med. 38:235-240, Dec., 1961

Massey, B. H.; and Chaudet, N. L.: Effects of systematic, heavy resistive exercise on range of joint movement in young male adults. Res. Quart. 27:41-51, Mar. 1956.

Master, Arthur M.: Effect of injury and effort on the normal and diseased heart. New York J. Med. 46:2634-2641, Dec. 1, 1946. (New York)

----: The electrocardiogram and "two-step" exercise: a test of cardiac function and coronary insufficiency. Amer. J. Med. Sci. 207:435-450, Apr., 1944.

----, Dack, Simon; and Jaffe, Harry L.: The relation of effort and trauma to acute coronary occlusion. Industr. Med. 9:359-364, July, 1940. (New York)

Master, Arthur M.; Dack, Simon; and Jaffe, Harry L.: Role of effort, trauma, work and occupation in onset and subsequent course of coronary artery occlusion. Med. Ann. D.C. 10:79-86, Mar., 1941. (New York)

----, Friedman, Rudolph; and Dack, Simon: The electrocardiogram after standard exercise as a functional test of the heart. Amer. Heart J. 24:777-793, Dec., 1942. (New York)

----, and Rosenfeld, I.: Monitored and post-exercise two-step test. Detection of silent coronary heart disease and differential diagnosis of chest pain. J.A.M.A. 190:494-500, Nov. 9, 1964. (New York)

----, ----, and Donoso, E.: The Master "2-step" exercise test. Bibl. Cardiol. (Suppl. to Cardiologia) No. 9:243-254, 1959. (New York)

Mateev; and Kiselkova, E.: Muskulnata aferentatsiia pri muskulna rabota i muskulna umora. (The afferent system of muscle in muscular work and muscular fatigue) (Bul). Izv. Inst. Fiziol. 6:19-33, 1963.

Matell, Georg: Time-courses of changes in ventilation and arterial gas tensions in man induced by moderate exercise. Acta Physiol. Scand. 58(Suppl. 206):1-53, 1963. (Stockholm)

Mathieu, Ésprit; and Urbain, V.: Des gaz du sang. Expériences physiologiques sur les circonstances qui en font varier la proportion dans le system artériel. Arch. Physiol. Norm. Pathol. 4:5-26, Jan.-Feb.; 190-203, March; 304-318, 447-469, May; 573-587, Sept.-Oct.; 710-731, Dec. 1872.

Matoush, LeRoy O.; Consolazio, C. Frank; Nelson, Richard A.; Isaac, Gerhard J.; and Torres, Juan B.: Effects of aspartic acid salts (Mg and K) on swimming performance of rats and dogs. J. Appl. Physiol. 19:262-264, Mar., 1964. (Denver)

Matsuoka, Kennosuke: Über die milchsäurebildung bei der chemischen Contractur des Muskels. Pflüger Arch. ges. Physiol. 204:51-71, 1924. (Kiel)

Matthes, K.; and Herberg, D.: (On the value of exercise test for the diagnosis of diffusion disorders) (Ger). Med. Thorac. 19:171-192, 1962.

Matthias, Eugen: Biologie der Leibesübungen. Leipzig, Quelle und Meyer, 1931.

Mauck, H. Page, Jr.; Shapiro, William; and Patterson, John L., Jr.: Pulmonary venous (wedge) pressure. Correlation with onset and disappearance of dyspnea in acute left ventricular heart failure. Amer. J. Cardiol. 13:301-309, Mar., 1964. (Richmond)

Maxfield, Mary E.: Use of heart rate for evaluating cardiac strain during training in women. J. Appl. Physiol. 19:1139-1144, Nov., 1964. (Wilmington)

----, and Brouha, Lucien: Validity of heart rate as an indicator of cardiac strain. J. Appl. Physiol. 18:1099-1104, Nov., 1963. (Wilmington)

May, P. R. A.: Pupillary abnormalities in schizophrenia and during muscular effort. J. Ment. Sci. 94:89-98, Jan., 1948. (Kent)

Mayer, Jean: Exercise and prevention of heart disease. Postgrad. Med. 34:601-604, Dec., 1963. (Boston)

----: Exercise and weight control. Postgrad. Med. 25:325-332, Feb., 1959. (Boston)

Mayer, Jean: Some aspects of obesity in children. Postgrad. Med. 34:83-88, July, 1963. (Boston)

----, Marshall, N. B.; Vitale, J. J.; Christensen, J. H.; Mashayekhi, M. B.; and Stare, F. J.: Exercise, food intake and body weight in normal rats and genetically obese adult mice. Amer. J. Physiol. 177:544-548, June, 1954. (Boston)

----, Zomzely, C.; and Stare, F. J.: Lack of effect of exercise on serum cholesterol levels in two types of experimental obesity. Experientia 13:250-251, June 15, 1957. (Boston)

Mazer, Milton; and Reisinger, John A.: An electrocardiographic study of cardiac aging based on records at rest and after exercise. Ann. Intern. Med. 21:645-652, Oct., 1944. (Washington)

Mazzella, G.: (Leukocytal peroxidases, oxidases and glycopolysaccharides after intense and prolonged muscular work) (It). Riv. Med. Aero. 23:117-122, Jan.-Mar., 1960.

Meakins, Jonathan; and Davies, H. Whitridge:. The influence of circulatory disturbances on the gaseous exchange in the blood. II. A method of estimating the circulation rate in man. Heart 9:191-198, Apr., 1922. (Edinburgh)

----, and ----: Observations on the gases in human arterial and venous blood. J. Path. Bact. 23:451-461, 1920. (Edinburgh)

----, and Gunson, E. B.: The pulse rate after a simple test exercise in cases of "irritable heart". Heart 6:285-292, May 20, 1917. (Hampstead)

Means, J. H.; and Newburgh, L. H.: The effect of caffeine upon the blood flow in normal human subjects. J. Pharmacol. Exp. Ther. 7:449-465, Nov., 1915. (Boston)

Mechelke, K.; and Nusser, E.: Über Blutdruck-und Pulsfrequenzänderungen während und nach körperlicher Arbeit bei Personen mit stabiler und labiler Blutdruckregelung. Deutsch. Arch. klin. Med. 202:599-633, Nov. 9, 1955. (Heidelberg)

Meek, Walter J.; and Eyster, J. A. E.: Cardiac size and output in man during rest and moderate exercise. Amer. J. Physiol. 63:400-401, Feb., 1922.

Meier, R.; and Meyerhof, Otto: Verbrennungswärme des Glycogens. Biochem. Zeits. 150:233-242, 1924.

Mellerowicz, H.; Meller, W.; and Mueller, J.: (Comparative research on increased work by interval training and continuous training (in connection with training work)) (Ger). Int. Zeits. angew. Physiol. 18:376-385, Apr., 1961.

Mellinkoff, Sherman M.; and Machella, Thomas E.: Effect of exercise upon liver following partial hepatectomy in albino rats. Proc. Soc. Exper. Biol. Med. 74:484-486, July, 1950. (Philadelphia)

Melville, Charles Henderson: Physiological effects of exercise. J. Roy. San. Inst. 38:373-381, 1912.

Mendelson, Myer: Deviant patterns of feeding behavior in man. Fed. Proc. 23:69-72, Jan.-Feb., 1964. (Philadelphia)

Mendez, Christobal: Book of bodily exercise (1553). Translated by F. Guerra. New Haven, Elizabeth Licht, 1960.

Menges, J.: (Thrombosis of effort) (Dut). Nederl. Milit. Geneesk. T. 16:37-44, Feb., 1963.

Mercier, J. N.: (The electrocardiogram after exertion. Indications and results) (Fr). Cah. Med. Interprof. 3:24-28, July, 1963.

Merklen, L.: Exercice musculaire et rythme du coeur. Paris Méd. 63:22-26, July 2, 1927.

Merrill, Arthur J.; and Cargill, Walter H.: The effect of exercise on the renal plasma flow and filtration rate of normal and cardiac subjects. J. Clin. Invest. 27:272-277, Mar., 1948. (Atlanta)

Merrill, J. P.; and Schupak, E.: Mechanisms of hypertension in renoprival man. Canad. Med. Ass. J. 90:328-332, Jan. 25, 1964. (Boston)

Merrill, Joseph M.; Callaway, James J.; and Blake, Thomas, M.: Concentration of hemoglobin in man during rest and exercise; relation to calculation of saturation of oxygen. Amer. J. Clin. Path. 30:209-210, Sept., 1958. (Nashville)

Merton, P. A.: Problems of muscular fatigue. Brit. Med. Bull. 12:219-221, Sept., 1956. (London)

----, and Pampiglione, G.: Strength and fatigue. Nature 166:527, Sept. 23, 1950. (London)

Messer, Joseph V.; Levine, Herbert J.; Wagman, Richard J.; and Gorlin, Richard: Effect of exercise on cardiac performance in human subjects with coronary artery disease. Circulation 28:404-414, Sept., 1963. (Boston)

----, Wagman, Richard J.; Levine, Herbert J.; Neill, William A.; Krasnow, Norman; and Gorlin, Richard: Patterns of human myocardial oxygen extraction during rest and exercise. J. Clin. Invest. 41:725-742, Apr., 1962. (Boston)

Metheny, Eleanor; Brouha, L.; Johnson, R. E.; and Forbes, W. H.: Some physiologic responses of women and men to moderate and strenuous exercise; a comparative study. Amer. J. Physiol. 137:318-326, Sept., 1942. (Boston)

Mettenleiter, M.: Untersuchungen über den Gaswechsel des tätigen Muskels beim Menschen. Deutsch. Arch. klin. Med. 117:517-539, July 20, 1915. (Munich)

Metz, B.; Sigwalt, D.; and Schaff, G.: Effets du travail et de la chaleur sur le rythme nycthéméral de la fréquence cardiaque chez l'homme normal. Comptes Rend. Soc. Biol. 152:526-529, Sept., 1958. (Strasbourg)

Meyer, Fritz: Über die vermehrte Produktion spezifischdynamischer Wärme im Anschluss an muskuläre Höchstleistungen. (Nach Versuchen am Hunde.) Arbeitsphysiol. 2:372-386, 1930. (Dortmund)

Meyer, M. H.; and Pella, G.: Effect of hard laboratory exercise on total and differential leukocyte count of young women. Res. Quart. 18:271-278, Dec., 1947.

Meyer, Nathaniel: The role of pyruvic acid in fatigue. New York J. Med. 45:1450-1451, July 1, 1945. (New York)

Meyerhof, Otto: Die Energieumwandlungen im Muskel. I. Über die Bezlehungen der Milchsäure zur Wärmebildung und Arbeitsleistung des Muskels in der Anaerobiose. Pflüger Arch. ges. Physiol. 182: 232-283, 1920. (Kiel)

----: Über die Energieumwandlungen im Muskeln. II. Das Schicksal der Milchsäure in der Erholungsperiode des Muskels. Pflüger Arch. ges. Physiol. 182:284-317, 1920. (Kiel)

----: Die Energieumwandlungen im Muskel. III. Kohlenhydrat und Milchsaureumsatz im Froschmuskel. Pflüger Arch. ges. Physiol. 185:11-32, 1920. (Kiel)

----: Die Energieumwandlungen im Muskel. IV. Mitteilung. Uber die Milchsaurebildung in der zerschnittenen Muskulatur. Pflüger Arch. ges. Physiol. 188:114-160, 1921. (Kiel)

----: Die Energieumwandlungen im Muskel. V. Mitteilung. Milchsäurebildung und mechanische Arbeit. Pflüger Arch. ges. Physiol. 191:128-183, 1921. (Kiel)

----: Die Energieumwandlungen im Muskel. VI. Mitteilung. Über den Ursprung der Kontraktionswarme. Pflüger Arch. ges. Physiol. 195:22-74, 1922. (Kiel)

----: Die Energieumwandlungen im Muskel. VII. Mitteilung. Weitere Untersuchungen über den Ursprung der Kontraktionswärme. Pflüger Arch. ges. Physiol. 204:295-331, 1924. (Kiel)

----: Über die Atmung der Froschmuskulatur. Pflüger Arch. ges. Physiol. 175:20-87, 1919. (Kiel)

----: Die Verbrennungswärme der Milchsäure. Biochem. Zeits. 129:594-604, 1922. (Kiel)

----: Zur Verbrennung der Milchsäure in der Erholungsperiode des Muskels. Pflüger Arch. ges. Physiol. 175:88-93, 1919. (Kiel)

----, and Meier, Rolf: Über den Milchsäurestoffwechsel im lebenden Tier. Pflüger Arch. ges. Physiol. 204:448-466, 1924. (Kiel)

Meylan, George L.: Effects of muscular exercise on heart. J. Med. Soc. New Jersey 2:332-335, May, 1906. (New York)

Mezey, A. G.; and Coppen, A. J.: Respiratory adaptation to exercise in anxious patients. Clin. Sci. 20:171-175, Apr., 1961. (London)

Michael, Ernest D., Jr.: Cardiovascular responses to training for underwater swimming. J. Sport Med. 3:218-220, Dec., 1963.

----, and Cureton, T. K.: Effects of physical training on cardiac output at ground level and at 15,000 feet simulated altitude. Res. Quart. 24:446-452, Dec., 1953.

----, Hutton, Kenneth E.; and Horvath, Steven M.: Cardiorespiratory responses during prolonged exercise. J. Appl. Physiol. 16:997-1000, Nov., 1961. (Philadelphia)

----, Thornton, R.; Rohter, F. D.; et al: Cardiovascular responses to breathholding while exercising. J. Sport Med. 4:28-31, Mar., 1964.

----, and Wolffe, Joseph B.: Comparison of step test and hand cranking test to indicate exercise tolerance of cardiovascular patients. Arch. Phys. Med. 44:327-331, June, 1963. (Santa Barbara, Calif. and Fairview Village, Pa.)

Michali, A. de: Contribution a l'étude de la fonction cardiorespiratoire au cours de l'exercice musculaire et de la phase de récupération chez les sujets normaux. Rev. Franc. Etud. Clin. Biol. 2:251-261, Mar., 1957.

Mies, H.; and Jovy, D.: Vegetatives System und körperliche Belastbarkeit Jugendlicher. Deutsch. med. Wschr. 86:2208-2213, Nov. 17, 1961. (Köln)

Miescher-Rüsch, F.: Bemerkungen zur Lehre von den Atembewegungen. Arch. Anat. Physiol. 1885:355-380, 1885.

Miettinen, M.; and Karvinen, E.: Effect of sauna bath on physical performance. J. Sport Med. 3:225-228, Dec., 1963.

Milic-Emili, G.; Cerretelli, P.; Petit, J. M.; and Falconi, C.: La consommation d'oxygène en fonction de l'intensité de l'exercice musculaire. Arch. Int. Physiol. 67:10-14, Feb., 1959. (Milan and Liege)

----, Petit, J. M.; and Delhez, L.: Les relations entre le travail méchanique ventilatoire pendant l'exercice musculaire et la capacité pulmonaire totale chez l'individu sain. Arch. Int. Physiol. 67:417-426, June, 1959. (Liege)

----, ----, and Deroanne, R.: The effects of respiratory rate on the mechanical work of breathing during muscular exercise. Int. Zeits. angew. Physiol. 18:330-340, 1960.

----, ----, and ----: The effects of respiratory rate on the mechanical work of breathing during muscular exercise. Arch. Int. Physiol. 68:528-531, May, 1960. (Liege)

----, ----, and ----: Mechanical work of breathing during exercise in trained and untrained subjects. J. Appl. Physiol. 17:43-46, Jan., 1962. (Liege)

Milla, E.; Bruni, L.; and dall'Ara, A. M.: La funzione renale nel lavoro muscolare. Boll. Soc. Ital. Biol. Sper. 23:725-726, July, 1947.

Millahn, H. P.; and Sollmann, H.: (The behavior of the stroke volume and pulse frequency after measured physical stress) (Ger). Int. Zeits. angew. Physiol. 19:143-148, 1962.

Miller, A. T., Jr.: Present status of the study of human fatigue. N. Carolina Med. J. 9:580-582, Nov., 1948. (Chapel Hill)

Miller, H.; Issekutz, B., Jr.; and Rodahl, K.: Effect of exercise on the metabolism of fatty acids in the dog. Amer. J. Physiol. 205:167-172, July, 1963. (Philadelphia)

Miller, Perry B.: Exercise-induced paroxysmal tachycardias. Geriatrics 19:185-190, Mar., 1964. (Brooks Air Force Base, Tex.)

----, Hartman, Bryce O.; Johnson, Robert L.; and Lamb, Lawrence E.: Modification of the effects of two weeks of bed rest upon circulatory functions in man. Aerospace Med. 35:931-939, Oct., 1964.

----, and Pollard, Lawrence W.: Paroxysmal tachycardia after exercise. Circulation 26:363-372, Sept., 1962. (Brooks Air Force Base, Tex.)

Minard, David: Work physiology. Arch. Environ. Health 8:427-436, Mar., 1964. (Pittsburgh)

Minarovjech, V.: K otázke vzniku struktúrnych zmien vyvolaných tréningom na pl'úcach potkanov. (Apropos of the origin of structural changes in rat lungs induced by training) (Cz). Bratisl. Lek. Listy 44:79-90, July 31, 1964.

Minc, S.: The civilized pattern of human activity and coronary heart disease. Med. J. Aust. 2: 87-91, July 16, 1960. (Perth)

Miraldi, C.; Montanaro, M.; and Rognone, L.: Su alcuni particolari aspetti dell'elettrocardiogramma. Boll. Soc. Ital. Cardiol. 8:206-211, 1963.

Missiuro, Wodzimierz: The influence of environmental stimuli and of intrinsic stimuli on the working capacity and on resistance to fatigue. Rumanian Med. Rev. 5:191-200, 1961. (Warsaw)

----, and Perlberg, A.: Untersuchungen über den Einfluss der Gymnastikunde auf den Gasstoffwechsel. Arbeitsphysiol. 9:514-527, 1937.

Mitchell, Jere H.: Mechanisms of adaptation of the left ventricle to muscular exercise. Pediatrics 32(Suppl.):660-670, Oct., 1963. (Dallas)

----, Remensnyder, John P.; and Sarnoff, Stanley J.: Vasomotor responses in a resting musculocutaneous area during muscular activity. Amer. J. Physiol. 205:37-40, July 1963. (Bethesda)

----, Sproule, Brian J.; and Chapman, Carleton B.: Factors influencing respiration during heavy exercise. J. Clin. Invest. 37:1693-1701, Dec., 1958. (Dallas)

----, ----, and ----: The physiological meaning of the maximal oxygen intake test. J. Clin. Invest. 37:538-547, Apr., 1958. (Dallas)

Mitchell, R. A.; Loeschcke, H. H.; Massion, W. H.; and Severinghaus, J. W.: Respiratory responses mediated through superficial chemosensitive areas on the medulla. J. Appl. Physiol. 18:523-533, May, 1963. (San Francisco)

----, ----, Severinghaus, J. W.; Richardson, B. W.; and Massion, W. H.: Regions of respiratory chemosensitivity on the surface of the medulla. Ann. N. Y. Acad. Sci. 109:661-681, June 24, 1963. (San Francisco)

Mitchell, Roger S.; Webb, N. Conant; and Filley, Giles F.: Chronic obstructive bronchopulmonary disease. III. Factors influencing prognosis. Amer. Rev. Resp. Dis. 89:878-896, June, 1964. (Denver)

Mitchem, J. C.; and Tuttle, W. W.: Influence of exercises, emotional stress, and age on static neuromuscular tremor magnitude. Res. Quart. 25:65-74, Mar., 1954.

Mitolo, M.: La chetonemia nell'allenamento all'esercizio fisico. Arch. E. Maragliano Pat. Clin. 6:239-264, Mar.-Apr., 1951.

----: L'endurance test come prova fisiologica di valutazione dell'allenamento all'eserciziofisico. Arch. Sci. Biol. 35:561-576, Nov.-Dec., 1951.

----, and Cotugno, V.: (Parameters of the potentials of striated muscle action in fatigue and training by physical exercise) (It). Boll. Soc. Ital. Biol. Sper. 36:1766-1770, Dec. 31, 1960.

---- Ruccia, D.; and Cotugno, V.: Fatica e lavoro del muscolo scheletrico nell'allenamento all'esercizio fisico nel vecchio. Gior. Geront. 12:1313-1320, Nov., 1964.

Mobitz, W.: Die Ermittelung des Herzschlagvolumens des Menschen durch Einatmung von Aethyljodiddampf; Konstanz der Ergebnisse und Werte beim Gesunden. Zeits. Kreislaufforsch. 19:480-490, July 15, 1927.

Moia, B.; and Batile, F. F.: El electrocardiograma antes y después del esfuerzo, previa ingestión de alimentos. Rev. Argent. Cardiol. 9:339-351, Jan.-Feb., 1943.

Molina, C.; and Giorgi, E.: Il metabolismo respiratorio del soggetti anziani durante l'esercizio muscolare. Med. Lavoro 42:315-325, Nov., 1951.

Molnar, George D.; Gastineau, Clifford F.; Rosevear, John W.; Helmholz, H. Frederic, Jr.; McGuckin, Warren F.; and Chenoweth, Wanda L.: Metabolic effects of exercise and of multiple-dose insulin regimens in hyperlabile diabetes mellitus. Metabolism 12:157-163, Feb., 1963. (Rochester, Minn.)

Monod, Hugues: Contributions à l'etude du travail statique. Thèse no. 721. Paris, Université Faculté de médecine, 1956.

----, Bouisset, S.; and Laville, A.: Étude d'un travail musculaire léger. III. Influence de la charge. Arch. Int. Physiol. 71:441-461, May, 1963. (Paris)

----, and Laville, A.: La contraction isométrique et le travail agricole. Concours Med. 86: 521-522, Jan. 25, 1964.

----, Lille, F.; and Bonde-Petersen, F.: Coût énergétique comparé des contractions statiques et dynamiques chez l'homme. Comptes Rend. Soc. Biol. 157:2152-2155, 1963. (Paris)

----, Saint-Saens, M.; Scherrer, J.; and Soula, C.: Étude du travail musculaire et de la fatigue. III. Le sang veineux efférent d'un muscle effectuant un travail dynamique chez l'homme. J. Physiologie 53:697-717, Sept.-Oct., 1961. (Paris)

----, ----, ----, and ----: Teneur en oxygène du sang efférent d'un muscle effectuant un travail dynamique. J. Physiologie 50:417-420, Mar., 1958.

Montastruc, P.; and Baisset, A.: (Influence of alcohol on water balance. Application to the diet of the athlete) (Fr). Bull. Soc. Sci. Hyg. Aliment. 51:88-96, 1963.

Montgomery, George E., Jr.; Wood, Earl H.; Burchell, Howard B.; Dry, Thomas J.; Parker, Robert L.; and Helmholz, H. Frederic, Jr.: Continuous observations of the arterial oxygen saturation at rest and during exercise in congenital heart disease. Amer. Heart J. 36:668-682, Nov., 1948. (Rochester, Minn.)

Montoye, Henry J.: Inter-relation of maximum pulse rate during moderate exercise, recovery pulse rate, and post-exercise blood lactate. Res. Quart. 24:453-458, Dec., 1953.

----: Summary of research on the relationship of exercise to heart disease. J. Sport Med. 2:35-43, Mar., 1962.

----, Collings, W. Doyne; and Stauffer, Gordon C.: Effects of conditioning on the ballistocardiogram of college basketball players. J. Appl. Physiol. 15:449-453, May, 1960. (East Lansing, Mich.)

----, Van Huss, Wayne D.; Brewer, Wilma D.; Jones, Evelyn M.; Ohlson, Margaret A.; Mahoney, Earl; and Olson, Herbert: The effects of exercise on blood cholesterol in middle-aged men. Amer. J. Clin. Nutr. 7:139-145, Mar.-Apr., 1959. (East Lansing, Mich.)

Moorhouse, Gretchen L.: The effect of repeated light exercise on the blood cells of albino rats. Amer. J. Hyg. 21:214-223, Jan., 1935. (Baltimore)

Morbelli, E.; and Mascaretti, L.: Cardiac output at rest and during graded exercise in normals and in patients with heart disease. A cardiac function test. Cardiologia 43:317-336, 1963.

----, and ----: Studio analitico delle curve di diluizione degli indicatori registrate durante lavori di intensita crescente nell'uomo sano. II. Le componenti di volume. Folia Cardiol. 23:327-353, July-Aug., 1964. (Milan)

----, ----, Manetti, M.; and Scime, A.: La funzionalita cardio-respiratoria in lavoro nel cuore polmonare cronico. Folia Cardiol. 23:423-436. Sept.-Oct., 1964. (Milan)

----, ----, Piane, C.; Castelluccio, A.; and Castelfranco, M.: (Cardiac output, oxygen consumption and arterial saturation during work of increasing intensity) (It). Atti Ital. Cardiol. 22:323-324, 1962.

Morehouse, L. E.; and Miller, A. T., Jr.: Physiology of exercise. St. Louis, C. V. Mosby, 1948.

Morgan, Donald P.; Kao, Fred; Lim, Thomas P. K.; and Grodins, Fred S.: Temperature and respiratory responses in exercise. Amer. J. Physiol. 183:454-458, Dec., 1955. (Chicago)

Morgan, John Edward: University oars; being a critical enquiry into the after health of the men who rowed in the Oxford and Cambridge boatrace, from the year 1829-1869. London, Macmillan and Co., 1873.

Moritz, F.: Ueber funktionelle Verkleinerung des Herzens. München. med. Wschr. 55:713-718, Apr. 7, 1908. (Strassburg)

----: Zur Frage von der akuten Dilatation des Herzens durch Ueberanstrengung. München. med. Wschr. 55:1331-1334, June 23, 1908. (Strassburg)

Morris, Norman; Osborn, S. B.; Wright, H. Payling; and Hart, A.: Effective uterine blood-flow during exercise in normal and pre-eclamptic pregnancies. Lancet 2:481-484, Sept. 8, 1956. (London)

Morse. Minerva; and Schultz, Frederic W.: The influence of kidney excretion upon the concentration of serum chloride and base of the dog during exercise. J. Biol. Chem. 119:lxxi-lxxii, June, 1937. (Chicago)

----, ----, and Cassels, Donald E.: Relation of age to physiological responses of the older boy (10-17 years) to exercise. J. Appl. Physiol. 1:683-709, Apr., 1949. (Chicago)

Mosco, D.: La velocita di circolo in riposo e subito dopo un esercizio fisico in una centuria d'individui sani (metodo alla lobelina). Endocr. Pat. Costit. 15:3-29, Feb., 1940.

Moskowitz, Merle J.: Running-wheel activity in the white rat as a function of combined food and water deprivation. J. Comp. Physiol. Psychol. 52:621-625, Oct., 1959. (Boston)

Mottu, T.: Puissance mécanique du coeur et rendement cardiovasculaire; notions appliquées a certains effets digitaliques et a l'effort. Arch. Mal. Coeur 49:50-56, Jan., 1956.

Moxness, Karen E.; Molnar, George D.; and McGuckin, Warren F.: Exercise and blood glucose concentration in intact and pancreatectomized dogs. Diabetes 13:37-43, Jan.-Feb., 1964. (Rochester, Minn.)

Muller, Albert: Über Schlagvolumen und Herzarbeit des Menschen. I. Darstellung und Kritik der Methode. Deutsch. Arch. klin. Med. 96:127-152, Apr. 28, 1909. (Vienna)

Müller, Erich A.: Ein Leistungs-Pulsindex als Mass der Leistungsfähigkeit. Arbeitsphysiol. 14: 271-284, 1950.

----: Die physiologischen Bedingungen des Muskeltrainings. Deutsch. med. Wschr. 85: 1311-1313, July 15, 1960. (Dortmund)

----: Regulation der Pulsfrequenz in der Erholungsphase nach ermüdender Muskelarbeit. Int. Zeits. angew. Physiol. 16:35-44, 1955.

----: Zur Vereinfachung des Respirationsversuches nach Douglas-Haldane. Arbeitsphysiol. 2: 18-22, 1930. (Berlin)

----, and Hettinger, T.: Die Energimehrbedarf bei Arbeitsbeginn. Arbeitsphysiol. 16:480-499, 1957.

----, and Karrasch, K.: Der Einfluss der Pausenanordnung auf die Ermüdung bei Schwerarbeit. Int. Zeits. angew. Physiol. 16:45-51, 1955.

Mueller, J.; and Kuechler, J.: (On the effect of sports activity on the serum enzyme level) (Ger). Zeits. Aerztl. Fortbild. 55:919-922, Aug. 15, 1961.

Muller, O.; and Veiel, E.: Beiträge zur Kreislaufphysiologie des Menschen besonders zur Lehre von der Blutverurteilung. Sammlung klin. Vortrage inn. Med. no. 194-196, p. 641-724, 1910.

Muir, G. G.; Chamberlain, D. A.; and Pedoe, D. Tunstall: Effects of B-sympathetic blockade on non-esterified-fatty-acid and carbohydrate metabolism at rest and during exercise. Lancet 2: 930-932, Oct. 31, 1964. (London)

Mulder, G. J.: Abänderung des Apparates, um die Köhlensäure bei Elementaranalysen aufzufangen. Zeits. anal. Chem. 1:2-9, 1862. (Utrecht)

Muller, Alex F.; Manning, Elizabeth L.; and Riondel, Anne M.: Influence of position and activity on the secretion of aldosterone. Lancet 1:711-713, Apr. 5, 1958. (Geneva)

Munter, Sussmann: Leibesubüngen bei den Juden von der ältesten Zeit bis auf die Gegenwart. Wien, Manter, 1926.

Muravov, I. V.; and Tkachev, F. T.: Fiziolohichr_yi analiz vplyru poperednikh m'iazovykh zusyl'na pratsezdalnist'nestomlenykh m'iaziv. (Physiologic analysis of the effect of previous muscular efforts on the working capacity of rested muscles) (Russ). Fiziol. Zh. 10:163-169, Mar.-Apr., 1964.

Musshoff, K.; Reindell, H.; and Klepzig, H.: Stroke volume, arterio-venous difference, cardiac output and physical working capacity, and their relationship to heart volume. Acta Cardiol. 14:427-452, 1959.

----, ----, Steim, H.; and Konig, K.: Die Sauerstoffaufnahme pro Herzschlag (O_2 - Puls) als Funktion des Schlagvolumens, der arteriovenösen Differenz des Minutenvolumens und des Herzvolumens. Zeits. Kreislaufforsch. 48:255-277, Mar., 1959. (Freiburg)

----, Schmidt, H. E. A.; Reindell, H.; König, K.; Bilger-Burchard, D.; Held, E.; and Keul, I.: Beziehungen zwischen Herzvolumen, Körpergewicht, körperlicher Leistungsfahigkeit und Blutvolumen bei gesunden Männern und Frauen unterschiedlicher Leistungsbreite. Acta Radiol. 57:377-400, Sept., 1962. (Freiburg)

Muth, H. A. V.; Wormald, P. N.; Bishop, J. M.; and Donald, K. W.: Further studies of blood flow in the resting arm during supine leg exercise. Clin. Sci. 17:603-610, Nov., 1958. (Birmingham, Eng.)

Muysers, K.; Siehoff, F.; Worth, G.; and Gasthaus, L.: (Recent results of respiratory physiological studies in coal miners with reference to silicosis, bronchitis and emphysema. V. End expiratory-arterial oxygen and carbon dioxide pressure differences at rest and during physical exertion) (Ger). Int. Arch. Gewerbepath. 19:589-612, Nov. 28, 1962.

Naimark, Arnold; Wasserman, Karlman; and McIlroy, Malcolm B.: Continuous measurement of ventilatory exchange ratio during exercise. J. Appl. Physiol. 19:644-652, July, 1964. (San Francisco and Palo Alto)

Namur, M.; Lagneau, D.; and Petit, J. M.: Influence des résistances au débit d'air sur la ventilation et sur la saturation artérielle en oxygène de l'homme normal pendant l'exercice musculaire. Arch. Int. Physiol. 68:608-617, Sept., 1960. (Liege)

Nasrallah, Salah; and Al-Khalidi, Usama: Nature of purines excreted in urine during muscular exercise. J. Appl. Physiol. 19:246-248, Mar., 1964. (Beirut)

Nathan, David A.; Samet, Philip; Center, Sol; and Wu, Chang You: Long-term correction of complete heart block. Clinical and physiologic studies of a new type of implantable synchronous pacer. Progr. Cardiov. Dis. 6:538-565 May, 1964. (Miami Beach and Coral Gables)

Naughton, John: The relationship of physical activity to the serum cholesterol concentration. J. Okla. Med. Ass. 57:540-541, Dec., 1964. (Oklahoma City)

----, and Balke, Bruno: Physical working capacity in medical personnel and the response of serum cholesterol to acute exercise and to training. Amer. J. Med. Sci. 247:286-292, Mar., 1964. (Oklahoma City)

----, ----, and Nagle, Francis: Refinements in method of evaluation and physical conditioning before and after myocardial infarction. Amer. J. Cardiol. 14:837-843, Dec., 1964. (Oklahoma City)

----, Sevelius, G.; and Balke, Bruno: Physiological responses of normal and pathological subjects to a modified work capacity test. J. Sport Med. 3:201-207, Dec., 1963. (Oklahoma City)

Navakamikian, A. O.; Lebedeva, V. V.; Blagoveshchenskaia, I. N.; et al: Analiz deistviia fizicheskoi nagruzki, vysokoi temperatury sredy i povyshennogo soderzhaniia kisloroda vo vdykhaemom vozdukhe na vozbudimost'zritel'nogo analizatora cheloveka. (Analysis of the effect of physical exercise, high environmental temperature and high oxygen content in inspired air on the excitability of the human visual analyzers) (Russ). Fiziol. Zh. SSSR Sechenov. 49:1036-1043, Sept., 1963.

Neciuk-Szczerbinski, Z.: Wplyw wysilku na przebieg gruźlicy doświadczainej u morskich świnek. (Effect of effort on the course of experimental tuberculosis in guinea pigs) (Pol). Gruzlica 31:889-900, Aug., 1963.

Nedbal, J.; and Seliger, V.: Electrophoretic analysis of exercise proteinuria. J. Appl. Physiol. 13:244-246, Sept., 1958.

Needham, Dorothy Mary: Energy production in muscle. Brit. Med. Bull. 12:194-198, Sept., 1956. (Cambridge, Eng.)

Neill, William A.; Krasnow, Norman; Levine, Herbert J.; and Gorlin, Richard: Myocardial anaerobic metabolism in intact dogs. Amer. J. Physiol. 204:427-432, Mar., 1963.

Newburger, Bernhard: Early postoperative walking. I. The influence of exercise on wound healing in rats. Surgery 13:692-695, May, 1943. (Cincinnati)

Newman, Faith; Smalley, B. F.; and Thomson, M. L.: Effect of exercise, body and lung size on CO diffusion in athletes and nonathletes. J. Appl. Physiol. 17:649-655, July, 1962. (London)

Newman, Henry W.: The effect of amphetamine sulfate on performance of normal and fatigued subjects. J. Pharmacol. Exp. Ther. 89:106-108, Feb., 1947. (San Francisco)

Newton, J. L.: The assessment of maximal oxygen intake. J. Sport Med. 3:164-169, June-Sept., 1963.

Nichols, John; Miller, A. T., Jr.; and Hiatt, E. P.: Influence of muscular exercise on uric acid excretion in man. J. Appl. Physiol. 3:501-507, Feb., 1951. (Chapel Hill)

Nicolai, G. F.; and Zuntz, N.: Füllung und Entleerung des Herzens bei Ruhe und Arbeit. Berlin. klin. Wschr. 51:821-824, 1914.

Nielsen, Bodil; and Nielsen, Marius: Body temperature during work at different environmental temperatures. Acta Physiol. Scand. 56:120-129, Oct., 1962. (Copenhagen)

Nielsen, Holger E.: Clinical investigations into the cardiac output of patients with compensated heart disease during rest and muscular work. Acta Med. Scand. 91:223-266, 1937. (Aalborg, Den.)

Nielsen, Marius: Untersuchungen über die Atemregulation beim Menschen besonders mit Hinblick auf die Art des chemischen Reizes. Scand. Arch. Physiol. 74(Suppl. 10):83-208, 1936.

----, and Smith, Helge: Studies on the regulation of respiration in acute hypoxia, with an appendix on respiratory control during prolonged hypoxia. Acta Physiol. Scand. 24:293-313, Feb. 12, 1951. (Copenhagen)

Nikkila, Esko A.; and Konttinen, Aarne: Effect of physical activity on postprandial levels of fats in serum. Lancet 1:1151-1154, June 2, 1962. (Helsinki)

----, Torsti, Pertti; and Penttila, O.: The effect of exercise on lipoprotein lipase activity of rat heart, adipose tissue and skeletal muscle. Metabolism 12:863-865, Sept., 1963. (Helsinki)

Niquet: (Changes in urinary secretion during exercise. Renal condition of fitness in sports) (Fr). Concours Med. 84:7197-7198, Dec. 29, 1962.

Nisell, Ove: The respiratory work and pressure during exercise, and their relation to dyspnea. Acta Med. Scand. 166:113-119, Feb. 17, 1960. (Stockholm)

----, Carlberger, Gunnar; and Bevegard, Sture: The mechanics of respiration in patients with mitral heart disease. Acta Med. Scand. 162:277-285, Nov. 10, 1958. (Stockholm)

Nitter-Hauge, S.: Hjertfrekvens, slagvolum og arteriovenos oksygendifferanse i hvile og ved arbeidsbelastning. Oversikt over publiserte funn fra friske mennesker. (Heart rate, heart output and arteriovenous oxygen difference at rest and on exertion. Review of published findings on healthy persons) (Nor). T. Norsk. Laegeforen. 83:1310-1316, Sept. 1, 1963.

----: Hjertefrekvens, slagvolum og arteriovenos oksygendifferanse i hvile og ved arbeidsbelastnint Oversikt over publiserte funn fra individer med hjerteog lungesykdommer. (Heart rate, heart output and arteriovenous oxygen difference at rest and on exertion. Review of published findings on persons with heart and lung diseases) (Nor). T. Norsk. Laegeforen. 83:1316-1322, Sept. 1, 1963.

Nitzescu, I.-I; and Mihalescu, Orthanse: Effet des injections intraveineuses de carbonate de soude sur la polyglobulie de l'exercice musculaire. Comptes Rend. Soc. Biol. 100:686-689, 1929. (Paris)

Noder, W.: Die allgemeinen Zustandsgleichungen des Kreislaufs. Zeits. Kreislaufforsch. 52:
1157-1159, Nov., 1963. (Bad Salzuflen)

----: Die Bestimmung des Herzminutenvolumens und des zentralen Blutvolumens bei korperlicher
Arbeit. Zeits. Kreislaufforsch. 52:1206-1210, Dec., 1963. (Bad Salzuflen)

----: Das Normalverhalten der Funktionsgrossen des Kreislauf unter korperlicher Arbeit. II. Die Abhängigkeit
des Herzminutenvolumens von der Korperoberflache. Arch. Kreislaufforsch. 45:19-28, Dec., 1964.

Nocker, J.; and Hartleb, O.: (Arteriosclerosis and physical work) (Ger). Schweiz. Zeits. Sportmed.
9:101-116, 1961.

----, Lohmann, D.; and Schleusing, G.: Einfluss von Training und Belastung auf den Mineralgehalt
von Herz und Skeletmuskel. Int. Zeits. angew. Physiol. 17:243-251, 1958.

Nordstrom-Ohrberg, Gunvor: Effect of digitalis glucosides on electrocardiogram and exercise test in
healthy subjects. Acta Med. Scand. 176(Suppl. 420):1-75, 1964. (Stockholm)

North, W.: The influence of bodily labour upon the discharge of nitrogen. Proc. Roy. Soc. 39:
443-503, Nov.-Dec., 1885.

North Carolina, U. of; Lab. of Applied Physiol.: Influence of physical characteristics, psychological
factors, and drugs on the capacity of man to work in the heat; progress report. Res. and Dev.
Division, U. S. Army Surgeon General's office. Contract No. DA-49-007-MD-949. Chapel
Hill, 1959.

Nova, M.; and Hubac, M.: Vzaimosviaz'mezhdu nekotorymi pakazateliami kardio-pul'monale' noĭ
funktsii pri trudovoi nagruzke podrostkov v period ikh razvitiia. (Relationship between some
indices of cardio-pulmonary activity in adolescents working during their developmental period) (Russ).
Gig. Tr. Prof. Zabol. 7:13-20, Oct., 1963.

Nowy, Herbert; Kikodse, Katharina; and Zollner, Nepomuk: Über Bestimmungen des Herzminutenvolumens
und zentralen Blutvolumens in Ruhe und bei korperlicher Arbeit mit Hilfe der Farbstoffmethode.
Zeits. Kreislaufforsch. 46:382-393, May, 1957. (Munich)

----, ----, and ----: Vergleichende Messungen des zentralen Blutvolumens und Herzminutenvolumens
im Liegen und im Stehen. Zeits. Kreislaufforsch. 46:393-398, May, 1957. (Munich)

Numajiri, K.: (A study on the recovery from muscular fatigue) (Jap). J. Sci. Labour 40:153-161,
Apr., 1964.

Nunney, D. N.: Fatigue, impairment, and psycho-motor learning. Percept. Motor Skills 16:369-375,
Apr., 1963.

Nylin, G.: The relation between heart volume and stroke volume in recumbent and erect positions.
Scand. Arch. Physiol. 69:237-246, 1934.

Ochwadt, Bruno; Bücherl, Emil; Kreuzer, Heinrich; and Loeschcke, Hans H.: Beeinflussung der Atemsteigerung bei Muskelarbeit durch partiellen neuromuskulären Block (Tubocurarin). Pflüger Arch. ges. Physiol. 269:613-621, Nov. 24, 1959. (Gottingen)

Odaira, T.: Studien über Gasstoffwechsel und Minutenvolum. Tohoku J. Exp. Med. 6:325-366, Sept., 1925.

Odum, Eugene P.; Rogers, David T.; and Hicks, David L.: Homeostasis of the nonfat components of migrating birds. Science 143:1037-1039, Mar. 6, 1964. (Athens, Ga.)

Ogston, D.; and Fullerton, H. W.: Changes in fibrinolytic activity produced by physical activity. Lancet 2:730-733, Sept. 30, 1961. (Aberdeen)

Okhrimenko, A. P.: Fiziologicheskie sdvigi v protsesse raboty u zhenshchin farforovogo savoda. (Physiological changes during work performance in women employed in a procelain factory) (Russ). Gig. Tr. Prof. Zabol. 7:9-13, Sept., 1963.

Olewine, Donald A.; Barrows, Charles H., Jr.; and Shock, Nathan W.: Effect of reduced dietary intake on random and voluntary activity in male rats. J. Geront. 19:230-233, Apr., 1964. (Baltimore)

Olmes de Carrasco, H.: Die Vollständigkeit arteriellen Sättigung beim Herzkranken unter körperlicher Arbeit. Klin. Wschr. 20:95-97, Jan. 25, 1941.

Oñate, J.; and Ramos, Guevara, H.: Cianosis e hipertensión arterial pulmonar. Correlación clínica en 33 enfermos. Rev. Esp. Tuberc. 32:557-562, Nov., 1963.

Opdyke, David F.: The influence of exercise on the heart. Phys. Ther. Rev. 30:462-468, Nov., 1950. (Cleveland)

Opie, Lionel H.; and Walfish, Paul G.: Plasma free fatty acid concentrations in obesity. New Eng. J. Med. 268:757-760, Apr. 4, 1963. (Toronto)

Orlowska, K.; and Jaworska, M.: Niektóre wskazniki ergospirometryczne u mlodziezy z bocznym skrzywieniem kregoslupa. (Some ergospirometric indices in adolescents with scoliosis) (Pol). Pediat. Pol. 39:421-423, Apr., 1964.

----, and Serzysko, W.: Ocena réwnoczesnego badania oksygramu, wentylacji minutowej i skladu powietrza wydechowego w dzasie krótkolrwalego wysilku. (Evaluation of the simultaneous determination of the oxigram, minute ventilation and expired air composition during effort of brief duration) (Pol). Pol. Arch. Med. Wewnet. 33:801-805, 1963.

Oskolkova, M. K.: Khronometriia faz serdechnoi sistoly u sdorovykh detei v pokoe i posle fizicheskoi nagruzki s pomoshch'iu polikardiograficheskogo issledovaniia. (Chronometry of the cardiac systole phases in healthy children during rest and after physical exertion using poly-cardiographic examination) (Russ). Vop. Okhr. Materin. Dets. 8:24-28, Dec., 1963.

Osten, H.: Die Bedeutung der Frequenztransposition fur die Registrierung atemmechanischer Analysen am offenen spirometersystem und ihre Ergebnisse. Klin. Wschr. 42:1136-1141, Nov. 15, 1964. (Bremen)

Ostrovskaia, A. A.: Izmeneniia pul'sa dykhaniia i arterial'nogo davleniia u detei rannego vozrasta posle fizicheskoi nagruzki. (Pulse, respiration and arterial pressure changes in young children after physical exercise) (Russ). Vop. Okhr. Materin. Dets. 8:41-46, Apr., 1963.

Ostyn, M.; and Styns, H. J.: (The influence of a blood donation on the work capacity of athletes) (Fr). Arch. Belg. Med. Soc. 17:375-387, May, 1959.

Ostyn, M.; and Willems, E.: (Orthostatic syncope after physical exertion) (Dut). Belg.
T. Geneesk. 16:420-425, May 1, 1960.

----, ----, and De Nayer, P. P.: Studie over de regeling van de terugkeer tot rustwarden van
diverse fysiologische parameters na lichamelijke inspanning. (Study on the regulation of
the return to resting values, of various physiological parameters after physical exertion)
(Dut). Verh. Kon. Vlaam. Acad. Geneesk. Belg. 25:431-457, 1963.

Otis, Arthur B.: Application of Gray's theory of respiratory control to the hyperpnea produced by
passive movements of the limbs. J. Appl. Physiol. 1:743-751, May, 1949. (Rochester,
N. Y.)

----: Physiology of respiration in relation to environment and to muscular exercise. J. Sport Med.
2:83-85, June, 1962. (Rochester, N.Y.)

----: The work of breathing. Physiol. Rev. 34:449-458, July, 1954. (Baltimore)

Otto, P.; Schmidt, E.; and Schmidt, F. W.: Enzymspiegel im Serum bei körperlicher Arbeit und
ambulanten Patienten. Klin. Wschr. 42:75-81, Jan. 15, 1964. (Marburg)

Overbeek, G. A.: Adrenals and fatigue. II. The cholinesterase activity of serum, brain and muscle
in normal and adrenalectomized rats. Arch. Int. Pharmacodyn. 79:314-322, May 1, 1949.
(Oss, Hol.)

Owen, Trevor: Fatigue, rest and exercise. Canad. Med. Ass. J. 47:41-45, July, 1942. (Toronto)

Owles, W. Harding: Alterations in the lactic acid content of the blood as a result of light exercise
and associated changes in the CO_2-combining power of the blood and in the alveolar CO_2 pressure.
J. Physiol. 69:214-237, Apr. 14, 1930. (Oxford)

Pachner, P.; Zaoralek, J.; and Kabat, A.: Miners' energy expenditure. Acta Med. Leg. Soc. 12:53-55, Jan.-June, 1959.

Pachon, V.; and Fabre, R.: Loi de constance du débit circulatoire en fonction de la puissance cardiaque. Application physiopathologique a l'homme. Comptes Rend. Soc. Biol. 105: 31-32, 1930. (Paris)

----, and ----: Loi de constance du débit circulatoire en fonction de la puissance cardiaque. Détermination expérimentale. Comptes Rend. Soc. Biol. 105:30-31, 1930. (Paris)

Panajotakos, Panos: Über die Phosphorverteilung in der Schenkelmuskulatur der Kröte. Hoppe-Seyler Zeits. physiol. Chem. 113:245-252, Apr. 5, 1921. (Frankfurt)

Panno, G.: (Influence of exertion on renal function in the aged) (It). Boll. Soc. Ital. Biol. Sper. 38:782-784, Aug. 31, 1962.

Pare, C. M. B.; and Sandler, M.: Amino-aciduria in march haemoglobinuria. Lancet 1:702-704, Apr. 3, 1954. (Shorncliffe, Eng.)

Parizkova, Jana: Impact of age, diet, and exercise on man's body composition. Ann. N. Y. Acad. Sci. 110:661-674, Sept. 26, 1963. (Prague)

----, and Poupa, O.: Some metabolic consequences of adaptation to muscular work. Brit. J. Nutr. 17:341-345, 1963. (Prague)

----, and Staňková, Libuše: Influence of physical activity on a treadmill on the metabolism of adipose tissue in rats. Brit. J. Nutr. 18:325-332, 1964. (Prague)

Park, Syuk Ryun; and Rodbard, Simon: Effects of load and duration of tension on pain induced by muscular contraction. Amer. J. Physiol. 203:735-738, Oct., 1962. (Buffalo)

Parker, John C.; Peters, Richard M.; and Barnett, Thomas B.: Carbon dioxide and the work of breathing. J. Clin. Invest. 42:1362-1372, Aug., 1963. (Chapel Hill)

Parker, P. A.: Acute effects of smoking on physical endurance and resting circulation. Res. Quart. 25:210-217, May, 1954.

Parkes, E. A.: On the elimination of nitrogen by the kidneys and intestines during rest and exercise, on a diet without nitrogen. Proc. Roy. Soc. 15:339-355, Jan. 24, 1867.

----: On the elimination of nitrogen during rest and exercise on a regulated diet of nitrogen. Proc. Roy. Soc. 16:44-59, June 20, 1867.

----: Further experiments on the effect of diet and exercise on the elimination of nitrogen. Proc. Roy. Soc. 19:349-361, March 2, 1871.

Parnas, J. K.; and Klisiecki, A.: Über den Ammoniakgehalt und die Ammoniakbildung im Blute. VI. Experimentelle Untersuchungen über die Faktoren, welche den Ammoniakgehalt des kreisenden Blutes beeinflussen, und über die Lokalisation der Ammoniakbildung und des Ammoniakschwandes beim Kaninchen. Biochem. Zeits. 173:224-248, 1926.

----, Mozolowski, W.; and Lewinski, W.: Über den Ammoniakgehalt und die Ammoniakbildung im Blute. IX. Der Zusammenhang des Blutammoniaks mit der Muskelarbeit. Biochem. Zeits. 188:15-23, 1927.

----, and Wagner, Richard: Über den Kohlenhydratumsatz isolierter Amphibienmuskeln und über die Beziehungen Zwischen Kohlenhydratschwund und Milchsäurebildung im Muskel. Biochem. Zeits. 61:387-427, 1914. (Strassburg)

Parrot, Jean-Louis; Dinanian, Jirayr; and Thouvenot, Joseph: Enregistrement continue de la fréquence cardiaque instantanée en vue de l'étude de l'exercice musculaire. Presse Méd. 67:671-673, Apr. 4, 1959. (Paris)

----, ----, and ----: L'exercice musculaire et la fréquence du coeur. Presse Méd. 68:1569-1571, Oct. 1, 1960. (Paris)

----, and Flavian, Nathalie: L'exercice musculaire et le vieillissement. Sem. Hôp. Paris 37: 3671-3675, Dec. 30, 1961. (Paris)

Parsonnet, Aaron E.; and Bernstein, Arthur: Heart strain: a critical review; the development of a physiologic concept. Ann. Intern. Med. 16:1123-1136, June, 1942. (Newark)

Parturier, G.; Fauqué; and Nénon: Valeur régulatrice de l'exercice musculaire sur les métabolismes chez les hépatobiliaires. Paris Med. 26:44-47, July 11, 1936.

Pasargiklian, M.; Ghiringhelli, G.; and Lombardo, G. G.: (A contribution to research on the physiology of respiration during rest and during physical exertion in young men) (Ger). Beitr. Klin. Tuberk. 123:111-131, 1960.

Passmore, R.: How many calories? Food requirements reconsidered in relation to activity. Lancet 2:853-854, Oct. 17, 1964. (Edinburgh)

----: A note on the relation of appetite to exercise. Lancet 1:29, Jan. 4, 1958. (Edinburgh)

----, and Durnin, J. V. G. A.: Human energy expenditure. Physiol. Rev. 35:801-840, Oct., 1955. (Edinburgh and Glasgow)

----, and Johnson, R. E.: Some metabolic changes following prolonged moderate exercise. Metabolism 9:452-455, May, 1960. (Edinburgh)

----, and Swindells, Yola E.: Observations on the respiratory quotients and weight gain of man after eating large quantities of carbohydrate. Brit. J. Nutr. 17:331-339, 1963. (Edinburgh)

Pastor, Paul J.: Threshold muscular fatigue level and strength decrement recovery of elbow flexor muscles resulting from varying degrees of muscular work. Arch. Phys. Med. 40:247-252, June, 1959. (Fresno)

Patel, R.: Urinary casts in exercise. Aust. Ann. Med. 13:170-173, May, 1964. (Dunedin, N.Z.)

Paterson, W. D.: Circulatory and respiratory changes in response to muscular exercise in man. J. Physiol. 66:323-345, Dec. 20, 1928. (Oxford)

Patterson, G. C.; and Shepherd, J. T.: The effects of continuous infusions into the brachial artery of adenosine triphosphate, histamine and acetylcholine on the amount and rate of blood debt repayment following rhythmic exercise of forearm muscles. Clin. Sci. 13:85-91, Feb., 1954. (Belfast)

Patterson, John L.; Graybiel, Ashton; Lenhardt, Harry F.; and Madsen, M. Jones: Evaluation and prediction of physical fitness, utilizing modified apparatus of the Harvard step test. Amer. J. Cardiol. 14:811-827, Dec., 1964. (Richmond)

Paulet, G.; and Van Den Driessche, J.: La masse sanguine pulmonaire au cours du travail musculaire. Comptes Rend. Soc. Biol. 154:2314-2316, 1960. (Rennes)

Pauli, H. G.: Beitrage zum Problem der Atemregulation unter Hohenadaptation. Pflüger Arch. ges. Physiol. 278:447-466, Dec. 23, 1964. (Bern)

Pautrat, Jean: L'épreuve d'effort et le diagnostic d'angine de poitrine. Presse Méd. 71: 1331-1332, May 25, 1963. (Paris)

Pavy, F. W.: The effect of prolonged muscular exercise on the system. Lancet 1:353-356, Mar. 4; 392-394, Mar. 11; 429-431, Mar. 18; 466-468, Mar. 25, 1876. (London)

----: The effect of prolonged muscular exercise upon the urine in relation to the source of muscular power. Lancet 2:741-743, Nov. 25; 815-818, Dec. 9; 848-850, Dec. 16; 887-889, Dec. 23, 1876; 1:42-44, Jan. 13, 1877. (London)

----: Report of analyses of urine during severe exercise in the case of Mr. Weston. Brit. Med. J. 1:298-299, Mar. 4; 315-316, Mar. 11, 1876. (London)

Pawlow, J. P.: Ueber den Einfluss des Vagus auf die Arbeit der linken Herzkammer. Arch. Anat. Physiol. (Physiol. Abt.):452-468, 1887.

Pearce, John M. S.; Pennington, R. J.; and Walton, John N.: Serum enzyme studies in muscle disease. I. Variations in serum creatine kinase activity in normal individuals. J. Neurol. Neurosurg. Psychiat. 27:1-4, Feb., 1964. (Newcastle-on-Tyne)

Pearce, R. G.: The history of the physiology of respiration. Cleveland Med. J. 13:262-270, Apr., 1914.

Pearson, Carl: Adams, Raymond D.; and Denny-Brown, D.: Traumatic necrosis of pretibial muscles. New Eng. J. Med. 239:213-217, Aug. 5, 1948. (Boston)

Peder, Hjalmar: Neue Versuche über die Bedeutung der Uebung für die Leistungsfähigkeit der Muskeln. Scand. Arch. Physiol. 27:315-340, 1912. (Helsinki)

Pelikán, V.; Kaláb, M.; Novosadová, J.; et al: Sledování metabolismu tryptofanu při sportovní námaze. (Determination of tryptophan metabolism during sports activity) (Cz). Cas. Lek. Cesk. 102: 967-969, Aug. 30, 1963.

Pelosse, J. L.; and Soulairac, A.: Évolution de l'excrétion urinaire des catécholamines en relation avec le rythme veille-sommeil et le travail chez des sujets nordscandinaves. Ann. Endocr. 25: 661-669, Nov.-Dec., 1964. (Paris)

Peltonen, L.; and Karvonen, M. J.: Effects of dietary cholesterol, dietary fat, and exercise on mouse plasma cholesterol. Ann. Med. Exp. Fenn. 34:246-252, 1956.

Pembrey, M. S.: The physiology of muscular work. Further Advances in Physiology, Pa. 208-257, 1909.

----: Respiration. In Text-book of Physiology, by E. A. Schafer. Edinburgh and London, Young J. Pentlord, 1898. Vol. 1, Pa. 698-712.

----, and Cook, F.: Observations upon "second wind". J. Physiol. 37:lxvii-lxviii, 1908.

----, and Todd, A. H.: The influence of exercise upon the pulse and blood-pressure. J. Physiol. 37:lxvi, 1908.

Pentecost, B. L.: The effect of exercise on the external iliac vein blood flow and local oxygen consumption in normal subjects, and in those with occlusive arterial disease. Clin. Sci. 27: 437-445, Dec., 1964. (London)

Penzoldt, F.; and Birgelen, H.: Ueber den Einfluss der Körperbewegung auf die Temperatur
    Gesunder und Kranker. München. med. Wschr. 46:469; 519; 555, 1899.

Peregrino, Jr.; and Lourdes-Oliveira, M. de: Menstruacão e exercicio fisico. Hospital (Rio) 25:
    751-759, May, 1944. (Rio de Janeiro)

Pereira, J. R.: Muscular exercise, lactic acid and the supply and utilization of oxygen. Part XII.
    A note on the technique of determining the resting oxygen intake while breathing concentrated
    oxygen mixtures. Proc. Roy. Soc. 98B:480-483, Oct. 1, 1925.

Peretti, G.; and Granati, A.: La gettata cardiaca durante il lavoro nelle miniere di carbone.
    Arch. Sci. Biol. 26:149-153, Apr., 1940.

Perkins, Peter; Constantine, Herbert; Luria, Milton N.; and Yu, Paul N.: The effect of exercise on
    venous admixture in valvular heart disease. Amer. J. Cardiol. 10:52-56, July, 1962.
    (Rochester, N.Y.)

Pernot, C.: (Exertion and myocardial infarct) (Fr). Arch. Mal. Prof. 24:553-556, June, 1963.

Pernow, Bengt: Methods for the analysis of the blood flow through the lower extremities in obliterative
    arterial diseases. Scand. J. Clin. Lab. Invest. 15(Suppl. 76):57-60, 1963. (Stockholm)

----, and Wahren, John: Lactate and pyruvate formation and oxygen utilization in the human forearm
    muscles during work of high intensity and varying duration. Acta Physiol. Scand. 56:267-285,
    Nov.-Dec., 1962. (Stockholm)

Perrault, Claude: Mécanique des animaux. Paris, 1680.

Perret, C.: Effet des hyperoxies itératives sur la ventilation lors de l'exercice musculaire: résultats
    préliminaires. Rev. Méd. Nancy 82:936-939, Aug.-Sept., 1957. (Lausanne)

----: Hyperoxie et régulation de la ventilation durant l'exercice musculaire. Helv. Physiol.
    Pharmacol. Acta 18:72-97, Mar., 1960. (Lausanne)

----, Haab, P.; Vulliet, J.; and Fleisch, A.: Intensité du travail et réponse ventilatoire aux
    hyperoxies itératives. J. Physiologie 49:349-352, Jan.-Mar., 1957. (Lausanne)

Pertuzon, E.: Influence de la vitesse réelle d'exécution sur le cout energetique du mouvement.
    J. Physiologie 56:422, May-June, 1964. (Lille)

Peters, Rudolph A.: The heat production of fatigue and its relation to the production of lactic
    acid in amphibian muscle. J. Physiol. 47:243-271, Nov. 7, 1913. (Cambridge, Eng.)

Petit, J. M.; Milic-Emili, G.; and Koch, R.: Le volume de réserve expiratoire pendant l'exercice
    musculaire chez l'homme sain. Arch. Int. Physiol. 67:350-357, June, 1959. (Nancy)

----, ----, and Sadoul, P.: L'influence de la position corporelle sur le travail ventilatoire dynamique pendant
    pendant l'exercice musculaire chez l'individu sain. Arch. Int. Physiol. 68:437-444, May, 1960.
    (Liege)

Petrun', N. M.: Izmenenie gazovogo sostava krovi u cheloveka, nakhodiashchegosia v razlichnykh
    usloviiakh vneshnei sredy. (Modification of the gaseous composition of the blood in men living
    under various conditions of the external environment) (Russ). Zdravookhr. Beloruss. 9:
    57-60, Apr., 1963.

Pettenkofer, Max: Ueber die Respiration. Ann. Chem. Pharm. 2(Suppl.):1-52, 1862-1863.

----: Ueber den Respirations- und Perspirations-Apparat im physiologischen Institute zu München. Sitzungsberichte der königl. bayerisch Acad. Wissensch. München, pages 296-304, July 21, 1860.

Pezzeri, V.; Venerando, A.; and Suraci, A.: Le modificazioni ematologiche nell'attivita muscolare, con particolare riguardo alla idoneita al lavoro. Rass. Mec. Industr. 32:390-394, May-Aug., 1963.

Pfleiderer, T.; and Kommerell, B.: Uber die Veranderung der Thrombocytenadhäsivität nach korperflicher Belastung. Verh. deutsch. Ges. inn. Med. 70:220-223, 1964.

Pfluger, Eduard Friedrich Wilhelm: Über die Kohlensäure des Blutes. Bonn, Max Cohen u. Sohn, 1864.

----: Ueber die Ursache der Athembewegungen, sowie der Dyspnöe und Apnöe. Pflüger Arch. ges. Physiol. 1:61-106, 1868. (Bonn)

Philp, R. B.; and Gowdey, C. W.: Decompression sickness in rats during exercise at simulated low altitudes after exposure to compressed air. Aerospace Med. 33:1433-1437, Dec., 1962. (London, Ont.)

Piacentini, V.; and Bollettino, A.: Il metabolismo respiratorio del bambini durante l'esercizio muscolare. La marcia e la corsa su terreno plano ed inclinato. Arbeitsphysiol. 12:272-286, 1942.

----, and ----: Sul comportamento della ventilazione polmonare durante d'esercizio muscolare nei bambini. Boll. Soc. Ital. Biol. Sper. 13:645, 1938.

Pickfold, Mary: Respiratory adaptation. Lancet 2:1225-1226, Dec. 11, 1954.

Piédallu, P.: A propos des effets circulatoires de l'exercice. J. Méd. Paris 46:32, 1927.

Pierson, William R.: Fatigue, work decrement, and endurance in a simple repetitive task. Brit. J. Med. Psychol. 36:279-282, 1963. (Burbank)

----: Isometric strength and occurrence of fatigue and work decrement. Percept. Motor Skills 17:470, Oct., 1963.

----, Cochran, William G.; Smith, Gene M.; and Beecher, Henry K.: Amphetamine sulfate and performance. A critique. A reply. J.A.M.A. 177:345-349, Aug. 5, 1961. (Los Angeles and Boston)

----, and Rasch, Philip J.: The injurious consequences of maximal isometric arm exercises. J. Amer. Phys. Ther. Ass. 43:582-583, Aug., 1963. (Los Angeles)

----, and ----: Isometric strength as a factor in functional muscle testing. Amer. J. Phys. Med. 42:205-207, Oct., 1963. (Los Angeles)

----, and ----: Strength development and performance capacity. J. Ass. Phys. Ment. Rehab. 17: 5-9, Jan.-Feb., 1963.

Piñero, H. G.: Fisiología del ejercicio y educación física cientifica. Rev. Soc. Méd. Argent. 12:71-123, 1904.

Pirnay, F.; Namur, M.; and Petit, J. M.: Variations cycliques respiratoires de la saturation en O$_2$ du sang artériel pendant l'exercice musculaire. Comptes Rend. Soc. Biol. 156:1204-1206 Oct. 30, 1962. (Liege)

Pitt, Aubrey; and Munro, J. A.: The clinical application of a physical working capacity test. Med. J. Aust. 1:472-476, Mar. 28, 1964. (Melbourne)

Pitteloud, J. J.: Effets de l'age et de l'entrainement sur les échanges respiratoires mésuré en état d'équilibre lors de l'exercice musculaire. Rev. Méd. Nancy 82:880-884, Aug.-Sept., 1957.

----, Forster, G.; and Gander, M.: La détermination de l'hémoglobine totale et sa signification dans l'estimation de la capacité de travail musculaire. Schweiz. med. Wschr. 94:811-816, June 13, 1964. (Zurich)

Pitts, Grover C.: Studies of gross body composition by direct dissection. Ann. N. Y. Acad. Sci. 110:11-22, Sept. 26, 1963. (Charlottesville)

Planet, N.; and Cardoso, D.-M.: Influence de l'exercice musculaire sur le phosphore et la créatine du sang. Comptes Rend. Soc. Biol. 112:1509-1510, 1933. (Paris)

Plas, F.: (The strained heart) (Fr). Gaz. Med. France 68:1637-1642, June 25, 1961.

----, and Chailley-Bert, P.: Electrocardiogramme du coeur au travail. Arch. Mal. Coeur 49:916-918, Oct., 1956.

----, and Pallardy, G.: Variations du volume cardiaque systolique et diastolique au cours et a la suite de l'effort. Presse Méd. 71:2436-2438, Nov. 30, 1963.

Plas, F. R.: Electrocardiographic changes during work and prolonged effort. J. Sport Med. 3:131-136, June-Sept., 1963.

Plouvier, S.: (Significance of impedence curves of the body to alternating currents of low frequency. Influence of muscular activity) (Fr). Agressologie 3:761-767, Sept.-Oct., 1962.

Podkaminsky, N. A.: Beiträge zur pathologischen Arbeitsphysiologie. I. Das Herz des Lästtragers im Röntgenbilde. Arbeitsphysiol. 1:306-356, 1929. (Kharkow)

----: Beiträge zur pathologischen Arbeitsphysiologie. II. "Kann schwere Körperarbeit ein Lungenemphysem hervorrufen?" Arbeitsphysiol. 1:577-585, 1929. (Kharkow)

Policreti, C.; Antonelli, F.; and Francesconi, A.: Osservazioni sull'influenza di diuerse sostanze psicotrope sulla capacita attentiva di un gruppo omogeneo di canottieri. Ann. Med. Nav. 68:803-808, Sept.-Oct., 1963.

Pollack, Albert A.; Taylor, Bowen E.; Myers, Thomas T.; and Wood, Earl H.: The effect of exercise and body position on the venous pressure at the ankle in patients having venous valvular defects. J. Clin. Invest. 28:559-563, May, 1949. (Rochester, Minn.)

----, and Wood, Earl H.: Venous pressure in the saphenous vein at the ankle in man during exercise and changes in posture. J. Appl. Physiol. 1:649-662, Mar., 1949. (Rochester, Minn.)

Pombo, J.: Valor semiológico de la pressión retroesternal o precordial provocada por el esfuerzo. Prensa Méd. Argent. 33:355-356, Feb. 15, 1946.

Pons, Eduardo R., Jr.; and Berg, Judith L.: The physiologic advantage of oxygen during exercise in patients with coronary artery insufficiency. Dis. Chest 39:551-556, May, 1961. (New York)

Poortmans, Jacques: La proteinurie physiologique au repos et a l'effort. Ann. Soc. Roy. Sci. Med. Natur. Brux. 17:89-188, 1964.

Poortmans, Jacques: Urinary excretion of the tryptophanrich pre-albumin after strenuous physical effort. Life Sci. 5:334-336, May, 1963. (Brussels)

----, S'Jongers, J. J.; Thys, A.; and Van Kerchove, E.: (The transaminase activity of the whole blood and serum during muscular effort) (Fr). Rev. Franc. Etud. Clin. Biol. 8: 173-175, Feb., 1963.

----, and Van Kerchove, E.: Dosage de la protéinure comparasion de deux méthodes. Clin. Chim. Acta 8:485-488, July, 1963. (Brussels)

----, and ----: La protéinurie d'effort. Clin. Chim. Acta 7:229-242, Mar., 1962. (Brussels)

----, ----, and Jaumain, P.: Aspects physiologiques et biochimiques de la proteinurie d'effort. Int. Zeits. angew. Physiol. 19:337-354, 1962.

Poruchikov, E. A.: O dinamike udarnogo i minutnogo ob'ema serdtsa posie fizicheskikh nagruzok razlichnoi intensivnosti. (On cardiac stroke and minute volume dynamics after physical exertion of varying intensity) (Russ). Fiziol. Zh. SSSR Sechenov. 49:1076-1083, Sept., 1963.

Postel, S.; Tobias, J. M.; Patt, H. M.; and Gerard, R. W.: The effect of exercise on mortality of animals poisoned with diphosgene. Proc. Soc. Exp. Biol. Med. 63:432-436, Nov., 1946. (Chicago)

Pratt, Carroll C.: The law of disuse. Psychol. Rev. 43:83-93, Jan., 1936. (Boston)

Preisler, E.; and Kabza, R.: Concentration changes of some human serum electrolytes and iron in consequence of physical efforts. Bull. Soc. Amis. Sci. Poznan (Med.) 13:85-93, 1964.

---- and Pankowska, U.: Les changements de concentration du cholestérol des lipides totaux et de la glucose dans le sérum sous l'influence d'efforts physiques de longue durée. Bull. Soc. Amis. Sci. Poznan (Med.) 12:61-70, 1963.

Price-Jones, Cecil: The effect of exercise on the growth of white rats. Quart. J. Exp. Physiol. 16: 61-67, Mar. 18, 1926. (London)

Prokop, Ludwig: Die Blut-und Schweissreaktion bei erschöpfender Arbeit. Medizinische, pp. 1622-1624, Dec. 20, 1952.

----, and Slapak, Leopold: Sport und Kreislauf. Wien, Moudrich, 1958.

Prosch, F.: The effect of exercise on heart rate. Res. Quart. 3:75-82, 1932.

Puccini, C.: Considerazioni sulla insufficienza e sulla occlusione coronarica da affaticamento acuto e da sforzo nella patologia infortunistica. Minerva Medicoleg. 75:133-140, July-Aug., 1955.

Pugh, L. G. C. E.; Gill, M. B.; Lahiri, S.; Milledge, J. S.; Ward, M. P.; and West, J. B.: Muscular exercise at great altitudes. J. Appl. Physiol. 19:431-440, May, 1964. (London)

Puyou, R. P. R. A.: Contribution expérimentale et critique a l'étude de l'effort. Bordeaux, Delmas, 1938.

Pyorala, K.: Lihastyön ja urheilun vaikutus verenkiertoon. (Effect of exercise and athletics on circulation) (Fin). Duodecim 80:101-109 1964.

Quensel, W.; and Kramer, K.: Untersuchungen über den Muskelstoffwechsel des Warmblüters. II. Mitteilung. Die Sauerstoffaufnahme des Muskels wahrend der tetanischen Kontraktion. Pflüger Arch. ges. Physiol. 241:698-716, Apr. 17, 1939. (Heidelberg)

Raab, W.: Loafer's heart. Arch. Intern. Med. 101:194-198, Feb., 1958. (Burlington, Vt.)

----: Neurogenic multifocal destruction of myocardial tissue (pathogenic mechanism and its prevention). Rev. Canad. Biol. 22:217-239, June, 1963.

----, De Paula e Silva, P.; Marchet, H.; Kimura, E.; and Starcheska, Y. K.: Cardiac adrenergic preponderance due to lack of physical exercise and its pathogenic implications. Amer. J. Cardiol. 5:300-320, Mar., 1960. (Burlington, Vt.)

Radcliff, F. J.; Baume, P. E.; and Jones, W. O.: Effect of venous stasis and muscular exercise on total serum-calcium concentration. Lancet 2:1249-1251, Dec. 15, 1962. (Sydney)

Ragan, Charles; and Briscoe, Anne M.: Effect of exercise on the metabolism of 40-calcium and of 47-calcium in man. J. Clin. Endocr. 24:385-392, May, 1964. (New York)

Raine, June; and Bishop, J. M.: The distribution of alveolar ventilation in mitral stenosis at rest and after exercise. Clin. Sci. 24:63-68, Feb., 1963. (Birmingham, Eng.)

Raisz, Lawrence G.; Au, William Y.; and Scheer, Robert L.: Studies on the renal concentrating mechanism. III. Effect of heavy exercise. J. Clin. Invest. 38:8-13, Jan., 1959. (Syracuse)

Ralfe, Charles Henry: Exercise and training. New York, D. Appleton and Co., 1879.

Ralston, H. J.: Comparison of energy expenditure during treadmill walking and floor walking. J. Appl. Physiol. 15:1156, Nov., 1960. (San Francisco and Berkeley)

Rao, M.: Il comportamento dei lipidi e dei polisaccaridi citoematici nel lavoro del diabetico. Folia Med. 37:496-499, June, 1954.

Rapport, David: The nature of the foodstuffs oxidized to provide energy in muscular exercise. III. The utilization of the "waste heat" of metabolism in muscular exercise. Amer. J. Physiol. 91:238-253, Dec., 1929. (Cleveland)

---- and Ralli, Elaine P.: The type of fuel used in muscular exercise. Proc. Soc. Exp. Biol. Med. 24:964-966, June, 1927. (Cleveland)

Rapport, D. L.: The systolic blood pressure following exercise; with remarks on cardiac capacity. Arch. Intern. Med. 19:981-989, June, 1917. (Boston)

Rasch, Philip J.; and Krieger, Frederick: The effect of progressively increased exercise on heart size. J. Amer. Osteopath. Ass. 56:286-288, Jan., 1957. (Los Angeles)

----, and Morehouse, Laurence E.: Effect of static and dynamic exercises on muscular strength and hypertrophy. J. Appl. Physiol. 11:29-34, July, 1957. (Los Angeles)

----, Pierson, W. R.; and Logan, G. A.: The effect of isometric exercise upon the strength of antagonistic muscles. Int. Zeits. angew. Physiol. 19:18-22, 1961.

----, and Wilson, I. Dodd: The correlation of selected laboratory tests of physical fitness with military endurance. Milit. Med. 129:256-258, Mar., 1964. (Camp Lejeune, N.C.)

Rastelli, G. C.; Hallermann, Franz J.; Fellows, James L.; and Swan, H. G. C.: Cardiac performance during exercise in dogs with constricted pulmonary artery. Circ. Res. 13:410-419, Nov., 1963. (Rochester, Minn.)

Ratnoff, Oscar D.; and Donaldson, Virginia H.: Physiologic and pathologic effects of increased fibrinolytic activity in man. With notes on the effects of exercise and certain inhibitors in fibrolysis. Amer. J. Cardiol. 6:378-386, Aug., 1960. (Cleveland)

Rautmann, Hermann: Zur allgemeinen Arbeitsphysiologie der Leibesübungen. Sportmedizin 1:
    2-4, Apr., 1929.

----: Das Herz Skiwettlaufers, Deutsch. med. Wschr. Sonderaugabe 62:42-44, 1936.

Rawlinson, W. A.; and Gould, M. K.: Biochemical adaptation as a response to exercise. 2.
    Adenosine triphosphatase and creatine phosphokinase activity in muscles of exercised rats.
    Biochem. J. 73:44-48, Sept., 1959. (Melbourne)

Ray, James T.; Martin, O. Edmund, Jr.; and Alluisi, Earl A.: Human performance as a function of
    the work-rest cycle; a review of selected studies. Special report for the Armed Forces-NRC
    Committee on Bio-Astronautics Panel on Psychology. National Academy of Sciences-National
    Research Council. Publication no. 882, 1961.

Razzak, Muhammad Abdel: Bigeminy on exertion. Circulation 28:32-34, July, 1963. (Cairo)

Read, John; and Fowler, K. T.: Effect of exercise on zonal distribution of pulmonary blood flow.
    J. Appl. Physiol. 19:672-678, July, 1964. (Sydney)

Redisch, W.; De Crinis, K.; Antonio, A.; Bogdanovitz, A.; and Steele, J. M.: Vasomotor responses
    to exercise in the extremities of subjects with vascular disease. Circulation 19:579-582, Apr.,
    1959. (New York)

Reed, Dwayne M.; and Kurland, Leonard T.: Muscle fasciculations in a healthy population. Arch.
    Neurol. 9:363-367, Oct., 1963. (Bethesda)

Reeves, John T.; Grover, Robert F.; Blount, S. Gilbert, Jr.; and Filley, Giles F.: Cardiac output response
    to standing and treadmill walking. J. Appl. Physiol. 16:283-286, Mar., 1961. (Denver)

----, ----, Filley, Giles F.; and Blount, S. Gilbert, Jr.: Circulatory changes in man during mild
    supine exercise. J. Appl. Physiol. 16:279-282, Mar., 1961. (Denver)

Reeves, T. Joseph; Hefner, Lloyd L.; Jones, William B.; Coghlan, Cecil; Prieto, Gustavo; and Carroll,
    John: The hemodynamic determinants of the rate of change in pressure in the left ventricle during
    isometric contraction. Amer. Heart J. 60:745-761, Nov., 1960. (Birmingham, Ala.)

Refsum, H. E.: Evaluation of cardio-pulmonary function by studying the recovery of the gaseous ex-
    change after exercise of short duration. Scand. J. Clin. Lab. Invest. 15(Suppl. 76):44-48, 1963.
    (Oslo)

----: Respiratory responses to acute exercise in induced metabolic acidosis. Acta Physiol. Scand. 52:
    32-35, May, 1961. (Oslo)

Regan, Timothy J.; Timmis, Gerald; Gray, Murray; Binak, Kenan; and Hellems, Harper K.: Myocardial
    oxygen consumption during exercise in fasting and lipemic subjects. J. Clin. Invest. 40:
    624-630, Apr., 1961. (Jersey City)

Regnault, V.; and Reiset, J.: Recherches chimiques sur la respiration des animaux des diverses
    classes. Ann. Chim. Phys. Sér. 3. 26:299-519, 1849.

Rehberg; and Wissemann: Die Alkalireserve im Blutplasma bei der militärischen Ausbildung und nach sportlichen
    Leistungen. Zeits. ges. exp. Med. 55:641-648, 1927. (Marburg)

Reichard, G. A.; Issekutz, Bela, Jr.; Kimbel, Philip; Putnam, Richard C.; Hochella, Norman J.; and
    Weinhouse, Sidney: Blood glucose metabolism in man during muscular work. J. Appl. Physiol.
    16:1001-1005, Nov., 1961. (Philadelphia)

Reijs, J. H. O.: Über die Veranderung der Kraft während Bewegung. Pflüger Arch. ges. Physiol.
    191:234-257, 1921. (s'-Gravenhage, Hol.)

Reindell, H.: Die Herzbeurteilung beim Sportsmann und die differentialdiagnostische Bewertung
    der Befunde im Ekg. und Kymogramme. Deutsch. med. Wschr. 65:1369-1373, Sept. 1,
    1939. (Freiburg)

----, Klepzig, H.; Musshoff, K.; Kirchhoff, H. W.; Steim, H.; Moser, F.; and Frisch, P.:
    Neuere Untersuchungsergebnisse über Beziehungen zwischen Grösse und Leistungsbreite des
    gesunden menschlichen Herzens, insbesondere des Sportherzens. Deutsch. med. Wschr. 82:
    613-619, Apr. 26, 1957. (Freiburg)

----, Roskamm, H.; and Steim, H.: (The heart and blood circulation in athletes) (Ger). Med.
    Welt 31:1557-1563, July 30, 1960.

Remensnyder, John P.; Mitchell, Jere H.; and Sarnoff, Stanley J.: Functional sympatholysis during
    muscular activity. Observations on influence of carotid sinus on oxygen uptake. Circ. Res.
    11:370-380, Sept. 1962. (Bethesda)

Remky, H.: L'adaptation de la circulation cérébrale aux efforts physiologiques; sa démonstration
    expérimentale par l'intermédiaire de la circulation rétinienne. Ann. Oculist. 188:849-858,
    Sept., 1955.

Remmers, August R., Jr.; and Kaljot, Victor: Serum transaminase levels: effect of strenuous and
    prolonged physical exercise on healthy young subjects. J.A.M.A. 185:968-970, Sept. 21,
    1963. (Fort Sill)

Remondino, P. C.: Use and abuse of medicine, religion, physical exercise, and bicycling. Nat.
    Pop. Rev., Chicago and San Diego 5:59-61, 1894.

Renker, K.; and Adam, J.: (Blood pressure fluctuations during the working period) (Ger). Zeits.
    aertzl. Fortbild. 54:903-905, Aug. 1, 1960.

Renner, K.: (Oxygen consumption in measured work and its relation to the requirement during rest)
    (Ger). Int. Zeits. angew. Physiol. 19:56-66, 1961.

Renold, Albert E.; Quigley, T. B.; Kennard Harrison E.; and Thorn, George W.: Reaction of the
    adrenal cortex to physical and emotional stress in college oarsmen. New Eng. J. Med. 244:754-757,
    May 17, 1951. (Boston)

Rice, Hugh A.; and Steinhaus, Arthur H.: Studies in the physiology of exercise. V. Acid-base changes in
    the serum of exercised dogs. Amer. J. Physiol. 96:529-537, Mar. 1931. (Chicago)

Richardson, Benjamin Ward: Observations on Mr. Edward Payson Weston after his walk of five thousand
    miles in one hundred days. A study of vital measurements. Asclepiad 1:166-176, 1884.

Riches, H. R. C.: Streptomycin reactions; relation to exercise. Lancet 1:540-541, Mar. 13,
    1954. (Frimley, Eng.)

Richter, K.; and Konitzer, K.: Veränderungen der Aldolaseaktivität im Blutserum bei Muskelarbeit. Klin. Wschr. 38:998-999, Oct. 1, 1960. (Berlin)

Rigan, Dennis: Exercise and cancer: a review. J. Amer. Osteopath. Ass. 62:596-599, Mar., 1963. (Ann Arbor)

Rihl, J.: Die Frequenz des Herzschlages. Handbuch der Norm. u. Path. Physiol. 7(Teil 1): 449-522, 1926.

Riley, R. L.; Himmelstein, A.; Motley, H. L.; Weiner, H. M.; and Cournand, A.: Studies of the pulmonary circulation at rest and during exercise in normal individuals and in patients with chronic pulmonary disease. Amer. J. Physiol. 152:372-382, Feb., 1948. (New York)

Rinetti, M.; Visioli, O.; Colombi, L.; and Barbaresi, F.: Myocardial lipids after intense muscular work. Cardiologia 45:269-275, 1964. (Parma)

Ring, Gordon C.: Adrenalin and the metabolism of exercise. Amer. J. Physiol. 97:375-385, May, 1931. (Boston)

Riss, Walter; Burstein, Stephen D.; Johnson, Robert W.; and Lutz, Arthur: Morphologic correlates of endocrine and running activity. J. Comp. Physiol. Psychol. 52:618-620, Oct., 1959. (New York)

Ritchie, Arthur David: The comparative physiology of muscular tissue. Cambridge, University Press, 1928.

Rizza, C. R.: Effect of exercise on the level of antihaemophilic globulin in human blood. J. Physiol. 156:128-135, Apr., 1961. (Oxford)

Robb, George P.; and Marks, Herbert H.: Latent coronary artery disease. Determination of its presence and severity by the exercise electrocardiogram. Amer. J. Cardiol. 13:603-618, May, 1964. (New York)

Robbe, Hjordis: Total amount of haemoglobin and physical working capacity in anaemia of pregnancy. Acta Obstet. Gynec. Scand. 37:312-347, 1958. (Stockholm)

Robertson, George H.: Pulse and blood pressure variations during exercise and their bearing on myocardial efficiency. Med. J. & Rec. 122:213-219, 1925. (Wanganui, N.Z.)

Robinson, Kathleen W.; and MacFarlane, W. V.: Urinary excretion of adrenal steroids during exercise in hot atmospheres. J. Appl. Physiol. 12:13-16, Jan., 1958. (Brisbane)

Robinson, Sid: Experimental studies of physical fitness in relation to age. Arbeitsphysiol. 10:251-323, 1938.

----: Temperature regulation in exercise. Pediatrics 32(Suppl.):691-702, Oct., 1963. (Bloomington)

----, Edwards, H. T.; and Dill, David B.: New records in human power. Science 85:409-410, Apr. 23, 1937. (Boston)

----, and Gerking, S. D.: Thermal balance of men working in severe heat. Amer. J. Physiol. 149: 476-488, May, 1947. (Bloomington)

Robinson, Sid; and Harmon, P. M.: The effects of training and of gelatin upon certain factors which limit muscular work. Amer. J. Physiol. 133:161-169, May, 1941. (Bloomington)

----, Pearcy, M.; Brueckman, F. R.; Nicholas, J. R.; and Miller, D. I.: Effects of atropine on heart rate and oxygen intake in working man. J. Appl. Physiol. 5:508-512, Mar., 1953. (Bloomington)

Roblot, Léon: Principes d'anatomie et de physiologie appliques a la gymnastique et aux sports. Septieme édition. Paris, Lamarre, 1925.

Rodman, Theodore; Gorczyca, Casimir A.; and Pastor, Bernard H.: The effect of digitalis on the cardiac output of the normal heart at rest and during exercise. Ann. Intern. Med. 55:620-631, Oct., 1961. (Philadelphia)

Röckemann, W.: Registrierung des Ventrikelinnenvolumens am isolierten Warmblüterherzen bei einstellbarer Belastungsfunktion. Arch. Kreislaufforsch. 44:274-287, Oct., 1964.

Roganti, M.; Barbieri, G. C.; and Guarienti, F.: Il test combinato sforzo-apnea nella diagnosi elettrocardiografica d'insufficienza coronarica. Cardiol. Prat. 14:367-375, Aug., 1963.

Rohde, C. P.; and Wachholder, K.: Weisses Blutbild und Muskelarbeit. Arbeitsphysiol. 15:165-174, 1953.

Rohmert, W.: (Determination of the recovery pause for static work of man) (Ger). Int. Zeits. angew. Physiol. 18:123-164, 1960.

----: (On the theory of recovery pauses in dynamic work) (Ger). Int. Zeits. angew. Physiol. 18:191-212, 1960.

Rohter, Frank D.; Rochelle, Rene H.; and Hyman, Chester: Exercise blood flow changes in the human forearm during physical training. J. Appl. Physiol. 18:789-793, July, 1963. (Santa Barbara and Los Angeles)

Romero-Brest, E.: Clasificación fisiológica de los ejercicios. Sem. Méd. 12:1-12, 1905.

----: Ejercicio fisico sobre el desarallo de los huesos. Sem. Méd. 11:1115-1125, 1904.

----: Ejercicio sobre el desarallo muscular. Sem. Méd. 6:1187-1194, 1904.

Roncoroni, Aquiles J.; Aramendia, Pedro; González, Roberto; and Taquini, Alberto C.: "Central" blood volume in exercise in normal subjects. Acta Physiol. Lat. Amer. 9:55-65, 1959. (Buenos Aires)

Rosa, Leslie Michael; Constantino, Jorge P.; and Harris, Raymond: Effects of physical exertion on the accelerogram in young, middle-aged and old subjects without clinical heart disease. J. Amer. Geriat. Soc. 11:287-298, Apr., 1963. (Chicago and Albany)

Rose, Donald L.; Radzyminski, Stanley F.; and Beatty, Ralph R.: Effect of brief maximal exercise on the strength of the quadriceps femoris. Arch. Phys. Med. 38:157-164, Mar., 1957. (Kansas City and Wadsworth, Kan.)

Rosen, I. T.; and White, H. L.: The relation of pulse pressure to stroke volume. Amer. J. Physiol. 78:168-184, Sept., 1926. (St. Louis)

Rosenbaum, Francis F. (Editor): Work and the heart. Transactions of the first Wisconsin conference on work and the heart. (with E. L. Belknap). New York, Paul Hoeber, 1959.

Rosenblueth, Arturo: Ventricular 'echoes'. Amer. J. Physiol. 195:53-60, Oct. , 1958.
(Mexico City)

Rosenblum, D. E. ; and Mendjuk, K. : Veränderungen in der Retikulocytenzahl im Menschenblute
bei bis zur Ermüdung geführter Muskeltätigkeit. Arbeitsphysiol. 2:395-408, Jan. 25, 1930.
(Smolensk)

Rosenfeld, Isadore; and Master, Arthur M. : Recording the electrocardiogram during the performance
of the Master two-step test: II. Circulation 29:212-218, Feb. , 1964. (New York)

----, ----, and Rosenfeld, Camilla: Recording the electrocardiogram during the performance
of the Master two-step test. I. Circulation 29:204-211, Feb. , 1964. (New York)

Roskamm, H. ; Reindell, H. ; Haubitz, W. ; Keul, J. ; and Koenig, K. : (Heart size and physical
efficiency in athletes during the course of varying training loads) (Ger). Schweiz. Zeits.
Sportmed. 10:121-129, 1962.

Roskamm, H. ; Reindell, H. ; Weissleder, H. ; et al: Zur Frage der Spatschäden nach intensivem
Hochleistungssport. Herzgrösse, Leistungsfähigkeit und EKG bei 92 chemaligen Hochleistungssportlern.
Med. Welt 41:2170-2180, Oct. 10, 1964.

Roslawski, A. ; and Zywień, T. : Przypadki zesztywniajacego zapalenia stawów kregoslupa (Z.Z.S.K.)
o bezbólowym przebiegu. (Cases of painless ankylosing spondylitis) (Pol). Reumatologia 1:
291-294, 1963.

Ross, Joseph C. ; Frayser, Regina; and Hickam, John B. : A study of the mechanism by which exercise
increases the pulmonary diffusing capacity for carbon monoxide. J. Clin. Invest. 38:916-932,
June, 1959. (Indianapolis and Durham)

----, Reinhart, Ronald W. ; Boxell, John F. ; and King, Leroy H. , Jr. : Relationship of increased breathholding diffusing capacity to ventilation in exercise. J. Appl. Physiol. 18:794-797, July,
1963. (Indianapolis)

Rost, R. ; and Schneider, K. W. : Formanalyse der Farbstoffverdunnungskuven unter korperlicher
Belastung und ihre Bedeutung für die Hämodynamik. Verh. deutsch. Ges. inn. Med. 70:
144-148, 1964.

Rothlin, M. E. ; and Alsleben, U. : Kreislaufzeit und Herzminutenvolumen unter körperlicher Belastung
bei Kreislaufgesunden jungen Männern. Schweiz. Zeits. Sportmed. 12:73-79, 1964.

Rothschuh, K. E. ; and Rave, O. : Physiologie der Ermüdung. Jahresk. aerztl. Fortbild. 33:1-11,
Sept. , 1942.

Rougier, Gilberte; and Babin, J. -P. : Étude de l'activité catalasique du sang humain au repos et au
cours du travail musculaire. J. Physiologie 56:436-437, May-June, 1964. (Bordeaux)

----, and ----: Répercussion chez l'homme des exercices musculaires répétés sur l'équilibre glycémique.
Comptes Rend. Soc. Biol. 158:1064-1067, 1964. (Bordeaux)

----, and Dupuy, G. : Sur les modifications du nombre des hématies consécutives à l'entraînement musculaire.
Arch. Mal. Prof. 20:176-177, Mar. -Apr. , 1959.

Rougier, Gilberte; Joly, R.; and Dupuy, G.: (The comparative effects on cardiac rhythm of work carried out at different altitudes) (Fr). Arch. Mal. Prof. 22:784-786, Dec., 1961.

----, and Linquette, Yvette: Menstruation et exercices physiques. Presse Méd. 70:1921-1923, Oct. 6, 1962.

----, and Osouf, P.: Effet des exercices musculaires répétés sur le métabolisme basal chez l'homme. J. Physiologie 52:216-217, Jan.-Feb., 1960. (Bordeaux)

Rovelli, E.; and Aghemo, P.: Physiological characteristics of the "step" exercise. Int. Zeits. angew. Physiol. 20:190-194, Oct. 16, 1963.

Rowe, D. S.; and Soothill, J. F.: The proteins of postural and exercise proteinuria. Clin. Sci. 21: 87-91, Aug., 1961. (Birmingham, Eng.)

Rowell, Loring B.; Blackmon, John R.; and Bruce, Robert A.: Indocyanine green clearance and estimated hepatic blood flow during mild to maximal exercise in upright man. J. Clin. Invest. 43:1677-1690, Aug., 1964. (Seattle)

----, Taylor, Henry L.; Wang, Yang; and Carlson, Walter S.: Saturation of arterial blood with oxygen during maximal exercise. J. Appl. Physiol. 19:284-286, Mar., 1964. (Minneapolis)

Rowland, Lewis P.; Fahn, Stanley; Hirschberg, Erich; and Harter, Donald H.: Myoglobinuria. Arch. Neurol. 10:537-562, June, 1964. (New York)

----, ----, and Schotland, Donald L.: McArdle's disease. Hereditary myopathy due to absence of muscle phosphorylase. Arch. Neurol. 9:325-342, Oct., 1963. (New York)

Royal Society: Food (War) Committee. Report on the food requirements of man and their variations according to age, sex, size and occupation. London, Harrison, 1919.

Royce, J.: Oxygen consumption during submaximal exercises of equal intensity and different duration. Int. Zeits. angew. Physiol. 19:218-221, 1962.

----: Oxygen intake curves reflecting circulatory factors in static work. Int. Zeits. angew. Physiol. 19:222-228, 1962.

Royle, N. D.: The vascular conditions of muscular exercise. Med. J. Aust. 1:472-474, Mar. 25, 1939. (Sydney)

Rozenblat, V. V.: Heart rate in man during natural muscular activity (data obtained by dynamic radiotelemetry). Fed. Proc. (Trans. Suppl.) 22:761-766, July-Aug., 1963. (Sverdlovsk)

----: O primenenii radiotelemetril v issledovaniiakh po fisiologii truda i sporta. (On the use of radiotelemetry in physiological research on work and sport) (Russ). Vestn. Akad. Med. Nauk. SSSR 19:66-71, 1964.

Rubenstein, E. H.; Braslavsky, M. B.; and Von der Walde, F. E.: Changes in arterial pressure during physical exercise. Acta Physiol. Lat. Amer. 13:130-137, 1963. (Buenos Aires)

Rudeloff, Max: Ueber den Einfluss körperlicher Uebungen auf den menschlichen Organismus, mit specieller Berücksichtigung der Militär-Gymnastik. Berlin, G. Lange und P. Lange, 1873.

Rütte, U. von: Der Einfluss der Schwangerschaftgymnastik auf den Geburtsschmerz. Gynaecologia 132:274-276, Nov., 1951. (Bern)

Rumball, C. Aubrey; and Acheson, E. D.: Electrocardiograms of healthy men after strenuous exercise. Brit. Heart J. 22:415-425, June, 1960.

----, and ----: Latent coronary heart disease detected by electrocardiogram before and after exercise. Brit. Med. J. 1:423-428, Feb. 16, 1963. (Oxford)

Rucsteenoja, R.: Studies on circulatory, respiratory, and thermal adaptation during heavy exercise. Acta Physiol. Scand. 31:248-262, July 18, 1954. (Helsinki)

----, and Karvonen, M. J.: Exercise studies on paraplegics and bilateral above-knee amputees. Ann. Med. Exp. Fenn. 34:57-62, 1956.

----, Linko, E.; Lind, J.; and Sollberger, A.: Heart volume changes at rest and during exercise. Acta Med. Scand. 162:263-275, Nov. 10, 1958. (Stockholm)

Rusch, H. P.; and Kline, B. E.: The effect of exercise on the growth of a mouse tumor. Cancer Res. 4:116-118, Feb., 1944. (Madison)

Rushmer, Robert F.: Constancy of stroke volume in ventricular responses to exertion. Amer. J. Physiol. 196:745-750, Apr., 1959. (Seattle)

----, and Smith, Orville A.: Cardiac control. Physiol. Rev. 39:41-68, Jan., 1959. (Seattle)

----, ----, and Franklin, Dean: Mechanisms of cardiac control in exercise. Circ. Res. 7:602-627, July, 1959. (Seattle)

----, ----, and Lasher, Earl P.: Neural mechanisms of cardiac control during exertion. Physiol. Rev. 40(Suppl. 4):27-34, Apr., 1960. (Seattle)

Rusin, V. I.: Vliianie dibazola i adaptatsii k myshechnoi rabote i kholodu na zhivotnykh s spukhol'in Erlikha. (The effect of dibazol and adaptation to muscular work and cold on animals with the Ehrlich tumor) (Russ). Vop. Onkol. 9:60-66, 1963.

Russek, Henry I.; and Howard, J. Campbell, Jr.: Glyceryl trinitrate in angina pectoris. Test of efficacy. J.A.M.A. 189:108-112, July 13, 1964. (Staten Island and Westfield, N.J.)

Russell, Richard D., Jr.; and Reeves, T. Joseph: The effect of digoxin in normal man on the cardiorespiratory response to severe effort. Amer. Heart J. 66:381-388, Sept., 1963. (Birmingham, Ala.)

Rutenfranz, Joseph: (On the behavior of the pulse frequency during work under pressure of time) (Ger). Int. Zeits. angew. Physiol. 18:264-279, 1960.

----, Hellbrügge, Theodor; and Keilhacker, Elisabeth: Über das Verhalten des Blutdruckes von Kindern und Jugendlichen bei körperlicher Aktivität und in Ruhe. I. Mitteilung. Veranderungen des Blutdruckes bei körperlicher Arbeit. Zeits. Kinderheilk. 85:317-342, Apr. 5, 1961.

----, ----, Stehr, Klemens; and Oberhoff, Peter: Über das Verhalten des Blutdruckes von Kindern und Jugendlichen bei körperlicher Aktivität und in Ruhe. III. Mitteilung: Die Abhängigkeit des Blutdruckes von der Tageszeit. Zeits. Kinderheilk. 89:227-244, Apr., 1964. (Munich)

Ryde, D. H.: The effect of strenuous exercise on women. J. Roy. Army Med. Corps 103:
    40-42, Jan., 1957.

Ryzhenko, G. M.: Vplyv riznykh vydiv navantazhennia na spivvidnoshennia mizh pokaznykami
    m'iazovoi pratsezdatnosti ta funktsional'nym stansm sertsevo-sudynnoi systemy u doshkil'nykiv.
    (Effect of different types of stress on the relations between the muscle capacity index and the
    functional state of the cardiovascular system in preschool children) (Uk). Pediat. Akush.
    Ginek. 6:29-30, 1963.

Sacker, Marvin A.; Akgun, Necati; Kimbel, Philip; and Lewis, David H.: The pathophysiology of scleroderma involving the heart and respiratory system. Ann. Intern. Med. 60:611-630, Apr., 1964. (Philadelphia)

Sacks, Jacob; and Smith, Jolynn F.: Effects of insulin and activity on pentose transport into muscle. Amer. J. Physiol. 192:287-289, Feb., 1958. (Fayetteville, Ark.)

Sadoul, P.; and Durand, D.: A propos du régime stable au cours de l'exercice musculaire chez l'homme sain. Comptes Rend. Soc. Biol. 151:1008-1009, 1957.

----, McIlhany, M. L.; Aubertin, N.; and Durand, D.: Les différentes variables respiratoires au cours de l'exercice de vingt minutes chez l'adulte sain. Rev. Med. Nancy 82:773-785, July, 1957.

----, Saunier, C.; and Milic-Emili, J.: Variations de l'équilibre acidobasique chez l'homme sain au cours de l'exercice musculaire. Comptes Rend. Soc. Biol. 152:993-995, 1958. (Nancy)

Sagild, Uffe; and Andersen, Vagn: Further studies on glucose metabolism in experimental potassium depletion. Effect of insulin, glucagon, and muscular exercise. Acta Med. Scand. 175:681-685, June, 1964. (Copenhagen)

Saito, C.; Mandai, H.; Yasaki, S.; and Takenaka, S.: Investigation into influence of bodily exercise on function of circulatory system; calculated change in the impulse conduction time and the ventricular contraction time after bodily exercise. Acta Sch. Med. Univ. Imp. Kioto 14: 353-364, 1932.

Saitta, G.: L'eliminazione dei 17-chetosteroidi urinari dopo sforzo negli atleti. Folia Med. 37: 345-352, May, 1954.

Salama, S. E.: Researches on exercise. J. Roy. Egypt. Med. Ass. 35:55-68, 1952.

Salminen, Simo; and Konttinen, Aarne: Effect of exercise on Na and K concentrations in human saliva and serum. J. Appl. Physiol. 18:812-814, July, 1963. (Helsinki)

Salomon, Siegfried: Premature systoles with myocardial injury produced by exercise test. Dis. Chest 43:439-440, Apr., 1963.

Saltin, Bengt: Aerobic and anaerobic work capacity after dehydration. J. Appl. Physiol. 19:1114-1118, Nov., 1964. (Stockholm)

----: Aerobic work capacity and circulation at exercise in man, with special reference to the effect of prolonged exercise and/or heat exposure. Acta Physiol. Scand. Suppl. 230:1-52, 1964. (Stockholm)

----: Circulatory response to submaximal and maximal exercise after thermal dehydration. J. Appl. Physiol. 19:1125-1132, Nov., 1964. (Stockholm)

----, and Stenberg, Jesper: Circulatory response to prolonged severe exercise. J. Appl. Physiol. 19:833-838, Sept., 1964. (Stockholm)

Salvetti, A.; Cella, P. L.; Arrigoni, P.; et al: Comportamento della fase di ripolarizzazione ventricolare dopo sforzo e dopo iperventilazione volontaria in giovani sani. Cuore Circ. 48:192-208, Aug., 1964.

Salvini, M.; Capodaglio, E.; and Felisi, A.: Valore e significato dell'ipossia arteriosa da sforzo controllata ossimetricamente. Folia Med. 38:777-789, Aug., 1955.

Sammartino, William F.; and Toole, James F.: Reversed vertebral artery flow. The effect of limb exercise and hypertensive agents. Arch. Neurol. 10:590-594, June, 1964. (Winston-Salem)

Sancetta, Salvatore M.; and Kleinerman, Jerome: Effect of mild steady state exercise on total pulmonary resistance of normal subjects and those with isolated aortic valvular lesions. Amer. Heart J. 53:404-414, Mar., 1957. (Cleveland)

----, and Rakita, Louis: Response of pulmonary artery pressure and total pulmonary resistance of untrained, convalescent man to prolonged mild steady state exercise. J. Clin. Invest. 36:1138-1149, July, 1957. (Cleveland)

Sandberg, Lars: Studies on electrocardiographic changes during exercise tests. Acta Med. Scand. 169(Suppl. 365):1-117, 1961. (Stockholm)

Sanders, Charles A.; Levinson, Gilbert E.; Abelmann, Walter H.; and Freinkel, Norbert: Effect of exercise on the peripheral utilization of glucose in man. New Eng. J. Med. 271:220-225, July 30, 1964. (Boston)

Sandow, Alexander; and Brust, Manfred: Effects of activity on contractions of normal and dystrophic mouse muscles. Amer. J. Physiol. 202:815-820, May, 1962. (New York)

Sannerstedt, R.; Rojs, G.; and Varnauskas, E.: Hemodynamic effect of angiotensin II in minute amounts. Observations on normal subjects at rest and during exercise. Scand. J. Clin. Lab. Invest. 15:159-166, 1963. (Goteborg)

Santler, R.: Zur Bedeutung des venösen Rückstromes. Zbl. Phlebol. 2:262-265, Nov. 15, 1963.

Sarajas, H. S. S.; Konttinen, Aarne; and Frick, M. H.: Thrombocytosis evoked by exercise. Nature 192:721-722, Nov. 25, 1961. (Helsinki)

Sargent, R. M.: Recovery from vigorous exercise of short duration. Proc. Roy. Soc. 100B:440-447, Dec. 10, 1926.

----: The relation between oxygen requirement and speed in running. Proc. Roy. Soc. 100B:10-22, June 1, 1926.

Sarkar, B.; Moitra, S. R.; and Karunes, B.: Bicycle ergometer. J. Exp. Med. Sci. 4:145-154, Mar., 1961.

Sasamoto, H.: Studies on electrocardiogram during exercise. Jap. Circ. J. 28:833-839, Nov., 1964.

Sassa, K.; and Miyazaki, H.: The influence of venous pressure upon the heart-rate. J. Physiol. 54:203-212, Dec. 7, 1920. (London)

Sato, M.: Investigation into influence of bodily exercise on function of circulatory system; relation between the production and the conduction of the impulse in the heart before and after exercise in healthy and diseased persons, and the influence of the exercise on the electrocardiogram. Acta Sch. Med. Univ. Imp. Kioto 11:457-517, 1929.

Schaff, G.; and Vogt, J. J.: Effets respectifs du travail musculaire et de la température ambiante sur la fréquence cardiaque au cours du travail a la chaleur. Comptes Rend. Soc. Biol. 155:2036-2039, 1961. (Strasbourg)

Schaff, G.; and Vogt, J. J.: Effets respectifs du travail musculaire et de la température ambiante sur la température rectale et la sudation au cours du travail a la chaleur. Comptes Rend. Soc. Biol. 155:1112-1116, 1961. (Strasbourg)

----, and ----: Evaluation indirecte de l'importance respective de la charge de travail musculaire et de la charge de chaleur ambiante à partir de leurs effets combinés sur la température rectale, la sudation et la fréquence cardiaque au cours du travil à la chaleur. Comptes Rend. Soc. Biol. 156:168-172, 1962. (Strasbourg)

----, ----, and Schieber, J. P.: Valeurs respectives de la température rectale, de la fréquence cardiaque et de la sudation en vue du repérage simultané de la charge de travail musculaire et de la charge de chaleur ambiante. J. Physiologie 53:468-469, Mar.-Apr., 1961. (Strasbourg)

Scharling, E. A.: Versuche über die Quantität der, von einem Menschen in 24 Stunden ausgeathmeten, Kohlensäure. Ann. Chem. Pharm. 45:214-242, 1843.

Schayer, Richard W.: Histamine and hyperaemia of muscular exercise. Nature 201:195, Jan. 11, 1964. (Rahway, N.J.)

Scheinberg, Peritz; Blackburn, L. Ione; Rich, Maurice; and Saslaw, Milton: Effects of vigorous physical exercise on cerebral circulation and metabolism. Amer. J. Med. 16:549-554, Apr., 1954. (Coral Gables)

----, ----, Saslaw, Milton; Rich, Maurice; and Baum, G.: Cerebral circulation and metabolism in pulmonary emphysema and fibrosis with observations on the effects of mild exercise. J. Clin. Invest. 32:720-728, Aug., 1953. (Coral Gables and Miami)

Schenck, Felix: Ueber den Einfluss der Muskelarbeit auf der Eiweisszersetzung im menschlichen Organismus. Naunyn Schmiedeberg. Arch. exp. Path. 2:21-32, Feb. 3, 1874. (Bern)

Schenck, Friedrich Wilhelm Julius: Physiologie der Uebung und Ermüdung. Rede, gehalten bei Uebernahme des Rektorats am 15 Oktober 1911. Marburg, N. G. Elwert, 1911.

Schenck, W. L.: Exercise; its physiologic functions. J.A.M.A. 22:417-421, 1894.

Schenk, Paul: Winterarbeit in der Bergen und unser Stoffwechsel. Sportarztliche Erfahrungen. Deutsch. med. Wschr. Sonderausgabe. 62:36-39, 1936. (Danzig)

----, and Craemer, Karl: Der Einfluss schwerer körperlicher Arbeit auf den menschlichen Stoffwechsel. Arbeitsphysiol. 2:163-186, 1930. (Marburg)

Scherrer, J.; and Monod, H.: Le travail musculaire local et la fatigue chez l'homme. J. Physiologie 52:419-501, Mar.-Apr., 1960. (Paris)

Scheuble, E.; and Müller, E. A.: Der Einfluss von Genussmitteln und Nahrungsaufnahme auf die Pulsfrequenz während der Arbeit. Arbeitsphysiol. 14:469-476, 1952.

Schimpf, K.: Über Änderungen der Gerinnungsfaktoren beim Menschen unter Warme- und Kälteeinfluss sowie während körperlicher Arbeit. Deutsch. Arch. klin. Med. 204: 472-478, Dec. 11, 1957. (Heidelberg)

Schirlitz, K.: Über caffein bei ermüdender Muskelarbeit. Arbeitsphysiol. 2:273-297, 1930. (Hamburg)

Schlang, H. A.: The effect of physical exercise on serum transaminase. Amer. J. Med. Sci. 242:338-341, Sept., 1961. (Jacksonville, Fla.)

Schlesinger, Eugen: Die Wirkung der Leibesubüngen auf den Körper des Kindes. Klin. Wschr. 8:1481-1484, Aug. 6, 1929. (Frankfurt)

Schlessinger, Bernard S.: Influences of exercise and diet on the blood lipids of military population. Milit. Med. 123:274-278, Oct., 1958. (Randolph Air Force Base, Tex.)

Schleusing, G.: Spiroergometrische Untersuchungen der Leistungsbreite bei angeborenen und erworbenen Herzfehlern. Zeits. Kreislaufforsch. 52:828-846, Aug., 1963. (Leipzig)

----, and Noecker, J.: (The effect of potassium deficiency and loading on extra- and intracellular mineral content of skeletal musculature in untrained and trained animals) (Ger). Med. Welt 31:1579-1583, July 30, 1960.

Schlüssel, H.; Schulte, M.; Heinrich, W.; and Hamacher, J.: Sport und Atherosklerose. Ein Tierexperimenteller Beitrag. Zeits. Kreislaufforsch. 48:734-745, Aug., 1959. (Koln)

Schlutz, Frederic W.; and Morse, Minerva: Factors influencing the concentrations of the serum protein, chloride and total fixed base of the dog during exercise. Amer. J. Physiol. 121: 293-309, Jan., 1938. (Chicago)

Schmid, E.; Bachmann, K.; Haas, H.; et al: Untersuchungen über die Harnausscheidung des Katecholaminmetaboliten 3-Methoxy-4-hydroxymandelsäure (Vanillinmandelsäure) bei verschiedenen Formen körperlicher und emotioneller Belastung. Verh. deutsch. Ges. inn. Med. 70: 443-445, 1964.

Schmid, L.: Excretion of tryptophan metabolites after physical effort. Nature 189:64-65, Jan. 7, 1961. (Prague)

Schmid, Zacharias Gottfried: De Mente sana in corpore sano. Halae Magdeb., Lit. Hendelianis, 1728.

Schmidt, Carl F.: Cardiac response to exercise. Circ. Res. 7:507-512, July, 1959. (Philadelphia)

----: Respiratory response to muscular exercise. Acta Med. Philipp. 11:27-48, Apr.-June, 1955.

Schmidt, Ferdinand August: Physiologie der Leibesubüngen. Dritte Auflage. Leipzig, Voigtländer, 1921.

----: Unser Körper. Handbuch der Anatomie, Physiologie und Hygiene der Leibesübungen. Leipzig, R. Voigtländer, 1899.

----, and Kohlrausch, Wolfgang: Physiology of exercise. Philadelphia, F. A. Davis, 1931.

Schmidt, Gerhardt: Über kolloidchemische Veränderungen bei der Ermüdung des Warmblütermuskels. Arbeitsphysiol. 1:136-153, 1929. (Frankfurt)

Schmidt, H. A. E.; Musshoff, K.; Reindell, H.; König, K.; Burchard, D.; Held, E.; and Keul, J.: Die Beziehungen zwischen Blutvolumen, Herzvolumen und körperlicher Leistung. Zeits. Kreislaufforsch. 51:165-176, Feb., 1962. (Freiburg)

Schmidt, R. H.: Über die Herzarbeit in der Frühschwangerschaft in der Ruhe und nach Arbeitsversuchen. Mschr. Geburtsh. Gynäk. 90:83-99, Jan., 1932.

Schmitt, M.; Vettes, B.; Minaire, Y.; et al: Etude de la depense energetique et de la lactacidemie au cours du travail musculaire et du frisson thermique. Comptes Rend. Soc. Biol. 158: 770-773, 1964.

Schnabel, Truman G., Jr.; Eliasch, Harold; Ek, Jan; and Werkö, Lars: Cardiovascular and renal studies during exertion in adult patients with left to right shunts entering the right atrium and great veins. Acta Med. Scand. 157:241-255, Apr. 18, 1957. (Stockholm)

Schnebel, William G.; and Elbel, Edwin R.: Reaction of pulse to successive periods of exercise. J. Appl. Physiol. 4:7-14, July, 1951. (Lawrence, Kan.)

Schneider, Edward C.: Blood changes and their significance in exercise and training. Amer. Phys. Educ. Rev. 32:178, Mar., 1927; 32:250, Apr., 1927.

----, Cheley, Glen E.; and Sisco, Dwight L.: The circulation of the blood in man at high altitudes. III. The effects of physical exertion on the pulse-rate, arterial, and venous pressures. Amer. J. Physiol. 40:380-417, May, 1916. (Colorado Springs)

----, and Clarke, Robert W.: Studies on muscular exercise under low barometric pressure. I. The consumption of oxygen and the oxygen debt. Amer. J. Physiol. 74:334-353, Oct., 1925. (Long Island)

----, and ----: Studies on muscular exercise under low barometric pressure. II. The frequency and volume of respiration. Amer. J. Physiol. 75:297-307, Jan., 1926. (Long Island)

----, and ----: Studies on muscular exercise under low barometric pressure. III. The output of carbon dioxide. Amer. J. Physiol. 85:65-77, May, 1928. (Long Island and Middletown, Conn.)

----, and ----: Studies of muscular exercise under low barometric pressure. IV. The pulse rate, arterial blood pressure and oxygen pulse. Amer. J. Physiol. 88:633-649, May, 1929. (Long Island)

----, and Crampton, C. B.: The cardio-vascular responses of pre-adolescent boys to muscular activity. Amer. J. Physiol. 114:473-482, Jan., 1936. (Middletown, Conn.)

----, and ----: The erythrocyte and hemoglobin increase in human blood during and after exercise. Amer. J. Physiol. 112:202-206, May, 1935. (Middletown, Conn.)

----, and ----: The respiratory responses of pre-adolescent boys to muscular activity. Amer. J. Physiol. 117:577-586, Dec., 1936. (Middletown, Conn.)

----, and Havens, Leon C.: Changes in the blood after muscular activity and during training. Amer. J. Physiol. 36:239-259, Feb., 1915. (Colorado Springs)

----, and Truesdell, Dorothy: The effects on the circulation and respiration of an increase in the carbon dioxide content of the blood in man. Amer. J. Physiol. 63:155-175, Dec., 1922. (Long Island)

----, and ----: A statistical study of the pulse rate and the arterial blood pressures in recumbency, standing, and after a standard exercise. Amer. J. Physiol. 61:429-474, Aug., 1922. (Long Island)

Schneider, Henry P.; Truex, Raymond C.; and Knowles, Jack O.: Comparative observations of the hearts of mongrel and greyhound dogs. Anat. Rec. 149:173-179, June, 1964. (Philadelphia)

Schneider, K. W.; Rieder, E.; Lösel, E.; et al: Kreislaufuntersuchungen mit der Farbstoffuerdünnungsmethode bei Trainierten unter körperlicher Belastung. Verh. deutsch. Ges. inn. Med. 70:140-144, 1964.

Schoenewald, G.: Über Beziehungen des Blutdrucks, besonders des Amplitundenfrequenzprodukts, zum Minutenvolumen des Herzens beim Menschen. Zeits. ges. exp. Med. 79:620-634, 1931.

Schönholzer, G.: Ermüdung, Erschöpfung, Tod. Schweiz. Zeits. Sportmed. 5:65-80, 1957. (Bern)

Scholander, P. F.; Irving, Laurence; and Grinnell, S. W.: Aerobic and anaerobic changes in seal muscles during diving. J. Biol. Chem. 142:431-440, Jan., 1942. (Swarthmore)

Schreiner, Bernard F., Jr.; Murphy, Gerald W.; Glick, Gerald; and Yu, Paul N.: Effect of exercise on the pulmonary blood volume in patients with acquired heart disease. Circulation 27:559-564, Apr., 1963. (Rochester, N.Y.)

Schröder, G.; Malmcrona, R.; Varnauskas, E.; and Werkö, Lars: Hemodynamics during rest and exercise before and after prolonged digitalization in normal subjects. Clin. Pharmacol. Ther. 3:425-431, July-Aug., 1962. (Goteborg)

----, and Werkö, Lars: Nethalide, a beta adrenergic blocking agent. Clin. Pharmacol. Ther. 5: 159-166, Mar.-Apr., 1964. (Goteborg)

Schroeder, W.: Die Kapillardruck-Stromstärke-Beziehungen in den Skelettmuskelgefässen des Menschen. Zeits. Kreislaufforsch. 53:47-53, Jan., 1964. (Frankfurt)

Schwartz, Arthur E.; Lawrence, Walter, Jr.; and Roberts, Kathleen F : Elevation of peripheral blood ammonia following muscular exercise. Proc. Soc. Exp. Biol. Med. 98:548-550, July, 1958. (New York)

Schwarz, H. G.: Die körperliche Leistungsfähigkeit Jugendlicher zur verschiedenen Tageszeiten. Zbl. Arbeitsmed. 13:186-192, Aug., 1963.

Schweizer, W.: Ueber die Anstrengungs-Toleranz im Alter. Schweiz. Zeits. Sportmed. 12: 98-104, 1964.

Scott, F. H.; Herrmann, E. T.; and Snell, A. M.: Factors influencing the interchange of fluid between blood and tissue spaces. II. Muscular activity. Amer. J. Physiol. 44:313-319, Oct., 1917. (Minneapolis)

Sedgwick, A. W.: Effect of actively increased muscle temperature on local muscular endurance. Res. Quart. Amer. Ass. Health Phys. Educ. 35:532-538, Dec., 1964.

Sedgwick, S. J.: Physical education. New York, J. D. Torrey, 1860.

Segers, M.; and Delille, P.: Modifications électrocardiographiques après effort chez des sujets jeunes et bien portants. Acta Belge Arte Med. Pharm. 110:635-644, Dec., 1957. (Brussels)

----, Jongers, J. J. s.; and Lewillie, L.: Étude des agents susceptibles de modifier les mécanismes d'adaptation de l'homme à l'effort. J. Physiologie 52:221, Jan.-Feb., 1960. (Brussels)

----, ----, and ----: Modifications cardio-circulatoires survenant au repos et à l'effort sous l'influence des agents du doping. Actualites Cardiol. Angeiol. Int. 12:195-204, July-Sept., 1963.

Seghizzi, P.; Di Gregorio, D.; and Andreuzzi, P.: (Observations on changes in the electrocardiogram during exertion in a group of normal young subjects) (It). Atti Soc. Ital. Cardiol. 2:86-88, June 1-3, 1962.

Seguin, Armand; and Lavoisier, A.: Sur la respiration des animaux. Hist. Acad. Sci. (1789):566-584, 1793. (Paris)

Seguin, F. L. J.: Quelques considérations sur l'influence de l'exercice sur nos organes. Paris, Thèse No. 188, Vol. 203, 1826.

Selye, Hans: Some blood chemical changes during recovery from exhaustive muscular exercise. Canad. J. Res. 17(Sect. D):109-112, May, 1939. (Montreal)

Sereni, E.: The effects of different salts on the heat-production of muscle. J. Physiol. 60:1-19, May 21, 1925. (London)

Serzysko, W.: Wartość kliniczna oksygramu wysilkowego. (Clinical value of the effort oxigram) (Pol). Pol. Arch. Med. Wewnet. 33:667-674, 1963.

Sessa, T.; Barile, R.; and Gazzero, F.: (On the incidence of atrial fibrillation in relation to occupational activity) (It). Atti Soc. Ital. Cardiol. 2:118-119, June 1-3, 1962.

Severin, Erik: Umwandlung des Musculus tibialis anterior in Narbengewebe nach Überanstrengung. Acta Chir. Scand. 89:426-432, 1943. (Stockholm)

Sexton, Alan W.: Value of longitudinal studies of exercise fitness tests. Pediatrics 32(Suppl.):730-736, Oct., 1963. (Denver)

Sharpey-Schafer, E. P.: Venous tone: effects of reflex changes, humoral agents and exercise. Brit. Med. Bull. 19:145-148, May, 1963. (London)

Shek, M. P.: Gipertermiia u sobak i ee zavisimost'ot vodnykh resursov organizma pri myshechnoi rabote v usloriiakh vysokoi temperatury sredy. (Hyperthermia in dogs and its relation to available body water during muscular work under conditions of high environmental temperature) (Russ). Fiziol. Zh. SSSR Sechenov. 49:542-547, May, 1963.

Shepherd, John T.: Circulatory changes in the lungs during exercise. Pediatrics 32(Suppl.):683-690, Oct., 1963. (Rochester, Minn.)

Shevchuk, M. G.; and Isakova, E. N.: Vliianie dozirovannoi fizicheskoi nagruzki na techenie i restitutsiiu infarkta miokarda v eksperimente. (The effect of measured physical exercise on the course and restitution of experimental myocardial infarct) (Russ). Pat. Fiziol. Eksp. Ter. 7:42-45, Nov.-Dec., 1963.

Shevelev, I. P.: Vliianie fizicheskikh uprazhnenii na nekotorye pokazateli funktsional'nogo sostoianiia vneshnego dykhaniia u shakhterov. (The influence of physical exertion on some indices of external respiratory function in miners) (Russ). Gig. Tr. Prof. Zabol. 7:13-17, Sept., 1963.

Shkhvatsabaia, Iuk: Issledovanie dlitel'nosti faz serdechnogo tsikla u sportsmenov v uslovilakh myshechnoĭ raboty. (Determination of the duration of phases of the cardiac cycle in athletes during muscular work) (Russ). Kardiologiia 4:62-68, Nov.-Dec., 1964.

Shock, Nathan W.: Physiological responses of adolescents to exercise. Texas Rep. Biol. Med. 4:368-386, Fall, 1946. (Baltimore and Berkeley)

Short, T. S.: The manner in which the effect of muscular exercise upon the heart and blood vessels alters the expectancy of life. Med. Exam. 9:361-365, 1899.

Shulack, Norman R.: Exhaustion syndrome in excited psychotic patients. Amer. J. Psychiat. 102:466-475, Jan., 1946. (Fort Benning, Ga.)

Shul'tsev, G. P.; and Teodori, M. I.: O'krovoizliianiiakh i nekrozakh v miokarde pri chrezmernoi fizicheskoi nagruzke (kliniko-anatomicheskie nabliudeniia. (On hemorrhages and necroses in the myocardium in excessive physical exertion (clinico-anatomical studies)) (Russ). Arkh. Pat. 25:33-38, 1963.

Siehoff, F.; Muysers, K.; and Worth, G.: Les gradients d'O_2 et de CO_2 de fin d'expiration chez les mineurs au repos, au cours d'un exercice musculaire et pendant la phase de récupération Poumon Coeur 19(Suppl.): 1385-1393, 1963.

Sigler, Louis H.: Can moderately heavy work cause an attack of acute coronary occlusion? Amer. J. Cardiol. 7:305-306, Feb., 1961. (Brooklyn)

----: Myocardial infarction due to physical strain. Amer. J. Cardiol. 7:458-463, Mar., 1961.

Siltanen, Pentti; and Kekki, Matti: Effect of exercise on the formed elements of urinary sediment. Acta Med. Scand. 164:151-157, June 6, 1959. (Helsinki)

----, and ----: Observations on the urinary excretion of amino-nitrogen at rest and during exercise as compared with the excretion of some main urinary constituents. Rev. Int. Serv. Santé Armées 35:209-213, May, 1962.

Silver, Harold M.; and Landowne, Milton: The relation of age to certain electrocardiographic responses of normal adults to standardized exercise. Circulation 8:510-520, Oct., 1953. (Bethesda and Baltimore)

Simic, B. S.: Contribution to the discussion on the question of calorie requirements of various categories of people. Ernaehrungsforschung 8:769-771, 1963.

Simko, V.; and Babala, J.: Physical activity and the fat metabolism in rats. Med. Exp. 10:286-291, 1964.

----, Ginter, E.; and Cerven, J.: The influence of physical work upon the resorption of triolein I-131 in rats. Med. Exp. 8:156-158, 1963.

Simonson, Ernst: Effect of moderate exercise on the electrocardiogram in healthy young and middle-aged men. J. Appl. Physiol. 5:584-588, Apr., 1953. (Minneapolis)

----: Industrial physiology. Ann. Rev. Physiol. 6:543-577, 1944. (Milwaukee)

----: Use of the electrocardiogram in exercise tests. Amer. Heart J. 66:552-565, Oct., 1963. (Minneapolis)

----: Die Wirkung verstärkter willkürlicher Atmung auf die Geschwindigkeit der Erholung nach körperlicher Arbeit. Arbeitsphysiol. 1:87-101, 1929. (Frankfurt)

----: Zur Physiologie des Energieumsatzes beim Menschen. I. Mitteilung. Beiträge zur Physiologie der Arbeit, der Restitution und der Atmung. Pflüger Arch. ges. Physiol. 214:380-402, 1926. (Greifswald)

Simonson, Ernst: Zur Physiologie des Energieumsatzes beim Menschen. II. Mitteilung. Zur
  Physiologie des Stehens. Pflüger Arch. ges. Physiol. 214:403-415, 1926. (Greifswald)

----: Zur Physiologie des Energieumsatzes beim Menschen. III. Mitteilung. Weitere Beiträge zur
  Physiologie der Erholung bei korperlicher Arbeit. Pflüger Arch. ges. Physiol. 215:716-742,
  1927. (Greifswald)

----: Zur Physiologie des Energieumsatzes beim Menschen. V. Mitteilung. Weitere Beitrage zur
  Physiologie der Atmung und der Übung. Pflüger Arch. ges. Physiol. 215:752-767, 1927.
  (Greifswald)

----, and Keys, Ancel: The electrocardiographic exercise test: changes in the scaler ECG and in
  the mean spatial QRS and T vectors in two types of exercise; effect of absolute and relative body
  weight and comment on normal standards. Amer. Heart J. 52:83-105, July, 1956. (Minneapolis)

----, Koff, Sheldon; Keys, Ancel; and Minckler, Jack: Contour of toe pulse, reactive hyperemia, and
  pulse transmission velocity: group and repeat variability, effect of age, exercise, and disease.
  Amer. Heart J. 50:230-279, Aug., 1955. (Minneapolis)

----, and Riesser, Otto: Zur Physiologie des Energieumsatzes beim Menschen. IV. Mitteilung.
  Zur Physiologie der Übung. Pflüger Arch. ges. Physiol. 215:743-751, 1927. (Greifswald)

Simonyi, J.; Gábor, G.; Kocsis, F.; et al: Haemodynamics in patients with cardiac neurosis.
  Cor Vasa 6:26-34, 1964.

Sjöstrand, Torgny: Blutverteilung und Regulation des Blutvolumens. Klin. Wschr. 34:561-569,
  June 1, 1956. (Stockholm)

----: The relationship between the stroke volume of the heart and the capacity of the vascular
  system. Acta Physiol. Scand. 42(Suppl. 145):126-127, 1957. (Stockholm)

----: Das Sportherz. Arzt u.Sport 80:963-966, 1955.

----: Über die Bedeutung der Lungen als Blutdepot beim Menschen. Acta Physiol. Scand. 2:
  231-248, Sept. 30, 1941. (Stockholm)

----: Volume and distribution of blood and their significance in regulating the circulation. Physiol.
  Rev. 33:202-228, Apr., 1953. (Stockholm)

Skinner, James S.; Holloszy, John O.; and Cureton, Thomas K.: Effects of a program of endurance
  exercises on physical work. Capacity and anthropometric measurements of fifteen middle-aged men.
  Amer. J. Cardiol. 14:747-752, Dec., 1964. (Urbana and Washington)

Skouby, Arne P.: A method for direct measurement of aortic pressure in the dog. (During work on a
  treadmill.) Acta Physiol. Scand. 10:366-373, Nov. 30, 1945. (Copenhagen)

Skubic, Vera; and Hilgendorf, Jane: Anticipatory, exercise, and recovery heart rates of girls as
  affected by four running events. J. Appl. Physiol. 19:853-856, Sept., 1964. (Santa Barbara)

Slabochova, Z.; Rath, R.; Placer, Z.; and Masek, J.: (The influence of physical exercise on the
  nitrogen balance of obese subjects) (Fr). Nutr. Dieta 4:251-260, 1962.

Slater-Hammel, A. T.: Influence of order of exercise bouts upon neuromuscular tremor. Res.
  Quart. 26:88-95, Mar., 1955.

Sloan, A. W.; and Allardyce, K. D.: The effect of exercise and of changes in posture on the blood platelet count in man. Quart. J. Exp. Physiol. 40:161-167, Apr., 1955. (Glasgow)

Sloman, Graeme; and Gandevia, Bryan: Ventilatory capacity and exercise ventilation in congenital and acquired cardiac disease. Brit. Heart J. 26:121-128, Jan., 1964. (Melbourne)

Slonim, N. Balfour; Gillespie, David G.; and Harold, William H.: Peak oxygen uptake of healthy young men as determined by a treadmill method. J. Appl. Physiol. 10:401-404, May, 1957. (Pensacola)

----, Ravin, A.; Balchum, O. J.; and Dressler, S. H.: The effect of mild exercise in the supine position on the pulmonary arterial pressure of five normal human subjects. J. Clin. Invest. 33:1022-1030, July, 1954. (Denver)

Smedley, W. P.: Isometric contraction. New Physician 13:198-199, June, 1964. (Danville)

Smith, Christianna; and Kumpf, Katharine F.: The effect of exercise on human erythrocytes. Amer. J. Med. Sci. 184:537-546, Oct., 1932. (South Hadley, Mass.)

Smith, Edward: Experimental inquiries into the chemical and other phenomena of respiration, and their modifications by various physical agencies. Phil. Trans. Roy. Soc. 149:681-714, 1859. (London)

----: Experiments on respiration. Second communication. On the action of foods upon the respiration during the primary processes of digestion. Phil. Trans. Roy. Soc. 149:715-742, 1859. (London)

----: Hourly pulsation and respiration in health. Brit. Med. J. 1:52, Jan. 19, 1856. (London)

----: Hourly pulsation and respiration in health. Med.-Chir. Soc. Trans. 39:35-58, 1856.

----: Inquiries into the quantity of air inspired throughout the day and night and under the influence of exercise, food, medicine, temperature, etc. Proc. Roy. Soc. 8:451-454, 1857.

----: Inquiries into the phenomena of respiration. Proc. Roy. Soc. 9:611-614, 1859.

----: On the immediate source of the carbon exhaled by the lungs. London, Edinburgh & Dublin Phil. Mag. & J. Sci., Fourth Series 18:429-436, Dec., 1859.

----: On the influence of exercise over the respiration and pulsation; with comments Edinburgh Med. J. 4:614-623, Jan. 1859. (London)

----: Remarks upon the most correct methods of inquiry in reference to pulsation, respiration, urinary products, weight of body, and food. Proc. Roy. Soc. 11:561-577, 1862.

----: The influence of the labour of the treadwheel over respiration and pulsation; and its relation to the waste of the system, and the dietary of the prisoners. Brit. Med. J. 1:591-592, July 11, 1857. (London)

----: The influence of the labour of the tread-wheel over respiration and pulsation, and its relation to the waste of the system, and the dietary of the prisoners. Med. Times Gaz. n.s. 14:601-603, June 13, 1857. (London)

----: The spirometer: its construction, indications and fallacies. Med. Circular 9:294, Dec. 17; 304, Dec. 24; 313-314, Dec. 31, 1856; 10:5, Jan. 7; 40, Jan. 28; 64-65, Feb. 11, 1857. (London)

Smith, Edward; and Milner, W. R.: Report on the action of prison diet and discipline on the bodily functions of prisoners. Part I. Rep. 31st Meeting British Ass. Adv. Sci. (Manchester). Pages 44-81, 1861.

----, and ----: Report on the action of prison diet and discipline on bodily functions of prisoners. London, Taylor and Francis, 1862.

Smith, Falconer; and Smith, Willie W.: Exercise effects on tolerance to radiation. Amer. J. Physiol. 165:662-666, June, 1951. (Bethesda)

Smith, J. A.; Robinson, Sid; and Pearcy, M.: Renal responses to exercise, heat and dehydration. J. Appl. Physiol. 4:659-665, Feb., 1952. (Bloomington)

Smith, Orville A., Jr.; King, Robert L.; Rushmer, Robert F.; and Ruch, T. C.: Techniques for determination of cardiovascular response to exercise in unanesthetized monkeys. J. Appl. Physiol. 17:718-721, July, 1962. (Seattle)

----, Rushmer, Robert F.; and Lasher, Earl P.: Similarity of cardiovascular responses to exercise and to diencephalic stimulation. Amer. J. Physiol. 198:1139-1142, June, 1960. (Seattle)

Smith, R. F.: Quantitative interpretation of the exercise electrocardiogram. Use of computer techniques in the cardiac evaluation of aviation personnel. Proj. MR 005. 13.7004, Subtask 8, Rep. No. 3. U. S. Naval Sch. Aviat. Med. 1-20, Nov. 4, 1964.

Smith, Robert Meade: The time required by the blood for making one complete circuit of the body. Trans. Coll. Physicians Phila., third series 7:133-152, 1884. (Philadelphia)

Smith, Willie W.; and Smith, Falconer: Effects of thyroid and radiation on sensitivity to hypoxia, basal rate of O_2 consumption and tolerance to exercise. Amer. J. Physiol. 165:651-661, June, 1951. (Bethesda)

Snapper, I.; and Grünbaum, A.: Ueber den Milchsäurestoffwechsel beim Sport. Deutsche med. Wschr. 54:1494-1495, Sept. 7, 1928. (Amsterdam)

Snellen, J. W.: External work in level and grade walking on a motor-driven treadmill. J. Appl. Physiol. 15:759-763, Sept., 1960. (Leiden)

Sobel, Harry: Physical activity and lipemia clearance. Amer. J. Clin. Nutr. 12:399, May, 1963. (Sepulveda, Calif.)

Soetens; DeNayer, P.; Niolette, Legros; and Delfosse, J.: Discussion de l'exposé sur la diététique de l'effort. Acta Belg. Arte Med. Pharm. Milit. 110:597-599, Dec., 1957.

Soiva, K.; Salmi, A.; Grönroos, M.; and Peltonen, Tuomas: Physical working capacity during pregnancy and effect of physical work tests on foetal heart rate. Ann. Chir. Gynaec. Fenn. 53:187-196, 1964. (Tampere, Fin.)

Soler, F. L.; and Soler, C. A.: Presión arterial durante la marcha; experiencias en perros. Prensa Méd. Argent. 28:1364-1374, June 25, 1941.

Solti, F.; and Foldesy, K.: (On sinoauricular block in the effort electrocardiogram in cardiovascular diseases) (Ger). Zeits. ges. inn. Med. 17:930-933, Oct. 15, 1962.

Somerville, Walter: Coronary artery disease: relation to effort. Med. Sci. Law 3:172-179,
    Apr., 1963.

----: The effect of benzedrine on mental or physical fatigue in soldiers. Canad. Med. Ass. J.
    55:470-476, Nov., 1946. (Suffield)

Sommer, Siegmund; and Hotovy, Rudolf: Der Einfluss von 2-Äthylamio-3-phenyl-norcamphan auf die
    muskuläre Leistung von Ratten. Arzneimittelforsch. 12:472-474, May, 1962. (Darmstadt)

Sonka, J.; Gregorová, I.; Slabochová, Z.; Rath, R.; and Zbirkova, A.: Einfluss verschiedener
    Reduktionsregime auf die Aktivität des Pentosenzyklus in den Erythrozyten. Endokrinologie 45:
    174-186, Nov., 1963. (Prague)

Sonnenblick, Edmund H.: Implications of muscle mechanics in the heart. Fed. Proc. 21:975-990,
    Novl-Dec., 1962. (Bethesda)

Sorbini, C. A.; Cinotti, G.; Giusti, C.; and Valori, C.: Il comportamento del consumo di ossigeno
    durante il lavoro in seguito a somministrazione di teofillina-etilendiamina in un gruppo di
    soggetti pneumopatici. Folia Cardiol. 22:445-459, Sept.-Oct., 1963. (Perugia and Pisa)

Soucy, R.; Grégoire, F.; Lepine, C.; Laberge, M. J.; and Lapalme, J.: Modification de la ventilation
    et de l'équilibre acidobasique observées au repos et à l'effort chez 159 malades atteints de
    pneumopathie chronique. Un. Méd. Canada 87:774-786, July, 1958.

Spain, David M.; and Bradess, Victoria A.: Occupational physical activity and the degree of coronary
    atherosclerosis in "normal" men. A postmortem study. Circulation 22:239-242, Aug., 1960.
    (Brooklyn and Westchester, N.Y.)

Speck, Carl: Kritische und experimentelle Untersuchungen über die Wirkung des veränderten
    Luftdrucks auf dem Athemprocess. Schriften Ges. Beförderung ges. Naturgewissensch. Marburg
    11:173-256, 1877.

----: Physiologie des menschlichen Athmens nach eigenen Untersuchungen. Leipzig, F. C. S. Vogel,
    1892.

----: Ueber den Einfluss der Muskelthätigkeit auf dem Athemprocess. Deutsch. Arch. klin. Med.
    45:461-528, Nov. 26, 1889. (Dillenburg)

----: Weitere Untersuchungen über die Wirkung körperlicher Anstrengung auf den menschlichen
    Organismus. Arch. Vereins Gemeinschaftl. Arbeiten Förderung Wissensch. Heilkunde, Göttingen
    6:161-324, 1863.

Spengler, J.: Untersuchungen über die Wirksamkeit Leistungssteigernder Pharmaka. Schweiz. Zeits.
    Sportmed. 5:97-124, 1957. (Zurich)

Spiller, William G.: Hyperreflexia of lower limbs after exercise. J.A.M.A. 87:639-640, Aug. 28,
    1926. (Philadelphia)

Spinazzola, A.: Sul comportamento del bilancio elettrolitico nel lavoro muscolare. Rass. Med. Sarda
    66:649-664, Jan.-Dec., 1964.

Springer, W. E.; Stephens, T. L.; and Streimer, I.: The metabolic cost of performing a specific
    exercise in a low-friction environment. Aerospace Med. 34:486-488, June, 1963. (Seattle)

Sproule, Brian J.; and Archer, Richard K.: Change in intravascular temperature during heavy
    exercise. J. Appl. Physiol. 14:983-984 Nov., 1959. (Dallas)

---- Mitchell, Jere H.; and Miller, William F.: Cardiopulmonary physiological responses
    to heavy exercise in patients with anemia. J. Clin. Invest. 39:378-388 Feb., 1960. (Dallas)

Sréter, Frank A.; and Friedman, Sydney M.: The effect of muscular exercise on plasma sodium and
    potassium in the rat. Canad. J. Biochem. Physiol. 36:333-338, Mar., 1958. (Vancouver)

----, and ----: The relation of water, sodium, and potassium distribution to work performance
    in old rats. Gerontologia 7:53-61 1963.

---- and ----: Sodium, potassium, and lactic acid after muscular exercise in the rat. Canad.
    J. Biochem. Physiol. 36:1193-1201, Nov., 1958. (Vancouver)

Stadler, E.: Einfluss der Muskelarbeit in Beruf und Sport auf Blutkreislauf. Samml. klin.
    Vorträge, Leipzig, n. F., No. 688 (Inn. Med. No. 224):673-692, 1913.

Staehelin, D.; Labhart, A.; Froesch, R.; and Kägi, H. R.: The effect of muscular exercise and hypoglycemia
    on the plasma level of 17-hydroxysteroids in normal adults and in patients with adrenogenital
    syndrome. Acta Endocr. 18:521-529, Apr., 1955. (Zurich)

Stare, Fredrick, J.: Comments on obesity with some practical suggestions. Worldwide Abstr. Gen.
    Med. 6:8-14, June, 1963. (Boston)

Stark, James: Case of over-driving in the human subject. Edinburgh Med. Surg. J. 74:77-82, July
    1. 1850. (Edinburgh)

Starke, R. D.; and Bartlett, R. G., Jr.: Oxygen consumption in normal subjects performing the
    modified Harvard step test. U. S. Naval Sch. Aviat. Med. Res. Rep. 14:7p, Feb. 28, 1962.

Starkweather, E. V.: Volume changes of arm during muscular exercise. Univ. Calif. Pub. Physiol.,
    Berkeley 18:187-200, 1913.

Starling, Ernest Henry: Circulatory changes associated with exercise. J. Roy. Army Med. Corps 34:
    258-272, 1920.

Starlinger, H.; and Bandino, R.: (The influence of work in high temperature on insulin and PAH
    clearance and on electrolytic and 17-21-dihydroxy-20-ketosteroid excretion in the urine)
    (Ger). Int. Zeits. angew. Physiol. 18:285-305, 1960.

----, and Berghoff, A.: (Studies on the usefulness of endogenous creatinine clearance in comparison
    to inulin clearance in experiments during rest and exertion on healthy subjects) (Ger). Int.
    Zeits. angew. Physiol. 19:194-200 1962.

Starr Isaac: An essay on the strength of the heart and on the effect of aging upon it. Amer. J.
    Cardiol. 14:771-783, Dec., 1964. (Philadelphia)

Start, K. B.: Load and local muscular isometric endurance with occluded blood supply. J. Appl.
    Physiol. 19:1135-1138, Nov., 1964. (Nedlands, Western Australia)

----, and Hines, J.: The effect of warm-up on the incidence of muscle injury during activities
    involving maximum strength, speed and endurance. J. Sport Med. 3:208-217, Dec., 1963.

Stead, E. A., Jr.; Warren, J. V.; Merrill, A. J.; and Brannon, E. S.: Cardiac output in male subjects as measured by the technique of right atrial catheterization. Normal values with observations on the effect of anxiety and tilting. J. Clin. Invest. 24:326-331, May, 1945. (Atlanta)

Stefanik, Patricia A.; Heald, Felix P., Jr.; and Mayer, Jean: Caloric intake in relation to energy output of obese and non-obese adolescent boys. Amer. J. Clin. Nutr. 7:55-62, Jan.-Feb., 1959. (Boston)

Stegemann, Jürgen: (Energy metabolism, efficiency and behavior of the pulse frequency in dogs running on a treadmill in comparison with the corresponding data in man) (Ger). Zeits. Biol. 113:369-381, Mar., 1963.

----: Ruheumsatz und Säurebasenglichgewicht. Int. Zeits. angew. Physiol. 20:363-375, Sept. 9, 1964. (Dortmund)

----: Zum Mechanismus der Pulsfrequenzeinstellung durch den Stoffwechsel. IV. Zur Frage der Lokalisation der stoffwechselempfindlichen Muskelreceptoren. Pflüger Arch. ges. Physiol. 276:511-524, Jan. 21, 1963. (Dortmund)

Steingass, G.; Falkenhahn, A. H.; and Kenter,H.: (Muscle training and stress effect on electrolyte metabolism in rats) (Ger). Zeits. ges. inn. Med. 18:292-298, Apr. 1, 1963.

Steinhaus, Arthur H.: Chronic effects of exercise. Physiol. Rev. 13:103-147, Jan., 1933. (Chicago)

----, Boyle, Robert W.; and Jenkins, Thomas A.: Studies in the physiology of exercise. IX. The chronic effects of running and swimming exercise on the hearts of growing dogs as determined electrocardiographically. Amer. J. Physiol. 99:503-511, Jan., 1932, (Chicago)

----, Hoyt, Loris A.; and Rice, Hugh A. Studies in the physiology of exercise. X. The effects of running and swimming on the organ weights of growing dogs. Amer. J. Physiol. 99:512-520, Jan., 1932. (Chicago)

----, and Jenkins, Thomas A.; Studies in the physiology of exercise. IV. Further data concerning exercise and basal metabolism in dogs. Amer. J. Physiol. 95:202-210, Oct., 1930. (Chicago)

----, Kirmiz, John P.; and Lauritsen, Knud: Studies in the physiology of exercise. VIII. The chronic effects of running and swimming on the hearts of growing dogs as revealed by roentgenography. Amer. J. Physiol. 99:487-502, Jan., 1932. (Chicago)

Steinmann, B.; and Voegeli, H.: Über die Wirkung des Rauchens auf das Kreislaufsystem; der Kreislauf nach Arbeit. Deutsch. Arch, klin. Med. 189:319-325, 1942.

Stengel, Alfred: The immediate and remote effects of athletics upon the heart and circulation. Amer. J. Med. Sci. 118:544-553, Nov., 1899. (Philadelphia)

Stepanov, A. S.; and Burkalow, M. L.: Electrophysiological investigation of fatigue in muscular activity. Fiziol. Zh. SSSR Sechenov. 47:43-47, 1961.

Stephens, Newman L.; Shafter, Harold A.; and Bliss, Harry A.: Hemodynamic and ventilatory effects of exercise in the upright position in patients with left-to-right shunts. Circulation 29:99-106, Jan., 1964. (Chicago)

Sterky, Göran: Physical work capacity in diabetic school-children. Acta Paediat. 52:1-10, Jan., 1963. (Stockholm)

Steven, G. A.: Swimming of dolphins. Sci. Progr. Twent. Cent. 38:524-525, 1950.

Stevenson, James A. F.; Feleki, Vera; Rechnitzer, Peter; and Beaton, John R.: Effect of exercise on coronary tree size in the rat. Circ. Res. 15:265-269, Sept., 1964. (London, Ont.)

Stewart, Corbet Page; Gaddie, Robert; and Dunlop, Derrick Melville: Fat metabolism in muscular exercise. Biochem. J. 25:733-748, 1931. (Edinburgh)

Stewart, G. N.: The pulmonary circulation time, the quantity of blood in the lungs and the output of the heart. Amer. J. Physiol. 58:20-44, Nov., 1921. (Cleveland)

----: Researches on the circulation time and on the influences which affect it. IV. The output of the heart. J. Physiol. 22:159-183, Nov. 20 1897. (Cleveland)

Stewart, Harold J.: The effect of exercise on the size of normal hearts and of enlarged hearts of dogs. J. Clin. Invest. 7:339-351, Aug., 1929. (New York)

Stokinger, Herbert E.; Wagner, William D.; and Wright, Paul G.: Studies of ozone toxicity. I. Potentiating effects of exercise and tolerance development. Arch. Industr. Health 14:158-162, Aug., 1956. (Cincinnati)

Stoner, H. B.; and Wilson, A.: The effect of muscular exercise on the serum cholinesterase level in normal adults and in patients with myasthenia gravis. J. Physiol. 102:1-4, June 30, 1943. (Sheffield)

Storey, Winnifred F.; and Butler, John: Evidence that the P_{CO2} of mixed venous blood is not a regulator of ventilation during exercise. J. Appl. Physiol. 18:345-348, Mar., 1963. (San Francisco)

Storstein, Ole: Fysisk aktivitet og hjerteinfarkt. (Physical activity and myocardial infarct) (Nor). Nord. Med. 65:281-283 Mar. 2, 1961. (Oslo)

----, and Gilje, O.: Oksygenmetning i variceblod effekt av gang og av komprimerende bandasje. (Measurement of oxygen in varicose blood. Effect of walking and of a confining bandage) (Nor). T. Norsk. Laegeforen. 83:1373-1374, Sept. 15, 1963.

Strandell, Tore: Circulatory studies on healthy old men, with special reference to the limitation of the maximal physical working capacity. Acta Med. Scand Suppl. 414:1-44, 1964. (Stockholm)

----: Electrocardiographic findings at rest, during and after exercise in healthy old men compared with young men. Acta Med. Scand. 174:479-499, Oct., 1963. (Stockholm)

----: Heart rate, arterial lactate concentration and oxygen uptake during exercise in old men compared with young men. Acta Physiol. Scand. 60:197-216, Mar., 1964. (Stockholm)

----: Heart volume and its relation to anthropometric data in old men compared with young men. Acta Med. Scand. 176:205-218, Aug., 1964. (Stockholm)

----: Total haemoglobin, blood volume and haemoglobin concentration at rest and circulatory adaptation during exercise in relation to some anthropometric data in old men compared with young men. Acta Med. Scand. 176:219-232, Aug., 1964. (Stockholm)

----, and Wahren, J.: Circulation in the calf at rest, after arterial occlusion and after exercise in normal subjects and in patients with intermittent claudication. Acta Med. Scand. 173: 99-105, Jan., 1963. (Stockholm)

Strandness, D. E. , Jr. ; and Bell, J. W. : An evaluation of the hemodynamic response of the claudicating extremity to exercise. Surg. Gynec. Obstet. 119:1237-1242, Dec. , 1964. (Seattle)

Strasburger, K. H. ; and Klepzig, H. : Der Einfluss einer Kombination Saluetikum-Reserpin auf den Belastungs-blutdruck des Menschen. Med. Welt 41:2079-2083, Oct. 12, 1963.

Straub, H. : Die Dynamik des Herzens. Handbuch. der Norm. Path. Physiol. 7(Teil 1):237, 1926.

Ström, Gunnar: The influence of anoxia on lactate utilization in man after prolonged muscular work. Acta Physiol. Scand. 17:440-451 Apr. 14, 1949. (Lund)

Strømme, S. ; Andersen, K. Lange; and Elsner, R. W. : Metabolic and thermal responses to muscular exertion in the cold. J. Appl. Physiol. 18:756-763, July, 1963. (Oslo)

Strumza, M. -V. ; and Traccan, J. : Travail musculaire en hypoxie et consommation d'oxygène. Comptes Rend. Soc. Biol. 154:1412-1415 1960. (Paris)

----, and Zeghers, J. : Rôle de l'hypocapnie dans l'exagération de la consommation d'oxygène lors d'un travail musculaire effectué en hypoxie. Comptes Rend. Soc. Biol. 157:1732-1735, 1963. (Paris)

Stuart-Harris, C. H. : Shortness of breath. Brit. Med. J. 1:1203-1209, May, 1964. (Sheffield)

Stunkard, Albert; and Pestka, Joan: The physical activity of obese girls. Amer. J. Dis. Child. 103:812-817, June, 1962. (Philadelphia)

Sturzenegger, E. ; Siegenthaler, W. ; and Lüthy, E. : Der Einfluss von Guanethidin auf den Blutdruck des Normotonikers unter körperlicher Belastung. Deutsch. med. Wschr. 85:1275-1277, July 9, 1960. (Zurich)

Styns, H. J. ; and Ostyn, M. : Note sur la modification du pH sanguin observée après effort physique chez l'homme. Comptes Rend. Soc. Biol. 151:415-416, Sept. 5, 1957. (Louvain)

Suggs, C. W. ; and Splinter, W. E. : Some physiological responses of man to workload and environment. J. Appl. Physiol. 16:413-420 May, 1961. (Raleigh)

Sugiura, Y. ; Yagyu, H. ; Sawano, M. ; et al: (Studies on body constitution and physical capacities of ground national defense force personnel. 1. The current status) (Jap). Nat. Def. Med. J. 10:562-568, Dec. , 1963.

----, ----, ----, et al: (Studies on the physical constitution and capacities of the ground self-defense force personnel. 2. Effects of training on physical capacities) (Jap). Nat. Def. Med. J. 1:57-60, Feb. , 1964.

Suskind, Mitzi; Bruce, Robert A. ; McDowell, Marion E. ; Yu, Paul N. G. ; and Lovejoy, Frank W. , Jr. : Normal variations in end-tidal air and arterial blood carbon dioxide and oxygen tensions during moderate exercise. J. Appl. Physiol. 3:282-290, Nov. , 1950. (Rochester, N.Y.)

Suzuki, Kiichiro: Oxygen consumption during and after exercise and its relation to the degree of fatigue as measured by the method of electric flicker. Tohuku J. Exp. Med. 52:9-16, May 31, 1950. (Sendai, Japan)

Suzuki, T. ; Yamashita, K. ; and Mitamura, T. : Muscular exercise and adrenal 17-hydroxycorticosteroid secrètion in dogs. Nature 181:715, Mar. 8, 1958. (Nagasaki)

Svorc, J.: and Chmelík, V.: Má pracovni zatizeni vliv na vznik recidiv inkontinence moče u žen? (Does work stress have an influence on the pathogenesis of recurring urinary incontinence in women?) (Cz). Cesk. Gynek. 28:513-516, Sept., 1963.

Swaiman, Kenneth F.; and Awad, Essam A.: Creatine phosphokinase and other serum enzyme activity after controlled exercise. Neurology 14:977-980, Nov., 1964. (Minneapolis)

Swan, H. J. C.; Marshall, Hiram W.; and Wood, Earl H.: The effect of exercise in the supine position on pulmonary vascular dynamics in patients with left-to-right shunts. J. Clin. Invest. 37:202-213, Feb., 1958. (Rochester, Minn.)

Syvorotkin, M. N.: Ob ostenke sokratitel'noi funktsii miokarda. (On evaluation of the contractile function of myocardium) (Russ). Kardiologiia 3:40-46, Sept.–Oct., 1963.

Szekely, P.: Venous pressure responses to exercise. Preliminary report. Amer. Heart J. 22:360-366, Sept., 1941. (London)

Tabakin, Burton S.; Hanson, John S.; Merriam, Thornton W., Jr.; and Caldwell, Edgar J.: Hemodynamic response of normal men to graded treadmill exercise. J. Appl. Physiol. 19:457-464, May, 1964. (Burlington, Vt.)

Taggart, Nan: Diet, activity and body-weight. A study of variations in a woman. Brit. J. Nutr. 16:223-235, 1962. (Aberdeen)

Takahashi, Haruo; Iwatsuki, Tohru; Ohashi, Ikuo; and Hotta, Shuji: Some observations of the ST depression in the exercise electrocardiogram. Jap. Heart J. 4:104-117, Mar., 1963. (Nagoya, Jap.)

Tamura, S. and Tsutsumi, S.: (Studies on glucuronic acid metabolism. 12. Effect of glucuronic acid on the onset of fatigue. 1. On variations in the glucuronic acid content of human urine and serum caused by physical exercise) (Jap). Folia Pharmacol. Jap. 59:70-77, Jan. 20, 1963.

Tangl, F.; and Zuntz, Nathan: Ueber die Einwirkung der Muskelarbeit auf den Blutdruck. Pfluger Arch. ges. Physiol. 70:544-558, 1898.

Tanner, J. M.; and Jones Maxwell: The psychological symptoms and physiological response to exercise of repatriated prisoners of war with neurosis. J. Neurol. Neurosurg. Psychiat. 11:61-71, Feb., 1948. (Dartford, Eng.)

Tavill, A. S.; Evanson, J. M.; Baker, S. B. DeC.; and Hewitt, Venise: Idiopathic paroxysmal myoglobinuria with acute renal failure and hypercalcemia. New Eng. J. Med. 271:283-287, Aug., 1964. (Manchester)

Taylor, A.: Some characteristics of exercise proteinuria. Clin. Sci. 19:209-217, May, 1960. (Porton Down, Eng.)

Taylor, Craig: Some properties of maximal and submaximal exercise with reference to physiologic variation and measurement of exercise tolerance. Amer. J. Physiol. 142:200-212, Sept., 1944. (Palo Alto)

----: Studies in exercise physiology. Amer. J. Physiol. 135:27-42, Dec., 1941. (Palo Alto)

---- and Franzen, R. H.: Measures of exercise tolerance. No. 57, Rep. Div. Res. U. S. Civil Aeronaut. Admin., Washington, 1946.

Taylor, Henry Longstreet: Coronary heart disease in physically active and sedentary populations. J. Sport Med. 2:73-82, June, 1962.

----, Anderson, Joseph T.; and Keys, Ancel: Physical activity, serum cholesterol and other lipids in man. Proc. Soc. Exp. Biol. Med. 95:383-386, June, 1957. (Minneapolis)

----, Buskirk, Elsworth; and Henschel, Austin: Maximal oxygen intake as an objective measure of cardio-respiratory performance. J. Appl. Physiol. 8:73-80, July, 1955. (Minneapolis)

----, Monti, M.; Puddu, V.; et al: Studio di alcune caratteristiche fisiche individuali correlate col possibile sviluppo della cardiopatia coronarica, nel personale delle ferrovie Italiane. Cuore Circ. 47:277-292, Dec., 1963.

----, and Stamler, J.: Exercise and cardiovascular disease. A review. Nat. Conf. Cardiov. Dis. 2:358-360, 1964.

----, Wang, Yang; Rowell, Loring; and Blomqvist, Gunnar: The standardization and interpretation of submaximal and maximal tests of working capacity. Pediatrics 32 (Suppl.):703-722, Oct., 1963. (Minneapolis)

Teillac, A.; and LeFrançois, R.: Analyse des réactions ventilatoires au cours des périodes d'adaptation et de récupération de l'exercice musculaire chez l'homme. J. Physiologie 54:417-418 Mar.-Apr., 1962. (Paris)

Tělupilová-Krestýnová, O.; and Šantavý, F.: Reduziertes Glutathion einiger Rattenorgane bei Arbeitsleistung (metabolismus des Glutathions und verwandter Stoffe IV). Pflüger Arch. ges. Physiol. 266:473-477, Apr. 15, 1958.

Tenney, S. M.: Concepts of threshold and sensitivity of ventilatory control. Ann. N. Y. Acad. Sci. 109:634-650, June 24, 1963. (Hanover, N.H.)

Teodori, M. I.; and Vlasov, K. F.: Infarkt miokarda i fizicheskie napriazheniia (Myocardial infarct and physical stress) (Russ). Ter. Arkh. 35:3-10 May, 1963.

Tepper, Wilhelm; and Effert, Sven: Ein neues Verfahren zur Venendruckmessung unter Belastung. Zeits. klin. Med. 146:509-515, Apr. 22, 1950. (Dusseldorf)

Tepperman, Jay; and Pearlman, David: Effects of exercise and anemia on coronary arteries of small animals as revealed by the corrosion-cast technique. Circ. Res. 9:576-584, May, 1961. (Syracuse)

Tessari, L.; and Parrini, L.: (Muscular work-induced variations of the serum lactic dehydrogenase in man) (It). Arch. Sci. Med. 112:94-98, Aug., 1961.

Thiebault, J.; Desbois; Jatre, D.; and Robert: (Blood electrolytes and muscular exercise) (Fr). Bull. Soc. Sci. Hyg. Aliment. 51:77-84, 1963.

Thörner, Walter: Über die Zellelemente des Blutes im Trainingzustand. Untersuchung an Olympiakämpfern in Amsterdam. Arbeitsphysiol. 2:116-128, 1930. (Bonn)

Thomas, Barbara M.; and Miller, A. T., Jr.: Adaptation to forced exercise in the rat. Amer. J. Physiol. 193:350-354, May, 1958. (Chapel Hill)

Thomas, Caroline Bedell: The cardiovascular response of normal young adults to exercise as determined by the double Master two-step test. Bull. Johns Hopkins Hosp. 89:181-207, Sept., 1951. (Baltimore)

Thomas, H. Duke; Boshell, Buris; Gaos, Carlos; and Reeves, T. J.: Cardiac output during exercise and anaerobic metabolism in man. J. Appl. Physiol. 19:839-848, Sept., 1964. (Birmingham, Ala.)

----, Gaos, Carlos; and Reeves, T. J.: Resting arteriovenous oxygen difference and exercise cardiac output. J. Appl. Physiol. 17:922-926, Nov., 1962. (Birmingham, Ala.)

Thompson, G. E. and Stevenson, J. A. F.: The effect of food deprivation on temperature regulation in exercise. Canad. J. Biochem. 41:528-530, Feb., 1963. (London, Ont.)

Thompson, Howard K., Jr.; Berry, J. Norman; and McIntosh, Henry D.: Circulatory responses to hyperventilation and exercise in normal subjects. Amer. Heart J. 63:106-114 Jan., 1962. (Durham)

Thompson, J. Ashburton: Physiological memoranda on E. P. Weston's third walk. Brit. Med. J. 1:297-298, Mar. 4, 1876.

Thorp, R. H.: Effect of exercise upon the response of rabbits to insulin. Quart. J. Pharm. Pharmacol. 17:75-88 Apr.-June, 1944.

Thouvenin, Antoine Charles: Influence de l'exercice musculaire sur la constitution. Paris, Thèse no. 85, vol. 624, 1858.

Thulesius, O.: A foot ergometer for graded muscular exercise. Scand. J. Clin. Lab. Invest. 15:550-552 1963. (Goteborg)

Tigerstedt, Carl: Zur Kenntnis der von dem linken Herzen herausgetriebenen Blutmenge in ihrer Abhängigkeit von verschiedenen Variabeln. Scand. Arch. Physiol. 22:115-190, 1909. (Helsinki)

Tigerstedt, Robert: Die Geschwindigkeit des Blutes in der Arterien. Ergebn. Physiol. 4:481-516, 1905. (Helsinki)

----: Studien über die Blutvertheilung im Körper. Scand. Arch. Physiol. 3:145-243, 1892. (Stockholm)

Tikhomirov, I. I.: Ob izmeneniiakh dykhaniia pri akklimatizatsii vo vnutrikontinental'nykh raĭonakh Antarktidy. (On changes in respiration following acclimatization in intracontinental regions of the antarctic) (Russ). Biull. Eksp. Biol. Med. 57:20-23 Jan., 1964.

----: Izmeneniia so storony serdechno-sosudistoĭ sistemy pri akklimatizatsii vo vnutrikontinental'nykh raionakh Antarktidy. (Changes in the cardiovascular system during acclimatization in intracontinental areas of Antarctica) (Russ). Biull. Eksp. Biol. Med. 56:28-31, Dec., 1963.

Tilles, Jeremiah G.; Elson, Shia H.; Shaka, James A.; Abelmann, Walter H.; Lerner, A. Martin; and Finland, Maxwell: Effects of exercise on Coxsackie A9 myocarditis in adult mice. Proc. Soc. Exp. Biol. Med. 117:777-782, Dec., 1964. (Boston)

Tinti, P.; Lucchini, C. R.; and Fumagalli, C.: Variazioni del pO_2, del pCO_2 e di alcuni metaboliti durant lo sforzo muscolare nel soggetto giovane el anziano. Gior. Geront. 12:1121-1132, Sept., 1964.

Titievskaia, R. L.: Ob izmenenii krovoobrashcheniia v verkhneĭ konechnosti pri staticheskom ee napriazhenii. (On changes in blood circulation in the upper limb during static loading) (Russ). Fiziol. Zh. SSSR Sechenov. 50:1129-1135, Sept., 1964.

Tlusty, L.; and Rehor, J.: Námahová tromboflebitida na horních končetináсh. (Exertion thrombophlebitis of the upper extremities) (Cz). Sborn. Ved. Prac. Lek. Fak. Karlov. Univ. 5(Suppl.):313-316, 1962.

Tochilov, K. S.; Morozova, M. M.; Osipova, O. V.; et al: K voprosu o fiziologicheskikh predposylkakh rezhima truda. (A propos of physiologic premises of work) (Russ). Nerv. Sist. 4:176-178, 1963.

Tomb, J. Walker: Fainting, shock and muscular activity. Med. J. Aust. 2:274-275, Sept. 9, 1944. (Sydney)

Tomkins, E. L.: The dangers of excessive physical exercise. New York Med. J. 52:589-595, Nov. 29, 1890. (Washington)

Tonnesen, K. H.: Clinical application of Na^{24}-clearance during standard exercise in chronic arterial thrombosis. Scand. J. Clin. Lab. Invest. 15(Suppl. 76):64-65, 1963. (Copenhagen)

Torelli, G.; and Brandi, G.: The components of nervous regulation of ventilation. J. Sport
    Med. 4:75-78, June 1964.

----, and ----: The hyperventilation in the first 15 seconds of muscular work. J. Sport Med. 4:
    25-27, Mar. 1964.

----, and ----: (Nervous regulation of ventilation in the initial phase of muscular work) (It).
    Boll. Soc. Ital. Biol. Sper. 36:1812-1814, Dec. 31, 1960.

----, and ----: (On hyperventilation of non-conditioning origin in the initial phase of muscular
    work) (It). Boll. Soc. Ital. Biol. Sper. 36:1814-1816, Dec. 31, 1960.

----, and ----: Regulation of the ventilation at the beginning of muscular exercise. Int. Zeits.
    angew. Physiol. 19:134-142, 1961.

----, ----, and Constantini, S.: (On hyperventilation of conditioning origin in the initial phase
    of muscular work) (It). Boll. Soc. Ital. Biol. Sper. 36:1816-1817, Dec. 31, 1960.

----, D'Angelo, E.; and Pini, A.: Considerazioni sui comportamento della ventilazione alla fine
    del lavoro muscolare. Boll. Soc. Ital. Biol. Sper. 39:1747-1750, Dec. 31, 1963.

----, ----, and ----: Relazione fra regolazione nervosa e chimica della ventilazione nelle fasi di
    adattamento e di equilibrio durante il lavoro muscolare. Boll. Soc. Ital. Biol. Sper. 39:
    1750-1753, Dec. 31, 1963.

Tornvall, Gunnar: Assessment of physical capabilities with special reference to the evaluation of
    maximal voluntary isometric muscle strength and maximal working capacity. An experimental
    study on civilian and military subject groups. Acta Physiol. Scand. 58(Suppl. 201):1-102,
    1963. (Stockholm)

Torreggiani, G. C.; Mariani, M.; and Micheli, G.: Il comportamento del tratto T-U e dell'onda
    U dopo sforzo in condizioni normali, nella cardiopatia ischemica e nell'ipertensione arteriosa.
    Folia Cardiol. 22:461-471, Sept.-Oct., 1963.

----, Sorbini, C.A.; and Mariani, M.: (Changes of electrical systole in the exertion electrocardio-
    gram) (It). Atti Soc. Ital. Cardiol. 2:97, June 1-3 1962.

Toth, F.; Kelemen, J.; and Szatai, I.: Die sog. "Überanstrengungsthrombose" der Vena axillaris.
    Fortschr. Roentgenstr. 99:484-492, Oct., 1963.

Tourniaire, A.; Blum, J.; Deyrieux, F.; et al: Crises angineuses spontanées indifferentes à l'effort. Lyon
    Med. 210:1303-1315 Dec. 22. 1963.

Traube, Moritz: Gegen die Herren Vogt und Voit. Arch. path. Anat. 23:196-201 1862. (Ratibor)

Travell, Janet: Use and abuse of muscles in housework. J. Amer. Med. Wom. Ass. 18:159-162,
    Feb., 1963. (Washington)

Trethewie, E. R.: Physiologic aspects of athletic endeavor. Med. J. Aust. 1:779-783, May 12, 1956.
    (Melbourne)

Tschirdewahn, B.; Kaltenbach, M.; and Klepzig, H.: Eine dosierbare Stufenbelastung fur Arm-
 und Beinarbeit im Vergleich mit dem Fahrradergometer. Arch. Kreislaufforsch. 42:45-63, Dec. 1963.

Turell, David J.: Primary myoglobinuria and exercise-induced secondary myoglobinuria: a report of 7
 cases seen at an army basic training center. Southern Med. J. 54:442-448, Apr., 1961.
 (Houston)

----, Austin, Robert C.; and Alexander, James K.: Cardiorespiratory response of very obese subjects to
 treadmill exercise. J. Lab. Clin. Med. 64:107-116, July, 1964. (Houston)

Tuttle, W. W.: The effect of exercises of graded intensity on the leukocyte count. Res. Quart. Amer.
 Phys. Educ. Ass. 6(Suppl.):37-45 Oct., 1935.

----, and Salit, Elizabeth Powell: The relation of resting heart rate to the increase in rate due to
 exercise. Amer. Heart J. 29:594-597, May, 1945. (Iowa City)

Tyler, David B.: The effect of amphetamine sulfate and some barbiturates on the fatigue produced
 by prolonged wakefulness. Amer. J. Physiol. 150:253-262, Aug., 1947. (Pasadena)

Uehlinger, A.; and Bühlmann, A.: Das Verhalten des Blutvolumens während kurzfristiger körperlicher Arbeit. Bestimmungen mit C^{51}-und I^{131}-Albumin. Cardiologia 38:357-370, 1961. (Zurich)

Ufland, J. M.: Einfluss des Lebensalters, Geschlechts, der Konstitution und des Berufs auf die Kraft verschiedener Muskelgruppen; uber den Einfluss des Lebensalters auf die Muskelkraft. Arbeitsphysiol. 6:653-663, 1933.

Ulmeanau, F. C.: Some considerations on the study of neural control in effort. J. Sport Med. 4:158-164, Sept., 1964.

----, and Mestes, E.: Ricerche sperimentali sulle modificazioni morfofisiologiche della circolazione nell'allenamento allo sforza di lunga durata. Minerva Med. 48:1319-1323, Apr. 18, 1957.

----, ----, and Rugendorff, E. W.: Experimental radiomicroangiographic investigations during effort. Rumanian Med. Rev. 5:273-274, 1961. (Bucharest)

Ulmer, W. T.; and Berta, G.: Herzminutenvolumen und Herz-index, Schlagvolumen und Schlagvolumen-index, Sauerstoffverbrauch und arterielle und venösen Blutgaswerte von gesunden Versuchspersonen in Ruhe und bei körperlicher Belastung. Pflüger Arch. ges. Physiol. 280:281-296, Sept. 14, 1964. (Bochum and Munster)

Urschel, Dan L.: The effect of exercise on the electrocardiogram in adolescent boys. J. Indiana Med. Ass. 37:561-563, Oct., 1944. (Mentone)

Uuspää, V. J.: The catecholamine content of the brain and heart of the hedgehog (Erinaceus Europaeus) during hibernation and in an active state. Ann. Med. Exp. Fenn. 41:340-348, 1963.

Vacca, C.: Sulla possibilitá che "stress" diuersi, specie l'ipossia, permettano la fuoriuscita di enzimi intracellulari per aumento della permeabilita'della membrana cellulare senza necrosi tissurale. Riv. Med. Aero. 26:443-453, July-Sept., 1963.

----, and Vacca, L.: (Experimental control of some interesting formulae based on a new concept of the humoral regulation of respiration, useful for the evaluation of pulmonary ventilation and cardiac output during muscular work, and as an index of cardiovascular function) (It). Riv. Med. Aero. 26:223-235, Apr.-June, 1963.

Valentin, H.; and Venrath, H.: Die Differenzierung der respiratorischen Arbeitsinsuffizienz von der kardialen Arbeitsinsuffizienz unter besonderer Berucksichtigung der Links- und Rechtsinsuffizienz des Herzens. Beitr. Klin. Tuberk. 107:35-63, 1952.

----, ----, Mallinckrodt, H. von; and Gürakar, M.: Die maximale Sauerstoffaufnahme in den verschiedenen Altersklassen. Eine praktisch wichtige Herz-Kreislauf-Funktions-prüfung im Vita-maxima-Bereich. Zeits. Alternsforsch. 9:291-309, Dec., 1955.

Van Beaumont, W.; and Bullard, Robert W.: Sweating: its rapid response to muscular work. Science 141:643-646, Aug. 16, 1963. (Bloomington)

Vance, John W.: Respiratory exchange during exercise in patients with diffuse obstructive pulmonary emphysema. Dis. Chest 42:191-197, Aug., 1962. (Buffalo)

Van de Berg, Leon; Deweese, James A.; and Rob, Charles G.: Arterial stenosis and its effect on muscle work as studied by ergomyography. Surg. Forum 14:296-298, 1963. (Rochester, N.Y.)

----, ----, and ----: The effect of arterial stenosis and sympathectomy on blood flow and the ergogram. Ann. Surg. 159:623-635, Apr., 1964. (Rochester, N.Y.)

Vanderhoff, Ellen R.; Imig, Charles J.; and Hines, H. M.: Effect of muscle strength and endurance development on blood flow. J. Appl. Physiol. 16:873-877, Sept., 1961. (Iowa City)

Vanhoutte, P.: L'adaptation cardio-vasculaire du chien anesthésié à un exercice musculaire imposé. Comptès Rend. Soc. Biol. 158:2489-2491, 1964. (Ghent)

Van Liere, Edward J.: The effect of exercise on the body. W. Virginia Med. J. 54:153-156, May, 1958. (Morgantown)

----, Hess, Helen H.; and Edwards, James E.: Effect of physical training on the propulsive motility of the small intestine. J. Appl. Physiol. 7:186-187, Sept., 1954. (Morgantown)

----, and Northrup, David W.: Cardiac hypertrophy produced by exercise in albino and in hooded rats. J. Appl. Physiol. 11:91-92, July, 1957. (Morgantown)

Van Linge, B.: The response of muscle to strenuous exercise. An experimental study in the rat. J. Bone Joint Surg. 44B:711-721, Aug., 1962. (Leiden)

van Muyden, N. H.: Das Kammerelektrokardiogramm nach Arbeit, bei Herzgesunden mit dem Spannungselektrokardiographen registriert. Zeits. klin. Med. 127:192-200, 1934. (Vienna)

Vannotti, A.: Adaptation of cell to effort, altitude and to pathological oxygen deficiency. Schweiz. med. Wschr. 76:899-903, 1946.

Van Pilsum, John F.; and Seljeskog, Edward L.: Long term endogenous creatinine clearance in man. Proc. Soc. Exp. Biol. Med. 97:270-272, Feb., 1958. (Minneapolis)

Vanroux, R.: (Study of the normal 50-year-old man during muscular effort) (Fr). Acta Tuberc. Belg. 52:389-397, Sept.-Oct., 1961.

Varnauskas, Eduardas: Studies in hypertensive cardiovascular disease with special reference to cardiac function. Scand. J. Clin. Lab. Invest. 7(Suppl. 17):1-117, 1955. (Stockholm)

Vasil'eva, V. V.; and Pravosudov, V. P.: Chastota serdechnykh sokrashchenii kak pokazatel'vozdeistviia fizicheskikh uprazhenii na serdtse. (The rate of cardiac contractions as an index of the effect of physical effort on the heart) (Russ). Tr. Leningr. Sanitarnogig. Med. Inst. 72:31-38, 1963.

Vaust, J.: La gymnastique musculaire electrique employée comme moyen de dévelloper la poitrine. Bull. Soc. Sci. Med. Nat. Bruxelles pp. 56-58, 1864.

Vauthrin, L. É. Stanislas: De l'influence des exercises physiques sur les fonctions digestives. Paris, Thèse No. 180, 1860.

Vedra, Bohumir and Horská, Svatava: Effect of daily activity on renal function and electrolyte excretion in healthy and toxemic third trimester pregnant women. Amer. J. Obstet. Gynec. 90:288-292, Oct. 1, 1964. (Prague)

Velasco-Sanfuentes, A.; Acevedo-Davenport, E.; and Casanueva del C., M.: Trombosis de la vena axilar por esfuerzo. Rev. Méd. Chile 71:779-780, Aug., 1943.

Venerando, A.; Rulli, V.; and Dal Monte, A.: Influenza dell'attivita fisica su alcune costanti enzimoplasmatiche. Gazz. Int. Med. Chir. 69:2160-2174, Dec. 15, 1964.

Venrath, H.; Bolt, W.; Hollmann, W.; Valentin, H.; and Kesteloot, H.: Untersuchungen zur Frage der Blutdepots beim Menschen. Zeits. Kreislaufforsch. 46:612-615, Aug., 1957. (Köln)

Vernon, H. M.; and Stolz, H. R.: The influence of forced breathing and of oxygen on athletic performance. Quart. J. Exp. Physiol. 4:243-248, 1911. (Oxford)

Verschure, J. C. M.; Gooszen, J. A. H.; Sjoukes, P.; Maas, Johanna W.; and Strengers, T.: Studies on histamine. V. Influence of physical exertion on blood histamine. Acta Allerg. 10:136-148, 1956. (Utrecht and Den Dolder)

Vetter, Klaus; and Horvath, Steven M.: Analysis of physiological tremor during rest and exhaustion. J. Appl. Physiol. 16:994-996, Nov., 1961. (Philadelphia)

Vierordt, C.: Ueber die Abhängigkeit des Kohlensäuregehaltes der ausgeathmeten Luft von der Häufigkeit der Athembewegungen. Arch. physiol. Heilk. 3:536-558 1845.

Vinnik, L. A.; and Filimonov, Iu I.: Vneshnee dykhanie pri dozirovannykh fizicheskikh nagruzkakh u bol'nykh tuberkulezom legkikh (veloérgometricheskie issledovaniia). (External respiration under controlled physical loading in patients with pulmonary tuberculosis (veloergometric studies)) (Russ). Probl. Tuberk. 42:27-34, 1964.

Virchow, H.: Der Muskelmann Maul. Berlin. klin. Wschr. 29:703, 1892.

Visioli, O.; Botti, G.; Barbaresi, F.; Chizzola, A.; Mastandrea, R.; and Monici, M.: L'ipertrofia cardiaca sperimentale da lavoro nel ratto. Studio anatomico. Folia Cardiol. 22:473-481, Sept.-Oct., 1963. (Parma)

----, Rinetti, M.; Barbaresi, F.; Mastandrea, R.; Rastelli, G.; and Trincas, L.: The free nucleotides in the myocardium of a rat undergoing intense muscular activity. Cardiologia 45:167-175, 1964. (Parma)

Visser, B. F.; Kreukniet, J.; and Maas, A. H., Jr.: Increase of whole blood lactic acid concentration during exercise as predicted from pH and pCO₂ determinations. Pflüger Arch. ges. Physiol. 281:300-304, Oct. 22, 1964. (Utrecht)

Vogel, J. H.; Weaver, W. F.; Rose, R. L.; Blount, S. G., Jr.; and Grover, R. F.: Pulmonary hypertension on exertion in normal man living at 10,150 feet (Leadville, Colorado). Med. Thorac. 19:461-477, 1962.

Vogel, Martin: Ernährung bei Leibesübungen. Deutsch. med. Wschr. 59:1254-1256, Aug. 11, 1933. (Dresden)

Volkov, B. S.: Ob éffektivnosti kralkovremennykh fizicheskikh uprazhnenii v seredine uchebnogo dnia uchashchikhsia 5-8x klassov. (On the effectiveness of short-term physical exercise in the middle of the school day for students of the 5th to 8th grades) (Russ). Gig. Sanit. 28:78-82, Nov., 1963.

Volkov, N. I.: Oxygen consumption and lactic acid content of blood during strenuous muscular exercise. Fed. Proc. (Trans. Suppl.) 22:118-122 Jan.-Feb., 1963. (Moscow)

----, and Zatsiorskii, V. M.: Kinetika laktata v krovi cheloveka pr napriazhennoi myshechoi rabote. (On the kinetics of lactate in human blood during intensive muscular activity) (Russ). Acta Biol. Med. German. 13:659-673, 1964.

Volkov, V. M.: Gazoobmen i vneshnee dykhanie u mal'chikov pri predel'nykh tsiklicheskikh skorostnykh uprazhneniiakh. (Gas exchange and external respiration in boys performing limited cyclic rapid exercises) (Russ). Fiziol. Zh. SSSR Sechenov. 49:1456-1460, Dec., 1963.

Vuori, A. K.: Study of changes in blood coagulation time immediately after mental irritation and physical exercise. Ann. Med. Int. Fenn. 37:167-181, 1948. (Also in Acta Med. Scand. 138(Suppl. 239): 296-300, 1950.)

Vuylsteek, K.: (The determination and appraisal of the effort test in man) (Fr). Bruxelles Med. 43:641-654, June 2, 1963.

Wachholder, Kurt: Müdigkeit ein allgemeines Stress-Symptom infolge der Ausschüttung von
    ACTH? Int. Zeits. angew. Physiol. 16:361-364, 1957.

----: Ueber vegetativ-nervöse Regulierung der Herzschlagzahl beim Gehen und Laufen. Schweiz.
    med. Wschr. 71:368-370, Mar. 22, 1941.

----: Zur Entstehung der Veränderungen des weissen Blutbildes bei und nach Muskelarbeit. Int. Zeits.
    angew. Physiol. 16:356-360, 1957.

----, Parchwitz, Erika; Egli, Hans; and Kesseler, Karlheinz: Der Einfluss körperlicher Arbeit auf die
    Zahl der Thrombocyten und auf deren Haftneigung. Acta Haemat. 18:59-79, July, 1957. (Bonn)

Wade, O. L.; Combes, B.; Childs, A. W.; Wheeler, H. O.; Cournand, A.; and Bradley, S. E.: The
    effect of exercise on the splanchnic blood flow and splanchnic blood volume in normal man. Clin.
    Sci. 15:457-463, Aug., 1956. (New York)

Wahlund, H.: Determination of physical working capacity; physiological and clinical study with special
    reference to standardization of cardio-pulmonary functional tests. Acta Med. Scand. Suppl. 215:
    1-78, 1948.

Wake, R. F.; Graham, B. F.; and McGrath, S. D.: A study of the eosinophil response to exercise in
    man. J. Aviation Med. 24:127-130, Apr., 1953. (Montreal)

Wald, George; Brouha, Lucien; and Johnson, Robert E.: Experimental human vitamin A deficiency and
    the ability to perform muscular exercise. Amer. J. Physiol. 137:551-556, Oct., 1942. (Boston)

----, and Jackson, Blanche: Activity and nutritional deprivation. Proc. Nat. Acad. Sci. 30:255-263,
    Sept., 1944. (Boston)

Walser, Albert: Über den Einfluss vegetativer Pharmaka auf den Ablauf der T-Zacken-Veränderungen
    im Arbeits-Elektrokardiogramm. Cardiologia 10:231-250, 1946. (Basel)

Walters, C. Etta: Study of the effects of prescribed strenuous exercises on the physical efficiency of
    women. Res. Quart. 24:102-111, Mar., 1953.

----, Garrison, Levon; Duncan, Howard J.; Hopkins, Franklin V.; and Snyder, Jack W.: The effects
    of therapeutic agents on muscular strength and endurance. Phys. Ther. Rev. 40:266-270, Apr., 1960.
    (Tallahassee)

Wang, Yang; Marshall, Robert J.; and Shepherd, John T.: The effect of changes in posture and of
    graded exercise on stroke volume in man. J. Clin. Invest. 39:1051-1061, July, 1960.
    (Rochester, Minn.)

----, ----, and ----: Stroke volume in the dog during graded exercise. Circ. Res. 8:558-563,
    May, 1960. (Rochester, Minn.)

----, ----, Taylor, Henry L.; and Shepherd, John T.: Cardiovascular response to exercise in
    sedentary men and athletes. Physiologist 3:173, Aug., 1960. (Minneapolis)

----, Shepherd, John T.; Marshall, Robert J.; Rowell, Loring; and Taylor, Henry L.: Cardiac
    response to exercise in unconditioned young men and in athletes. Circulation 24:1064, Oct.,
    1961. (Minneapolis)

Warner, Homer R.; Swan, H. J. C.; Connolly, Daniel C.; Tompkins, Robert G.; and Wood, Earl
    H.: Quantitation of beat-to-beat changes in stroke volume from the aortic pulse contour in
    man. J. Appl. Physiol. 5:495-507, Mar., 1953. (Rochester, Minn.)

----, and Toronto, Alan F.: Regulation of cardiac output through stroke volume. Circ. Res. 8:
    549-552, May, 1960. (Salt Lake City)

Warren, John Collins: Physical education and the preservation of health. Boston, W. T. Ticknor
    and Co., 1846.

Wasserman, Karlman; and McIlroy, Malcolm B.: Detecting the threshold of anaerobic metabolism in
    cardiac patients during exercise. Amer. J. Cardiol. 14:844-852, Dec., 1964. (Palo Alto and
    San Francisco)

Waterland, Joan C.; and Hellebrandt, F. A.: Involuntary patterning associated with willed movement
    performed against progressively increasing resistance. Amer. J. Phys. Med. 43:13-30, Feb., 1964.
    (Madison)

----, and Munson, Nancy: Involuntary patterning evoked by exercise stress. Radioulnar pronation and
    supination. J. Amer. Phys. Ther. Ass. 44:91-97, Feb., 1964. (Madison)

Wathen, Ronald L.; Rostorfer, Howard H.; Robinson, Sid; Newton, Jerry L.; and Bailie, Michael D.:
    Changes in blood gases and acid-base balance in the exercising dog. J. Appl. Physiol. 17:656-660,
    July, 1962. (Bloomington)

Watkins, Arthur L.; Cobb, Stanley; Finesinger, Jacob E.; Brazier, Mary A. B.; Shands, Harley C.; and
    Pincus, Gregory: Psychiatric and physiologic studies on fatigue: preliminary report. Arch. Phys.
    Med. 28:199-206, Apr., 1947. (Boston)

Weaver, Elaine Knowles; and Elliot, Doris E.: Factors affecting energy expended in homemaking tasks.
    J. Amer. Diet. Ass. 39:205-208, Sept., 1961. (Columbus, Ohio)

Wechselmann, Amely Camilla: Untersuchungen über den Lactacidogengehalt des Froschmuskels.
    Hoppe-Seyler Zeits. physiol. Chem. 113:146-173, Mar. 30, 1921. (Frankfurt)

Wechsler, W.: (Electron microscope findings in experimental inactivity of skeletal musculature)
    (Ger). Verh. deutsch. Ges. Path. 46:300-305, 1962.

Weichardt, Wolfgang: Ueber Ermudungstoxine und deren Antitoxine. Erst Mitteilung. München.
    med. Wschr. 51:12-13 Jan. 5, 1904. (Berlin)

----: Ueber das Ermüdungstoxin und -antitoxin. Zweite Mitteilung. München. med. Wschr. 51:
    2121-2126, Nov. 29, 1904. (Berlin)

Weidmann, R.; and Klepzig, H.: Über die Wirkung von blutdrucksenkenden Medikamenten auf den
    Belastungsblutdruck. Zeits. Kreislaufforsch. 49:723-731, Aug., 1960. (Königstein)

----, and ----: Die Veranderungen des Kreislaufs und der körperlichen Leistungsfähigkeit beim
    Menschen nach Gaben von 2-Athyl-amino-3-phenyl-norcamphan. Zeits. Kreislaufforsch.
    49:1103-1108, Dec., 1960. (Konigstein)

Weis-Fogh, T.: Biology and physics of locust flight. 8. Lift and metabolic rate of flying locusts. J. Exp. Biol. 41:257-271, June, 1964.

----: Diffusion in insect wing muscle, the most active tissue known. J. Exp. Biol. 41:229-256, June, 1964.

Weiss, S.: Ueber die Bedeutung des erhöhten respiratorischen Quotienten bei forcierter Atmung und erhohter Muskelarbeit. Biochem. Zeits. 101:7-32, 1920. (Budapest)

Weisse, Allen B.; Calton, Farrell M.; Kuida, Hiroshi; and Hecht, Hans H.: Hemodynamic effects of normovolemic polycythemia in dogs at rest and during exercise. Amer. J. Physiol. 207:1361-1366, Dec., 1964. (Salt Lake City)

Weissler, Arnold M.; Leonard, James J.; and Warren, James V.: Effects of posture and atropine on the cardiac output. J. Clin. Invest. 36:1656-1662, Dec., 1957. (Durham)

Wells, J. B.; Parizkova, J.; and Jokl, E.: Exercise, excess fat and body weight. J. Ass. Phys. Ment. Rehab. 16:35-40, Mar.-Apr., 1962.

Wendland, John P.: Effect of muscular exercise on dark adaptation. Amer. J. Ophthal. 31:1429-1436, Nov., 1948. (Minneapolis)

Wenzig, Kurt: Zur Frage der Wiederbelebung mit Sauerstoff. Arbeitsphysiol. 4:503-507, 1931. (Dortmund-Munster)

Werkö, Lars: The influence of positive pressure breathing on the circulation in man. Acta Med. Scand. Suppl. 193:3-125, 1947. (New York and Stockholm)

Werner, E.; and Möhlmann, E.: Die freien Fettsauren im Serum bei Kindern unter dem Einfluss korperlicher Belastung. Zeits. Kinderheilk. 89:160-169, Mar. 4, 1964.

Wetherbee, Donald G.; Brown, Morton G.; and Holzman, Daniel: Ventricular rate response following exercise during auricular fibrillation and after conversion to normal sinus rhythm. Amer. J. Med. Sci. 223:667-670, June, 1952. (Framingham)

Whalen, W. J.: The relation of work and oxygen consumption in isolated strips of cat and rat myocardium. J. Physiol. 157:1-17, June, 1961. (Iowa City)

----, and Collins, L. C.: Work and oxygen consumption in the frog sartorius muscle. J. Cell. Comp. Physiol. 61:293-299, June, 1963. (Iowa City)

Whalley, John; Howden, Jean; and Goetzl, Franz R.: On the influence of enforced exercise upon voluntary food intake of rats. Permanente Found. Med. Bull. 9:114-118, Oct., 1951. (Oakland)

Whitaker, D. M.; Blinks, L. R.; Berg, W. E.; Twitty, V. C.; and Harris, Morgan: Muscular activity and bubble formation in animals decompressed to simulated altitudes. J. Gen. Physiol. 28:213-223, Jan., 1945. (Palo Alto)

White, H. L.; and Rolf, Doris: Effects of exercise and of some other influences on the renal circulation in man. Amer. J. Physiol. 152:505-516, Mar., 1948. (St. Louis)

Widdicombe, J. G.: Respiratory reflexes in man and other mammalian species. Clin. Sci. 21:163-170, Oct., 1961. (London)

Widimsky, Jiri; Berglund, Erik; and Malmberg, Rolf: Effect of repeated exercise on the lesser circulation. J. Appl. Physiol. 18:983-986, Sept., 1963. (Göteborg)

Wiedemann, G.: Die Beeinflussung der Blutkörperchensenkungsgeschwindigkeit durch Belastung unter besonderer Berücksichtigung der Lungentuberkulose. Tuberkulosearzt 4:465-470, Aug., 1950.

Wierzuchowski, M.: Cieżka praca miesnowa podczas dozylnego karmienia glikoza z rozmaila predkościa. (Heavy muscular work during intravenous glucose infusion at various rates) (Pol). Acta Physiol. Pol. 15:729-758, Nov.-Dec., 1964.

Wilber, Charles G.: The effect of violent exercise on tissue glycogen in albino mice. Life Sci. 8:564-568, Aug., 1963. (Kent, Ohio and Washington)

Wilcox, Ethelwyn B.; Galloway, Leora S.; and Taylor, Frances: Effect of protein, milk intake, and exercise on athletes. J. Amer. Diet. Ass. 44:95-99, Feb., 1964. (Logan, Utah)

Wilkie, D. R.: The relation between force and velocity in human muscle. J. Physiol. 110:249-280, Dec. 31, 1949. (London)

Willebrand, E. A. von: Ueber Blutveränderungen durch Muskelarbeit. Scand. Arch. Physiol. 14:176-187, 1903. (Helsingfors)

Williams, Armistead D.; and De Niord, Richard N.: The disappearance of pulses after exercise in patients having the Leriche syndrome. Virginia Med. Monthly 90:281-282, June, 1963. (Williamsburg and Lynchburg)

Williams, C. B.; Bredell, G. A. G.; Wyndham, C. H.; Strydom, N. B.; Morrison, J. F.; Peter, J.; Fleming, P. W.; and Ward, J. S.: Circulatory and metabolic reactions to work in heat. J. Appl. Physiol. 17:625-638, July, 1962. (Johannesburg)

Williams, John F., Jr.; and Behnke, Roy H.: The effect of pulmonary emphysema upon cardiopulmonary hemodynamics at rest and during exercise. Ann. Intern. Med. 60:824-842, May, 1964. (Indianapolis)

----, White, Douglas H.; and Behnke, Roy H.: Cardiopulmonary hemodynamics during exercise in patients with pulmonary emphysema. Amer. J. Cardiol. 10:46-51, July, 1962. (Indianapolis)

----, ----, and ----: Changes in pulmonary hemodynamics produced by isoproterenol infusion in emphysematous patients. Circulation 28:396-403, Sept., 1963. (Indianapolis)

Williams, M. Henry, Jr.; Zohman, Lenore R.; and Ratner, Arnold C.: Hemodynamic effects of cardiac glycosides on normal human subjects during rest and exercise. J. Appl. Physiol. 13:417-421, Nov., 1958. (Valhalla)

Williamson, Charles Spencer: The effects of exercise on the normal and pathological heart: based upon the study of one hundred cases. Amer. J. Med. Sci. 149:492-503, Apr., 1915. (Chicago)

Wilmore, Jack H.; and Horvath, Steven M.: Alterations in peripheral blood flow consequent to maximal exercise. Amer. Heart J. 66:353-362, Sept., 1963. (Santa Barbara)

Wilson, D. Wright; Long, W. L.; Thompson, H. C.; and Thurlow, Sylva: Changes in the composition of the urine after muscular exercise. J. Biol. Chem. 65:755-771, Oct., 1925. (Philadelphia)

Wilson, D. Wright; Long, W. L.; Thompson, H. C.; and Thurlow, Sylva: Changes in the composition of the urine after muscular exercise. Proc. Soc. Exp. Biol. Med. 21:425-426, May, 1924. (Philadelphia)

Wilson, May G.: Circulatory reactions in normal children after exercise. Arch. Pediat. 37:368-371, June, 1920. (New York)

Wilson, Michael F.: Left ventricular diameter, posture, and exercise. Circ. Res. 11:90-95, July, 1962. (Lexington)

Wilson, Vernon H.: Femoral venous blood oxygen studies upon normal and abnormal subjects at rest and after exercise. S. Afr. J. Med. Sci. 15:115-119, Dec., 1950. (Johannesburg)

----: Serial femoral venous blood oxygen studies at rest, after exercise and during recovery from exercise in normal subjects and in patients with heart failure. S. Afr. J. Med. Sci. 19:161-164, Dec., 1954. (Johannesburg)

Winter, Charles A.; and Flataker, Lars: Work performance of trained rats as affected by corticoadrenal steroids and by adrenalectomy. Amer. J. Physiol. 199:863-866, Nov., 1960. (West Point)

Winter, W.: Physiologische Unterstützung mit Antacid bei Ermüdung und Erschöpfung unter körperlicher Belastung. Med. Klin. 53:2195-2196, Dec. 19, 1958.

Winterstein, Hans: Die Regulierung der Atmung durch das Blut. Pflüger Arch. ges. Physiol. 138:167-184, Feb. 9, 1911. (Rostock)

Witzleb, E.; Bartels, H.; Budde, H.; and Mochizucki, M.: Der Einfluss des arteriellen O_2-Drucks auf die chemoreceptorischen Aktionspotentiale im Carotissinusnerven. Pflüger Arch. ges. Physiol. 261:211-218, July 12, 1955. (Hamburg and Gottingen)

Wolf, J. G.: Effects of posture and muscular exercise on electrocardiogram. Res. Quart. 24:475-490, Dec., 1953.

Wolf-Heidegger, G.: Über den Einfluss systematisch betriebener Leibesübungen auf den Thoraxumfang der Frau. Schweiz. med. Wschr. 83:917-919, Sept. 26, 1953. (Basel)

Wolffe, Joseph B.: The heart of the athlete. J. Lancet 77:76-78, Mar., 1957. (Fairview Village, Pa.)

Wood, J. Edwin: The mechanism of the increased venous pressure with exercise in congestive heart failure. J. Clin. Invest. 41:2020-2024, Nov., 1962. (Augusta)

----, and Bass, David E.: Responses of the veins and arterioles of the forearm to walking during acclimatization to heat in man. J. Clin. Invest. 39:825-833, June, 1960. (Natick and Boston)

Workman, John M.; and Armstrong, Bruce W.: A nomogram for predicting treadmill-walking oxygen consumption. J. Appl. Physiol. 19:150-151, Jan., 1964. (Baltimore)

----, and ----: Oxygen cost of treadmill walking. J. Appl. Physiol. 18:798-803, July, 1963. (Baltimore)

Worth, G.; Muysers, K.; and Siehoff, F.: Zur Problematik der Normwerte der arteriellen O_2- und CO_2-Partialdrucke sowie der alveolo-arteriellen O_2- und CO_2-Druckgradienten im Rahmen arbeitsmedizinischer Fragen. Med. Thorac. 20:223-234, 1963.

Wright, Elizabeth A.: Correlation of respiration and heart beat during exercise. Boston Med. & Surg. J. 162:417-424, Mar. 31, 1910. (Boston)

Wright, George W.: Maximum oxygen consumption for work periods of six minutes' duration in normal and pathological subjects. Science 112:423-424, Oct. 13, 1950.

Wuschech, H.; Köhler, W.; Friedel, W.; et al: Zur Verhalten der freien Fettsauren und des Blutzuckers bei Sporttreibenden nach dosierter Fahrradergometerbelastung. Deutsch. Gesundh. 19:1668-1670, Sept. 3, 1964.

Wyndham, C. H.; Merwe-Bouwer, W. van der; Devine, M. G.; and Paterson, H. E.: Effect of exercise and environment on urine secretion after a water load. J. Appl. Physiol. 5:285-289, Dec., 1952. (Johannesburg)

----, Strydom, N. B.; Maritz, J. S.; Morrison, J. F.; Peter, J.; and Potgieter, Z. U.: Maximum oxygen intake and maximum heart rate during strenuous work. J. Appl. Physiol. 14:927-936, Nov., 1959. (Johannesburg)

----, ----, Morrison, J. F.; Du Toit, F. D.; and Kraan, J. G.: Responses of unacclimatized men under stress of heat and work. J. Appl. Physiol. 6:681-686, May, 1954. (Johannesburg)

----, ----, ----, ----, and ----: Thermal responses of men with high initial temperatures to stress of heat and work. J. Appl. Physiol. 6:687-690, May, 1954. (Johannesburg)

----, ----, ----, Peter, J.; Williams, C. G.; Bredell, G. A. G.; and Joffe, A.: Differences between ethnic groups in physical working capacity. J. Appl. Physiol. 18:361-366, Mar., 1963. (Johannesburg)

----, ----, Williams, C. G.; and von Rahden, M.: A physiological basis for the 'optimum' level of energy expenditure. Nature 195:1210-1212, Sept. 22, 1962. (Johannesburg)

----, Walker, S. E.; and Morrison, J. F.: 24-hour metabolisms of sedentary people. S. Afr. J. Lab. Clin. Med. 10:1-7, Apr. 4, 1964. (Witwatersrand and Johannesburg)

Yagyu, M.; Sawano, M.; Sugiura, U.; et al: (The present status of physical constitution and capacities of the ground self-defence force personnel) (Jap). Nat. Def. Med. J. 11:61-62, Feb., 1964.

Yang, T. L.; and Endroczi, E.: The effect of work performed in hypothermia and hyperthermia on pituitary-adrenocortical function. Acta Physiol. Acad. Sci. Hung. 18:131-136, 1960.

Yo, B.: Influence of bodily exercise upon blood pressure. (Abstract) Far East Sci. Bull. 2:89, Dec., 1942.

Yoder, J. T.; Kingrey, B. W.; and Dragstedt, L. R. II: Physical fitness in the confined dog: criteria and monitoring of muscular performance. Amer. J. Vet. Res. 25:727-738, May, 1964. (Ames and Des Moines)

Young, Allan C.: Dead space at rest and during exercise. J. Appl. Physiol. 8:91-94, July, 1955. (Seattle)

Young, D. R.: Effect of body composition and weight gain on performance in the adult dog. J. Appl. Physiol. 15:493-495, May, 1960. (Chicago)

----: Effect of food deprivation on treadmill running in dogs. J. Appl. Physiol. 14:1018-1022, Nov., 1959. (Chicago)

----, Mosher, R.; Erve, P.; and Spector, H.: Body temperature and heat exchange during treadmill running in dogs. J. Appl. Physiol. 14:839-843, Sept., 1959. (Chicago)

----, ----, ----, and ----: Energy metabolism and gas exchange during treadmill running in dogs. J. Appl. Physiol. 14:834-838, Sept., 1959. (Chicago)

----, and Price, R.: Utilization of body energy reserves during work in dogs. J. Appl. Physiol. 16:351-354, Mar., 1961. (Chicago)

----, ----, Elder, N. E.; and Adachi, R. R.: Energy and electrolyte metabolism and adrenal responses during work in dogs. J. Appl. Physiol. 17:669-674, July, 1962. (Chicago)

----, Schafer, N. S.; and Price, R.: Effect of nutrient supplements during work on performance capacity in dogs. J. Appl. Physiol. 15:1022-1026, November, 1960. (Chicago)

Young, W. J.; and Breinl, A.; Harris, J. J.; and Osborne, W. A.: Effect of exercise and humid heat upon pulse rate, blood pressure, body temperature and blood concentration. Proc. Roy. Soc. 91B:111-126, Jan. 1, 1920. (Townsville, Australia)

Yu, Paul N. G.; Yim, Bernard J. B.; and Stanfield, C. Alphens: Hyperventilation syndrome. Changes in the electrocardiogram, blood gases, and electrolytes during voluntary hyperventilation, possible mechanisms and clinical implications. Arch. Intern. Med. 103:902-913, June, 1959. (Rochester, N.Y.)

Zachu-Christiansen, B.: The rise in serum uric acid during muscular exercise. Scand. J. Clin. Lab. Invest. 11:57-60, 1959. (Copenhagen)

Zambrano, A.: Variazioni dell'attivita fosfatasica del siero di sangue di soggetti normali e di soggetti diabetici sottoposti a lavoro. Folia Med. 35:143-151, Mar., 1952.

Zander, R.: Einfluss der Körperübungen auf Herz und Lungen. Gesundh. in Wort und Bild, Berlin, 1904.

Zannini, D.: Sull'attitudine al lavoro in condizioni di sovraccarico calorico. Rass. Med. Industr. 32: 409-411, May-Aug., 1963.

Záruba, K.: Effect of severe physical exercise on the kidneys. Med. Exp. 11:233-238, 1964.

Zöllner, Nepomuk; and König, Erwin: Veränderungen des Belastungsvenendruckes durch die Wirkung von Herzglykosiden. Zeits. Kreislaufforsch. 47:31-39, Jan., 1958. (Munich)

Zubek, John P.: Counteracting effects of physical exercises performed during prolonged perceptual deprivation. Science 142:504-506, Oct. 25, 1963. (Winnipeg)

Zuntz, Nathan: Einfluss der Geschwindigkeit, der Körpertemperatur und der Uebung auf den Stoffverbrauch bei Ruhe und bei Muskelarbeit. Pflüger Arch. ges. Physiol. 95:192-208, Mar. 30, 1903. (Berlin)

----: Die Ergebnisse der jungsten Arbeiten über Herzthatigkeit und Kreislauf. Deutsch. Zeits. Thiermed. 18:261-277, April 28, 1892.

----: Die Ernährung des Herzens und ihre Beziehung zu seiner Arbeitsleistung. Deutsch. med. Wschr. 18:109-111, Feb. 11, 1892. (Berlin)

----: Ueber Beziehung zwischen Arbeit und Stoffwechsel bei Thieren nach Versuchen der Professoren Lehmann und Zuntz. Tagebl. Versamml. deutsch. Naturf. Aerzte. 61:70, 1889.

----: Ueber den Stoffverbrauch des Hundes bei Muskelarbeit. Pflüger Arch. ges. Physiol. 68:191-211, 1897.

----: Ueber die Warmeregulierung bei Muskelarbeit. Berlin. klin. Wschr. 33:709, 1896.

----: Wirkungen des Gehens, Bergsteigens, und anderer Muskelbewegungen auf den Stoffwechsel. Deutsch. med. Zeitung 9:281-283, 1890.

----, and Geppert, J.: Nochmals über den Einfluss der Muskeltätigkeit auf der Atmung. Deutsch. Arch. klin. Med. 48:444-445, Aug. 6, 1891.

----, ----- Ueber die Natur der normalen Atemreize und den Ort ihrer Wirkung. Pflüger Arch. ges. Physiol. 38:337-338, 1886.

----, and Hagemann, Oscar: Untersuchungen über den Stoffwechsel des Pferdes bei Ruhe und Arbeit. Neue Folge unter Mitwirkung von Curt Lehmann und Johannes Frentzel. Berlin, P. Parey, 1898.

----, and Lehmann, Curt: Remarks on the chemistry of respiration in the horse during rest and work. J. Physiol. 11:396-398, 1890. (Berlin)

----, and Loewy, Adolf (Editors): Lehrbuch der Physiologie des Menschen. Unter Mitwirkung der Herren du Bois-Reymond, Cohnheim (et al). Second edition. Leipzig, F. C. W. Vogel, 1909.

Zuntz, Nathan; and Schumberg, W. A. E. F.: Studien zu einer Physiologie des Menschen. Berlin; A. Hirschwald; 1901.

Part Two   Subject Index

A

Accelerogram

effects of physical exertion in young, middle-aged and old subjects, without clinical heart disease
(Rosa and others) J. Amer. Geriat. Soc. 11:287-298, 1963

Acetone bodies

in blood of diabetic children after exercise (Akerblom & Maijala) Ann. Paediat. Fenn. 10:36-41,
1964

Acetylene

and dye injection methods to determine cardiac output (Asmussen and Nielsen) Acta Physiol. Scand.
27:230, 1953

use in determination of cardiac output (Grollman) Amer. J. Physiol. 88:432-443, 1929

Acid-base equilibrium

.acidosis, mechanism, during muscular effort (Bugyi) Poumon Coeur 15:1021-1023, 1959

acidosis, metabolic, induced, respiratory response to acute exercise (Refsum) Acta Physiol. Scand.
52:32-35, 1961

arterial blood gas analysis using Fleish's metabograph; determination of ventilation and acid-base balance
in heavy work (Abelin and Scherrer) Schweiz. med. Wschr. 90:369-374, 1960

arterial blood, and pH during exercise, effect of temperature (Holmgren and McIllroy) J. Appl. Physiol.
19:243-245, 1964

arterial gas tensions and ventilation, time-courses of changes in, induced by exercise (Matell) Acta Physiol.
Scand. 58(Suppl. 206):1-53, 1963

in blood and cerebrospinal fluid during muscular exercise (Leusen and others) J. Physiologie 52:151-152,
1960

and blood gases, changes in exercise, dog (Wathen and others) J. Appl. Physiol. 17:656-660, 1962

and blood gases, changes during muscular activity (De Lanne and others) J. Appl. Physiol. 14:328-332,
1959

changes during muscular exercise, healthy adult (Sadoul and others) Comptes Rend. Soc. Biol. 152:993-995,
1958

changes following short periods of vigorous muscular exercise (Barr and others) J. Biol. Chem. 55:495-523,
1923.

changes in serum of exercised dogs (Rice and Steinhaus) Amer. J. Physiol. 96:529-537, 1931

changes, interpretation, and application to exercise (Hastings and Steinhaus) Amer. J. Physiol. 96:538-540,
1931

Acid-base equilibrium (Cont.)

 central and chemoreflex components in respiratory activity during acid-base displacements in blood
  (Hesser) Acta Physiol. Scand. 18(Suppl. 64):5-69; appendix, 1949

 development and duration of changes after exercise (Barr and Himwich) J. Biol. Chem. 55:539-555, 1923

 hydrogen-ion concentration and CO_2 pressure in cerebrospinal fluid, influence on respiration (Loeschcke
  and others) Pflüger Arch. ges. Physiol. 266:569-585, 1958

 hydrogen-ion concentration, effect on recovery process in muscle (Hartree and Hill) J. Physiol. 58:470-
  479, 1924

 neutrality regulation, theory, animal organism (Henderson) Amer. J. Physiol. 21:427-448, 1908; Ergebn.
  Physiol. 8:254-325, 1909

 pH changes in striated muscle after contraction, man and rabbit (Maison and others) Amer. J. Physiol. 121:
  311-324, 1938

 pH, influence of muscular effort (Coster and others) Comptes Rend. Soc. Biol. 106:1937-1939, 1962

 physical-chemical system of blood; relation to respiration and circulation (Hochrein and others) Naunyn
  Schmiedeberg Arch. exp. Path. 143:129-146, 1929.

 physical-chemical system of blood; relation to respiration and circulation; ionic changes at rest and work
  (Edwards and others) Naunyn Schmiedeberg Arch. exp. Path. 143:161-169, 1929

 and resting metabolism (Stegemann) Int. Zeits. angew. Physiol. 20:363-375, 1964

 urine, changes after physical exercise (Goiffon and Chauvois) Comptes Rend. Soc. Biol. 100:330-332,
  1929

 and ventilation (Lowe) Bull. Millard Fillmore Hosp. 10:11-12, 1963

 and ventilation during heavy work, Fleisch metabograph (Abelin and Scherrer) Schweiz. med. Wschr. 90:
  369-374, 1960

 and ventilation, rest and effort, chronic pneumopathy (Soucy and others) Union Méd. Canada 87:774-786,
  1958

Acid phosphatase

 activity, adrenal medulla, histochemistry, effect of muscular work and denervation, rat (Eranko and Harkonen)
  Ann. Med. Exp. Fenn. 40:129-133, 1962

ACTH

 distribution, relation to fatigue, a general stress-symptom (Wachholder) Internat. Zeits. Angewand. Physiol.
  16:361-364, 1957

Adaptation

 circulation, cerebral, to physiological effort (Remky) Ann. Ocul. 188:849-858, 1955

 circulatory, respiratory, and thermal, during heavy exercise (Ruosteenoja) Acta Physiol. Scand. 31:248-262,
  1954

 dark, effect of muscular exercise (Wendland) Amer. J. Ophthal. 31:1429-1436, 1948.

Adaptation (Cont.)

    to effort, effect on nitrogen balance (Gontzea and others) Arch. Sci. Physiol. 16:127-138, 1962

    to effort, mechanisms (Segers and others) J. Physiologie 52:221, 1960

    to forced exercise, rat (Thomas and Miller) Amer. J. Physiol. 193:350-354, 1958

    to muscular work, metabolic consequences (Pařízková and Poupa) Brit. J. Nutr. 17:325-332, 1964

    respiratory (Pickfold) Lancet 2:1225-1226, 1954

    ventilatory reaction, muscular exercise (Teillac and LeFrancois) J. Physiologie 54:417-418, 1962

    visual, to darkness, expediting (Kekcheyev) Nature 151:617-618, 1943

Adenopathy

    of muscular work (Chevallier) Rev. Med. Moyen Orient 18:7-10, 1961

Adenosine triphosphatase

    activity in skeletal and heart muscle of rats (Hearn and Gollnick) Int. Zeits. angew. Physiol. 19:23-26,
        1961

    administration in fatigue, rats submitted to hard physical work (Greco) Gazz. Int. Med. Chir. 69:795-798,
        1964

    administration, and respiratory recovery, trained subjects (Lazzari) Gazz. Int. Med. Chir. 69:674-678, 1964

    blood picture, influence on, untrained subjects (Lazzari) Gazz. Int. Med. Chir. 69(Suppl.):3726-3731, 1963

    and creatine phosphokinase activity in muscles of exercised rats (Rawlinson and Gould) Biochem. J. 73:
        44-48, 1959

Adipose tissue

    metabolism, influence of treadmill work on, rats (Pařízková and Stankova) British J. Nutr. 18:325-332, 1964

Adolescence

    cardiopulmonary system during (Birčák and Nikš) Bratisl. Lek. Listy 2:701-709, 1963; (Birčák and others)
        Bratisl. Lek. Listy 2:541-558, 637-648, 1963

    development of children and adolescents, suitability of physical work (Janda) Rev. Czech. Med. 9:82-93,
        1963

    girls, obese and non-obese, attitudes towards physical activity, food and family (Bullen and others) Amer. J.
        Clin. Nutr. 12:1-11, 1963; 14:211-223, 1964

    physical exercise, physical stress, and heart volume (Keul and others) Int. Zeits. angew. Physiol. 19:287-
        329, 1962

    physiological response to exercise (Shock) Texas Rep. Biol. Med. 4:368-386, 1946

Adrenal cortex

    emotion and exercise (Editorial) Brit. Med. J. 2:496-497, 1958

    functional reserve capacity following exhaustive exercise (Diczfalusy and others) J. Clin. Endocrinol. 22:
        78-86, 1962

    reaction to physical and emotional stress, oarsmen (Renold and others) New Eng. J. Med. 244:754-757, 1951

    reactions to heavy physical exertion and Thorn test in analysis of physical insufficiency syndromes (Koster and
        others) Acta Med. Scand. 150:63-79, 1954

Adrenal cortical extract

   effects of infusion on exercise tolerance, blood constituents, and adrenal cortex, dog (Ettinger and Jeffs)
      Endocrinology 32:351-355, 1943

Adrenal cycle

   in motor and mental activity (Halberg and others) Experientia 17:282-284, 1961

Adrenal gland

   adaptation and physical exertion (De Nayer and Ostyn) Acta Belg. Arte Med. Pharm. Milit. 110:621-630,
      1957

   and fatigue, cholinesterase activity, rats (Overbeek), Arch. Int. Pharmacodyn. 79:314-322, 1949

   histological diagnostic function, guinea pigs, in swimming, exercise and in hunger (Creutzfeldt and others)
      Beitr. path. Anat. 113:428-449, 1953

   physiology (Asher) Zeits. Biol. 58:274-304, 1912

   secondary school children during physical exercise (Dzhuganian) Pediatriia 43:77-81, 1964

   secretion and electrolyte metabolism and energy expenditure in work, dogs (Young and others) J. Appl.
      Physiol. 17:669-674, 1962

   secretion, effect on muscular fatigue (Cannon and Nice) Amer. J. Physiol. 32:44-60, 1913

Adrenal hormones, see Adrenocorticosteroids; Epinephrine; Norepinephrine

Adrenal medulla

   acid phosphatase activity, effect of muscular work and denervation, rat. (Eränkö and Härkönen) Ann.
      Med. Exp. Fenn. 40:129-133, 1962

   and cortex, volume changes in exercise, and after injection of certain substances (Hajdu and Korényi) Arch.
      Int. Pharmacodyn. 67:373-389, 1942

   emergency function in pain and major functions (Cannon) Amer. J. Physiol. 33:356-372, 1914

   long-term effects of muscular work on, mouse (Eränkö and Härkönen) Endocrinology 69:186-187, 1961;
      rat (Eränkö and others) Acta Endocrinol. 39:285-287, 1962

Adrenalectomy

   and corticoadrenal steroids, effect on work performance, rats (Winter and Flataker) Amer. J. Physiol. 199:
      863-866, 1960

Adrenaline, see Epinephrine

Adrenocortical function

   effect of regular muscular activity, rats (Frenkl and Csalay) J. Sport Med. 2:207-211, 1962

Adrenocortical-pituitary activity

   effect of prolonged physical exercise, aged (Erez) Ter. Arkh. 36:15-19, 1964

Adrenocorticosteroids

   adrenal 17-hydoxycorticosteroid secretion, and muscular exercise, dogs (Suzuki and others) Nature 181:715,
      1958

Adrenocorticosteroids (Cont.)

    and adrenalectomy, effect on work performance, rats (Winter and Flataker) Amer. J. Physiol. <u>199</u>:
        863-866, 1960

    and aldosterone in prolonged effort of sport (Bugard and others) Rev. Path. Gen. <u>61</u>:159-175, 1961

    blood concentration, influence of muscular work (Kägi) Helv. Med. Acta <u>22</u>:258-267, 1955

    chemistry and pharmacology (Junkmann and Witzel) Zeits. Vitamin Hormon Fermentforsch. <u>13</u>:
        49-128, 129-208, 209-304, 1963

    endogenous, elimination, effects of hepatectomy, total abdominal evisceration and adrenalectomy, cat
        (Bojesen and Egense) Acta Endocr. <u>33</u>:347-369, 1960

    and mucoproteins, urinary excretion, during rest and exercise (Hatch and others) J. Appl. Physiol. <u>9</u>:465-468,
        1956

    plasma level during physical effort (Crabbé and others) Acta Endocr. <u>22</u>:119-124, 1956

    plasma level of 17-hydoxycorticosteroids, effect of muscular exercise and hypoglycemia, adrenogenital
        syndrome (Staehelin and others) Acta Endocr. <u>18</u>:521-529, 1955

    proteosynthesis, proteolysis, during work, influence of relation to age (Gattuso and others) Sicilia
        Sanit. <u>1</u>:71-73, 1963

    17-21-dihydroxy-20-ketosteroid excretion in urine, influence of work in high temperatures (Starlinger
        and Bandino) Int. Zeits. angew. Physiol. <u>18</u>:285-305, 1960

    release, after physical exertion (Derevenco, P. and Derevenco, V.) Endokrinologie <u>45</u>:25-33, 1963

    urinary excretion of adrenal steroids during exercise in hot atmosphere (Robinson and MacFarlane) J. Appl.
        Physiol. <u>12</u>:13-16, 1958

Adrenogenital syndrome

    effect of muscular exercise and hypoglycaemia on plasma level of 17-hydroxysteroids (Staehelin and others)
        Acta Endocr. <u>18</u>:521-529, 1955

Adynamia

    episodica hereditaria, four cases and clinical studies (Herman and McDowell) Amer. J. Med. <u>35</u>:749-767,
        1963

    and isolation, changes in nervous reactions after long stay conditions (Agadzhanian and others) Zh. Vyssh.
        Nerv. Deiat. Pavlov <u>13</u>:953-962, 1963

Age

    and aerobic work capacity, relation to (Åstrand) Acta Physiol. Scand. <u>49</u>(Suppl. 169):1-92, 1960

    and altitude, work tolerance (Dill and others) J. Appl. Physiol. <u>19</u>:483-488, 1964; Rep. 63-33, U.S.
        Civil Aeromed. Res. Inst. 1-8, 1963

    capaeity for physical work, and cardiovascular responses to exercise, influence of aging on (Dawson and
        Hellebrandt) Amer. J. Physiol. <u>143</u>:420-427, 1945

Age (Cont.)

    chronological and physiological, evaluation of work capacity (Balke) Report 63-18 U.S. Civil
        Aeromed. Res. Inst. 1-6, 1963

    and exercise electrocardiogram response, relation to, normal adults (Silver and Landowne) Circulation
        8:510-520, 1953

    exercise performance, influence on (Dill) Pediatrics 32(Suppl.):737-741, 1963

    and exercise, responses to (Dill and others) J. Appl. Physiol. 12:195-196, 1958

    and experience, effect on bar pressing and activity, rat (Desroches and others) J. Geront. 19:168-172,
        1964

    heart, effect of aging on (Starr) Amer. J. Cardiol. 14:771-783, 1964

    and physical fitness (Robinson) Arbeitsphysiol. 10:251-323, 1938

    physiological aging, and exercise (Leake) Geriatrics 19:227, 1964

    physiological, determination (Hensley and others) J. Geront. 19:317-321, 1964

    and sex, and human physical fitness (Åstrand) Physiol. Rev. 36:307-335, 1956

    and sex, relation to physical working capacity (Åstrand) Copenhagen, Munksgaard, 1952

    see also Middle-age

Age, old

    adaptation to strenuous exercise (Iakovlev and others) Fisiol. Zh. SSSR Sechenov. 49:1067-1070, 1963

    advocation of outdoor sport (Graham) Med. News 61:403-404, 1892

    effect of exertion on renal function (Panno) Boll. Soc. Ital. Biol. Sper. 38:782-784, 1962

    serum and muscle creatine in, rats (Gsell and others) Gerontologia 9:42-51, 1964

    ventilatory and circulatory reactions, static effort, normal air and inhalation of oxygen (Binet and Bochet)
        Rev. Franc. Geront. 10:7-19, 1964

Air

    end-tidal, arterial blood carbon dioxide and oxygen tensions, normal variations, moderate exercise (Suskind
        and others) J. Appl. Physiol. 3:282-290, 1950

    expired, composition, minute ventilation, and oxigram, during effort of brief duration (Orlowska and
        Serzysko) Pol. Arch. Med. Wewnet. 33:801-805, 1963

    expired, nature (Zuntz and Geppert) Pflüger Arch. ges. Physiol. 38:337-338, 1886

    moisture and carbonic acid, determination (Haldane and Pembrey) London, Edinburgh and Dublin Phil.
        Mag. and J. Sci., 5th Series 29:306-331, 1890

    passages, capacity, under varying physiological conditions (Douglas and Haldane) J. Physiol. 45:235-238,
        1912

    resistance, to runner (Hill) Proc. Roy. Soc. 102B:380-385, 1928

    see also Oxygen; Respiration

Albumin

    decomposition in human organs, influence of muscular work (Schenck) Naunyn Schmiedeberg Arch.

        exp. Path. 2:21-32, 1874

Albuminuria

    of effort (Jundell and Fries) Nord. Med. Ark. 44; Afd. II:1-154, 1911

    following exercise, relation to speed of work (Hellebrandt and others) Amer. J. Physiol. 101:365-

        375, 1932

    following exercise, in women, relation to negative phase in pulse pressure (Hellebrandt) Amer. J.

        Physiol. 101:357-364, 1932

    and lactic acid in sweat, relation, in muscle work (Koriakina and Krestownikoff) Arbeitsphysiol. 2:

        421-426, 1930

    and micturition, frequency in service patients (Mair) Lancet 1:427-428, 1943

Alcohol

    blood content, influence of muscular work (Hebbelinck) Arch. Int. Pharmacodyn. 119:521-523, 1959

    ethanol, effect on circulatory, metabolic, and neurohormonal function during muscular work (Garlind and

        others) Acta Pharmacol. Toxicol. 17:106-114, 1960

    ethyl, effect on cardiac rate during muscular work (Hebbelinck) Arch. Int. Pharmacodyn. 140:61-67,

        1962

    ethyl, effect on respiratory gas exchange during rest and exercise (Hebbelinck) Arch. Int. Pharmacodyn.

        126:214-218, 1960

    ethyl, radioactive, metabolism, influence of muscular exercise, mice (Hebbelinck) Arch. Int.

        Pharmacodyn. 119:495-496, 1959

    habitual alcoholics, heavy work under influence of alcohol (Atzler and Meyer) Arbeitsphysiol. 4:

        410-432, 1931

    water balance, and diet of athletes, influence on (Montastruc and Baisset) Bull. Soc. Sci. Hyg. Aliment.

        51:88-96, 1963

Aldolase activity

    in heart and skeletal muscle, exercised rats (Hearn and Wainio) Amer. J. Physiol. 190:206-208, 1957

    serum, change during muscular work (Richter and Konitzer) Klin. Wschr. 38:998-999, 1960

    serum, effect of muscular work, trained and untrained men (Cantone and Cerretelli) Int. Zeits. angew.

        Physiol. 18:107-111, 1960

    and succinic dehydrogenase activities of skeletal muscle, exercised rats (Hearn) J. Lancet 77:80, 1957

Aldosterone

    and corticoids in prolonged effort of sport (Bugard and others) Rev. Path. Gen. 61:159-175, 1961

    secretion, influence of position and activity (Muller and others) Lancet 1:711-713, 1958

    and sweat electrolytes (McConahay and others) J. Appl. Physiol. 19:575-579, 1964

    and vasopressin, effect on distribution of water, sodium and potassium, and on work performance, rats

    (Friedberg and others) Gerontologia 7:65-76, 1963

Alkali reserve

blood, static work (Marschak) Arbeitsphysiol. 4:1-19, 1931

metabolic recovery rates from exercise after alteration (Berg) Amer. J. Physiol. 152:465-469, 1948

plasma, in military training and sports performance (Rehberg and Wissemann) Zeits. ges. exp. Med.
55:641-648, 1927

Altitude

and age, work tolerance (Dill and others) J. Appl. Physiol. 19:483-488, 1964; Rep. 63-33, U.S. Civil
Aeromed. Res. Inst. 1-8, 1963

and cardiac performance (Balke) Amer. J. Cardiol. 14:796-810, 1964

different, comparative effects on cardiac rhythm (Rougier and others) Arch. Mal. Prof. 22:784-786,
1961

endurance running of Peromyscus maniculatus, effect on (Hock) J. Appl. Physiol. 16:435-438, 1961

energy exchange, rest and exercise (Aykut and others) Arch. Int. Physiol. 68:285-298, 1960

and exercise, comparison, with respect to decompression sickness (Cook and others) War Med. 6:182-187,
1944

and exercise, effect on growth and decay of aviator's bends (Henry) J. Aviation Med. 27:250-259, 1956

high, bends, moderate exercise as cause (MacKenzie and Riesen) J.A.M.A. 124:499-501, 1944

high, cardiac output during physical training (Michael and Cureton) Res. Quart. 24:446-452, 1953

high, circulation; pulse-rate, arterial, and venous pressure, effects of exertion (Schneider and others)
Amer. J. Physiol. 40:380-417, 1916

high, decreased atmospheric pressure, thorax enlargement and lung volume increase in different work
(Bühlmann) Helv. Physiol. Pharmacol. Acta 8:286-296, 1950

high, influence on pulse rate (Mangili and others) Helv. Physiol. Pharmacol. Acta 22:66-69, 1964

high, low barometric pressure, muscular exercise, parts I-IV (Schneider and Clark) Amer. J. Physiol.
74:334-353, 1925; 75:297-307, 1926; 85:65-77, 1928; 88:633-649, 1929

high, moderate exercise causing bends (MacKenzie and Riesen) J.A.M.A. 124:499-501, 1944

high, and muscular exercise (Pugh and others) J. Appl. Physiol. 19:431-440, 1964

high, and physical strain, effects on heart and circulation (Dill) Amer. Heart J. 23:441-454, 1942

high, physiological processes of body, effect on; work done in Peruvian Andes (Barcroft and others)
Philos. Trans. Roy. Soc. 211B:351-480, 1923

high, Pike's Peak, physiological observations, with special reference to low barometric pressures (Douglas
and others) Phil. Trans. 203B:185-318, 1913

high, reduced atmospheric pressure and work fatigue (Margaria) Arbeitsphysiol. 2:261-272, 1929

high, and regulation of respiration (Pauli) Pflüger Arch. ges. Physiol. 278:447-466, 1964

high, regulation of ventilation (Dejours and others) Rev. Franc. Etud. Clin. Biol. 4:115-127, 1959

high, variable atmospheric pressure, effect on respiration (Speck) Schriften Ges. Beförderung ges.
Naturgewissensch. Marburg 11:173-256, 1877

high, winter work in the mountains, metabolism (Schenk) Deutsch. med. Wschr. Sonderausgabe
62:36-39, 1936

Altitude (Cont.)

  low, oxygen stimulus for ventilation, rest and exercise (Dejours and others) Rev. Franc. Etud.
      Clin. Biol. 3:105-123, 1958

  medium, work test (Bünlmann and Hofstetter) Helvet. Physiol. Pharmacol. acta 9:222-226, 1951

  pulmonary ventilation (Lahiri) Indian J. Physiol. Pharmacol. 8:31-39, 1964

  simulated, effects on pulmonary ventilation, maximal inspiratory (peak) flow and pressure in relation
      to oxygen requirements (Hall and Wilson) J. Aviation Med. 15:160-166, 1944

  simulated, muscle activity and bubble formation, decompressed animals (Whitaker and others) J.
      Gen. Physiol. 28:213-223, 1945

  tolerance and exercise training, rats: blood, tissue, enzyme and isoenzyme changes (Altland and
      others) Aerospace Med. 35:1034-1039, 1964

Alveolar air

  arterial oxygen pressure difference, measurements with different methods at rest and work (Bartels and
      others) Pflüger Arch. ges. Physiol. 261:133-151, 1955; (Friehoff) Poumon Coeur 16:987-992, 1960

  capillary diffusion of carbon monoxide, progressively increasing muscular exercise in mitral disease
      (Chiavaro and others) Boll. Soc. Ital. Cardiol. 8:634-638, 1963

  carbonic acid pressure, normal (Fitzgerald and Haldane) J. Physiol. 32:486-494, 1905

  composition (Agostini and others) Boll. Soc. Ital. Biol. Sper. 34:674-676, 1958

  normal alveolar carbonic acid pressure (Fitzgerald and Haldane) J. Physiol. 32:486-494, 1905

  oxygen, partial pressure and respiratory response to carbon dioxide, relation between (Lloyd and
      others) Quart. J. Exp. Physiol. 43:214-227, 1958

  and physiological dead space, at rest and during muscular exercise (Asmussen and Nielsen) Acta
      Physiol. Scand. 38:1-21, 1956

Amino acids

  free, and free fatty acids, arterial concentrations, at rest and work (Carlsten and others) Scand. J.
      Clin. Lab. Invest. 14:185-191, 1962

  see also Aspartic acid

Amino-aciduria

  in march haemoglobinuria (Pare and Sandler) Lancet 1:702-704, 1954

γ -Amino-butyric acid

  content in brain after a single and prolonged physical effort (Janota-Lukaszewska and Romanowski)
      Acta Physiol. Pol. 15:187-191, 1964

Ammonia, blood

  concentration, effect of exercise (Allen & Conn) Yale J. Biol. Med. 33:133-144, Oct. 1960

  of epileptics (Luck and others) Brit. J. Exp. Path. 6:276-279, 1925

  exercise and aspartic acid administration, effect on rat (Barnes and others) Amer. J. Physiol. 207:1242-1246,
      1964

  levels after muscular work (Kalk and Bonis) Zeits. klin. Med. 123:731-741, 1933

Ammonia, blood (Cont.)

    in muscular work (Parnas and others) Biochem. Zeits. 188:15-23, 1927

    peripheral, elevation, following muscular exercise (Schwartz and others) Proc. Soc. Exp. Biol. Med.
        98:548-550, 1958

    rabbits (Parnas and Klisiecki) Biochem. Zeits. 173:224-248, 1926

Ammonium, quaternary salts

    derived from strychnine and its amino oxide, action on muscular contraction (Hazard and others) J.
        Physiologie 49:198-202, 1957

Amphetamine

    forced exercise, effect on toxicity, and noradrenaline amount in the brain (Beauvallet and Solier) Comptes
        Rend. Soc. Biol. 158:2306-2309, 1964

    mental or physical fatigue, soldiers, effect on (Somerville) Canad. Med. Ass. J. 55:470-476, 1946

    physical and psychological efficiency, effects on (Alwall) Acta Med. Scand. 114:33-58, 1943

    prolonged exercise, effect during (Bovet and Luigi) Comptes Rend. Acad. Sci. 256:3901-3904, 1963

    sulphate, effect on performance of normal and fatigued subjects (Newman) J. Pharmacol. Exp. Ther.
        89:106-108, 1947

    sulphate and performance, a critique: reply (Pierson and others) J.A.M.A. 177:345-349, 1961

    sulphate, effect on physical performance (Golding and Bernard) J. Sport Med. 3:221-224, 1963

    sulphate and some barbiturates, effect on fatigue produced by prolonged wakefulness (Tyler) Amer. J.
        Physiol. 150:253-262, 1947

    toxicity, and body temperature, effect of forced exercise (Hardinge and Peterson) J. Pharmacol. Exp.
        Ther. 145:47-51, 1964

    toxicity, effects of exercise and limitation of movement (Hardinge and Peterson) J. Pharmacol. Exp.
        Ther. 141:260-265, 1963

Amputation

    above-knee, exercise in (Ruosteenoja and Karvonen) Ann. Med. Exp. Fenn. 34:57-62, 1956

    double, circulation and respiration during physical work after (Drews and Rosenkranz) Zeits. Kreislaufforsch.
        51:611-621, 1962

Anaerobic

    anaerobiosis in rest and work, aerobic recovery (Asmussen) Acta Physiol. Scand. 11:197-210, 1946

    anaerobiosis, secondary anoxia and catalases (Ghiringhelli and Molina) Med. Lavoro 43:463-467, 1952

    changes and aerobic changes, in seal muscles during diving (Scholander and others) J. Biol. Chem. 142:
        431-440, 1942

    metabolism, and cardiac output during exercise (Thomas and others) J. Appl. Physiol. 19:839-848, 1964

    metabolism, threshold, detecting in cardiac patients during exercise (Wasserman and McIlroy) Amer. J.
        Cardiol. 14:844-852, 1964

Anaerobic (Cont.)

processes involved in muscular activity (Hartree and Hill) J. Physiol. 58:127-137, 1923

and aerobic work capacity after dehydration (Saltin) J. Appl. Physiol. 19:1114-1118, 1964

see also Oxygen

Analeptics

theophylline, and glucosides; influence on cardiac output in congestive heart failure (Berséus) Acta
Med. Scand. 113(Suppl. 145):1-76, 1943

Anaphylaxis

after effort (Kral) Bruxelles Méd. 28:571-583, 1948

Anemia

cardiopulmonary physiological responses to heavy exercise (Sproule and others) J. Clin. Invest. 39:
378-388, 1960

and exercise, effects on coronary arteries, small animals, corrosion-cast technique (Tepperman and Pearlman)
Circ. Res. 9:576-584, 1961

oxygen in venous blood in (Lundsgaard) J. Exp. Med. 30:147-158, 1919

Aneurysm

popliteal, with femoral osteochondroma (Anastasi and others) Arch. Surg. 87:636-639, Oct. 1963

Angina pectoris

crises, spontaneous, indifferent of effort (Tourniaire and others) Lyon Med. 210:1303-1315, 1963

effort, effect on diagnosis (Pautrat) Presse Med. 71:1331-1332, 1963

of effort, effect of intravenous cytochrome C on capacity for effort without pain (Bakst and Rinzler) Proc.
Soc. Exp. Biol. Med. 67:531-533, 1948

exercise electrocardiogram, two step, double-blind use in diagnosis (Friedberg and others) Circulation 26:
1254-1260, 1962

exercise, hemodynamic responses to (Foster and Reeves) J. Clin. Invest. 43:1758-1768, 1964

exercise test and anoxia test in diagnosis (Kimura and others) Jap. Heart J. 4:313-322, 1963

glyceryl trinitrate in, test of efficacy (Russek and Howard) J.A.M.A. 189:108-112, 1964

propranolol in, effect of (Hamer and others) Brit. Med. J. 2:720-723, 1964

radioelectrocardiography during exercise, use of multiple leads (Bellet and others) Circulation 29:366-375,
1964

segontin in, evaluation of oxygen deficiency and exercise load (Kimura and others) J. Ther. 46:162-165,
1964

sympathectomy, effects on electrocardiogram and effort tolerance (Apthorp and others) Brit. Heart J.
26:218-226, 1964

with syncope (Golden) Amer. Heart J. 28:689-698, 1944

Angiotensin II

> in minute amounts, hemodynamic effect, normal subjects, rest and exercise (Sannerstedt and others)
> Scand. J. Clin. Lab. Invest. 15:159-166, 1963

Anoxia

> and exercise, effects on electrocardiogram (Baum and others) J. Aviation Med. 16:422-428, 1945
>
> and histamine formation (Graham and others) J. Physiol. 172:174-188, 1964
>
> lactate utilization after prolonged muscular work, influence on (Ström) Acta Physiol. Scand. 17:440-451,
> 1949
>
> secondary, and catalases, in work carried out in anaerobiosis (Ghiringhelli and Molina) Med. Lavoro 43:
> 463-467, 1952

Antacids

> physiological support with, during fatigue and exhaustion during physical load (Winter) Med. Klin.
> 53:2195-2196, 1958

Anterior tibial compartment syndrome

> anterior crural ischemia, clinical entity (Blum) Arch. Surg. 74:59-64, 1957
>
> march gangrene; ischaemic myositis of leg muscles from exercise (Blandy and Fuller) J. Bone Joint Surg.
> 39B:679-693, 1957
>
> ischaemic, of anterior tibial muscles due to fatigue (Hughes) J. Bone Joint Surg. 30B:581-594, 1948
>
> strenuous exercise as cause (Leach and others) Milit. Med. 129:610-613, 1964; Arch. Surg. 88:187-192,
> 1964; (Carter and others) Lancet 2:928-934, 1949
>
> traumatic necrosis (Pearson and others) New Eng. J. Med. 239:213-217, 1948

Anthropologic measurements

> and capacity, middle-aged men (Skinner and others) Amer. J. Cardiol. 14:747-752, 1964
>
> difference in 4 groups of young men with different physical activity (Keller and Kopf) Int. Zeits. angew.
> Physiol. 19:110-119, 1961

Antihemophilic A factor (F. VIII)

> changes, and in bleeding time in muscular exercise and adrenaline infusion (Egeberg) Scand. J. Clin.
> Lab. Invest. 15:539-549, 1963
>
> increase associated with muscular exercise (Egeberg) Scand. J. Clin. Lab. Invest. 15:202-203, 1963
>
> variations during muscular exercise (Goudemand and others) Ann. Inst. Pasteur Lille 14:203-215, 1963; Nouv.
> Rev. Franc. Hemat. 4:315-319, 1964

Anxiety states

> and normal controls, comparison of exercise response (Jones and Mellersh) Psychosom. Med. 8:180-187,
> 1946
>
> see also Neurosis

Aorta, coarctation, see Coarctation of aorta

Aortic valvular lesions

    isolated, effect of exercise (Sancetta and Kleinerman) Amer. Heart J. 53:404-414, 1957

Aptitude tests

    functional, statistical study of three (Martin) Acta Belg. Arte Med. Pharm. Milit. 110:669-678,

        1957

    step-ladder trial (Grandpierre and others) Rev. Méd. Nancy 82:865-871, 1957

Arm

    blood circulation during static loading (Titievskaia) Fiziol. Zh. SSSR Sechenov 50:1129-1135, 1964

    muscles, effect of fatigue on contraction (Long and Lupton) J. Physiol. 58:334-337, 1924

    vasomotor responses during leg exercises (Blair and others) Circ. Res. 9:264-274, 1961

    volume changes, muscular exercise (Starkweather) Univ. Calif. Pub. Physiol., Berkeley 18:187-200,

        1913

    see also Forearm

Arrhythmia

    atrial flutter and sinus rhythm, haemodynamic response to exercise during (Åstrand and others) Acta Med.

        Scand. 173:121-127, 1963

    atrial, transitory flutter, and atrioventricular dissociation after exertion (Jacono and Juliani) Riforma

        Med. 76:429-431, 1962

    sinus, in children, changes with injections of adrenaline, noradrenaline, pilocarpine, and atropine

        (Kanematsu) Acta Paediat. Jap. 68:101-106, 1964

    see also Fibrillation, atrial

Arterial insufficiency

    muscle work, effect on, ergomyography (Van de Berg and others) Surg. Forum 14:296-298, 1963

    occluded blood supply, load, and local muscular isometric endurance (Start) J. Appl. Physiol 19:1135-1138,

        1964

    and sympathectomy effect on blood flow, ergogram (Van de Berg and others) Ann. Surg. 159:623-635, 1964

    see also Angina pectoris; Claudication; Coronary disease

Arteries

    blood velocity (Tigerstedt) Ergebn. Physiol. 4:481-516, 1905

    distension, and velocity of sphygmic wave, during muscular exercise (Gobbato and others) Minerva

        Cardioangiol. 12:251-256, 1964

    large, conditions during muscular exercise, oscillometric measurements (Christensen) Acta Med. Scand.

        121:319-332, 1945

Arteries (Cont.)

oxygen and carbon dioxide partial pressure, also alveolar-arterial oxygen and carbon dioxide (Worth

and others) Med. Thorac. 20:223-234, 1963

tension, recovery time, hypoxic test (Lazzari) Gazz. Int. Med. Chir. 69:304-308, 1964

see also names of specific arteries

Arteriosclerosis

atherogenesis, effect of prolonged exercise, rabbit (Brainard) Proc. Soc. Exp. Biol. Med. 100:

244-246, 1959

atheromatosis, effect of nicotine in cholesterol loaded rats (Grandjean and Abelin) Schweiz. Zeits. Sportmed.

12:132-144, 1964

atheromatosis, experimental, influence of physical exertion, rabbit (Brechter and Forsby) Beits. Ernährungswiss.

3:95-110, 1962

atheromatosis, induced by cholesterol feeding, effect of nicotine on, rats (Grandjean and Abelin) Schweiz. Zeits.

Sport Med. 12:132-144, 1964

blood flow through lower extremities in obliterative arterial disease, analysis of (Pernow) Scand. J. Clin.

Lab. Invest. 15(Suppl. 76):57-60, 1963

cholesterol-induced, effect of physical exercise, rabbits (Gudbrandsen) USAF Arctic Aeromed. Lab. TR

60-2:1-85, 1961

and cholinesterase metabolism and physical activity (Karvonen) Schweiz. Zeits. Sportmed. 9:90-100,

1961

coronary, degree in 'normal', and occupational physical activity, postmortem study (Spain and Bradess)

Circulation 22:239-242, 1960

exercise and iliac vein blood flow, and local oxygen consumption in occlusive arterial disease, effect of

(Pentecost) Clin. Sci. 27:437-445, 1964

experimental, accelerating effects of muscular exercise (McAllister and others) Arch. Surg. 80:54-60, 1960

experimental cholesterol, physical activity in, rabbits (Kobernick and Niwayama) Amer. J. Path. 36:393-409,

1960; (Kobernick and others) Proc. Soc. Exp. Biol. Med. 96:623-628, 1957

histochemistry, lesions of aorta, exercised and sedentary rabbits, parts I and II (Kobernick and Hashimoto)

Lab. Invest. 12:638-647, 685-696, 1963

and physical labour (Kerimov and others) Azerbaidzh. Med. Zh. 2:42-48, 1964; (Nöcker and Hartleb)

Schweiz. Zeits. Sportmed. 9:101-116, 1961

and sport, animals (Schlüssel) Zeits. Kreislaufforsch 48:734-745, 1959

tonoscillography after exercise as early diagnosis of peripheral arterial disease (Ejrup) Acta Med. Scand.

138(Suppl. 239):347-355, 1950

Arterio-venous difference, see Oxygen content, blood

Aspartic acid

administration and effects of exercise on blood ammonia, rat (Barnes and others) Amer. J. Physiol.
207:1242-1246, 1964

salts, effects on swimming performance, rats and dogs (Matoush and others) J. Appl. Physiol. 19:
262-264, 1964

salts, inhibitory effects against march fatigue (Fujioka and others) Nat. Def. Med. J. 10:525-528,
1963

Asthma

and gas metabolism in physical exertion (Herbst) Deutsch. Arch. klin. Med. 162:129-143, 1928

Asystole

cardiac, in normal young men following physical effort (Eichna and others) Amer. Heart J. 33:254-262,
1947

Athletes

alcohol, influence on water balance (Montastruc and Baisset) Bull. Soc. Sci. Hyg. Aliment. 51:88-96,
1963

blood donation, influence on work capacity of (Ostyn and Styns) Arch. Belg. Med. Soc. 17:375-387,
1959

breakfast and no breakfast and of caffeine, effect of and in non-athlete (Hyde and others) Amer. J. Physiol.
43:371-394, 1917

cardiac cycle, determination of duration of phases in muscular work (Shkhvatsabaia) Kardiologiia 4:62-68,
1964

cardiac output during training (Freedman and others) J. Appl. Physiol. 8:37-47, 1955

cardiac response to exercise (Wang and others) Circulation 24:1064, 1961

cardiovascular response to exercise (Wang and others) Physiologist 3:173, 1960

circulatory studies, rest and heavy exercise (Bevegård and others) Acta Physiol. Scand. 57:26-50, 1963

comparative clinical, electrocardiographic and biochemical observations, before and after intensive
exertion (Loutsides and others) Rev. Méd. Moyen Orient 19:433-437, 1962

exercise, body and lung size, effect on CO diffusion (Newman and others) J. Appl. Physiol. 17:649-655,
1962

former, relationship between heart volume, total hemoglobin, and physical working capacity in (Holmgren
and Strandell) Acta Med. Scand. 163:149-160, 1959

heart (Wolffe) J. Lancet 77:76-78, 1957

heart and blood circulation (Reindell and others) Med. Welt 31:1557-1563, 1960

heart size and physical efficiency (Roskamm and others) Schweiz. Zeits. Sportmed. 10:121-129, 1962

Athletes (Cont.)

lipid, requirements (Bour) Bull. Soc. Sci. Hyg. Aliment. 51:63-76, 1963

male, anaerobic metabolic responses to acute maximal exercise (Bruce and others) Amer. Heart J.
67:643-650, 1964

metabolic modifications during prolonged exertion (Chailley-Bert and others) Rev. Path. Gen. 61:
143-157, 1961

metabolism, compared with normal of similar height and weight (Benedict and Smith) J. Biol. Chem.
20:243-252, 1915

Olympic, observations (Best and Partridge) Proc. Roy. Soc. 105B:323-332, 1929

oxygen, influence of (Hill and Flack) J. Physiol. 38:xxviii-xxxvi, 1909; (Hill and others) Brit. Med. J.
2:499-500, 1908

protein, milk intake and exercise, effect of (Wilcox and others) J. Amer. Diet. Ass. 44:95-99, 1964

trained, level and composition of blood serum proteins during exhausting and graded exercise (Bojanovský
and Filip) Rev. Czech. Med. 2:339-345, 1953

see also Basketball; Climbing; Cyclists; Oarsmen; Rowing; Running; Skiers; Swimming

Athletics

circulation, effect on (Pyorala) Duodecim 80:101-109, 1964

endeavour, physiologic aspects (Trethewie) Med. J. Austr. 1:779-783, 1956

evaluation, and maximal exertion test (Greco) Gaz. Int. Med. Chir. 69:309-313, 1964

forced breathing and oxygen, influence of (Vernon and Stolz) Quart. J. Exp. Physiol. 4:243-248, 1911

heart and circulation, immediate and remote effect on (Stengel) Amer. J. Med. Sci. 118:544-553, 1899

and heart, electrocardiography and radiology (Cooper and others) Med. J. Austr. 1:569-579, 1937

Lancet Commission on Lancet 1:999-1001; 2:218-219, 1880

pseudonephritis, alteration of urine in athletics (Gardner) J.A.M.A. 161:1613-1617, 1956

records, physiological basis (Hill) Scientific Monthly 21:409-428, 1925; Nature 116:544-548, 1925

Atrial septal defect

blood lactate concentration, in absolute and relative work load (Holmgren and Ström) Acta Med.
Scand. 163:185-193, 1959

physical working capacity and haemodynamics during exercise (Jonsson and others) Acta Med. Scand. 159:
275-294, 1957

pulmonary diffusing capacity during rest and exercise (Bedell and Adams) J. Clin. Invest. 41:1908-1914, 1962

Atrioventricular block

complete congenital, response to exercise (Ikkos and Hanson) Circulation 22:583-590, 1960

Atrium

acute overloading, response to stress (Cortes) Amer. J. Med. Sci. 246:443-450, 1963

right atrial cathertization, cardiac output measured by (Stead and others) J. Clin. Invest. 24:323-
331, 1945

Atropine

cardiac output, effect on (Weissler and others) J. Clin. Invest. 36:1656-1662, 1957

and cardiac output, stroke volume and central venous pressure, changes in (Berry and others) Amer.
Heart J. 58:204-213, 1959

and catecholamines, effect on cardiovascular response to exercise, dogs (Keck and others) Circ. Res.
9:566-570, 1961

heart rate and oxygen intake, effect on (Robinson and others) J. Appl. Physiol. 5:508-512, 1953

heat and work, effects on heart rate and sweat production (Craig) J. Appl. Physiol. 4:826-833, 1952

and reserpine, effect on pulmonary diffusing capacity during exercise (Krumholz and Ross) J. Appl.
Physiol. 19:465-468, 1964

Auditory threshold

measurement before and after strenuous physical exercise (Boys and Curry) Ann. Otol. 65:190-197, 1956

Autonomic nervous system

and body loading in juveniles (Mies and Jovy) Deutsch. med. Wschr. 86:2208-2213, 1961

cardiac adrenergic preponderance due to lack of physical exercise, pathogenic implications (Raab) Amer.
J. Cardiol. 5:300-320, 1960

effects of temperature, calcium and activity on phospholipid metabolism in a sympathetic ganglion
(Larrabee and others) J. Neurochem. 10:549-570, 1963

influence on contraction of heart, under normal circulatory conditions (Kjellberg and others) Acta
Physiol. Scand. 24:350-360, 1952

muscular exercise, influence on bulbar centers (Martin and Gruber) Amer. J. Physiol. 32:315-328, 1913

Auto-transfusion

of "work-blood", effect on pulmonary ventilation (Asmussen and Nielsen) Acta Physiol. Scand. 20:79-87,
1950

Axillary vein, thrombosis

caused by overexertion (Velasco-Sanfuentes and others) Rev. Med. Chile 71:771-780, 1943; (Toth and others)
Fortschr. Roentgenstr. 99:484-492, 1963; (Keener and others) U. S. Naval Med. Bull. 40:
687-692, 1942; (Adrower) Minerva Med. 54:2243-2245, 1963; (Tlusty and Rehor) Sborn. Ved. Prac.
Lek. Fak. Karlov. Univ. 5(Suppl.):313-316, 1962

B

Ballistocardiogram

after muscular work, quantitative evaluation (Busnengo) Riv. Med. Aero. 23:385-396, 1960

changes after exercise (Makinson) Circulation 2:186-196, 1950

effects of conditioning of basketball players on (Montoye and others) J. Appl. Physiol. 15:449-453, 1960

Bar pressing

> and activity, effect of age and experience, rat (Desroches and others) J. Geront. <u>19</u>:168-172, 1964

Basketball

> effects of conditioning on ballistocardiogram (Montoye and others) J. Appl. Physiol. <u>15</u>:449-453, 1960

Bed rest

> circulatory functions during, modifications of effects after two weeks (Miller and others) Aerospace Med. <u>35</u>:931-939, 1964

> prolonged, cardiodynamic and metabolic effects (Birkhead and others) Techn. Docum. Rep. No. AMRL-TDR-64-61, USAF 6570, Aerospace Med. Res. Lab. 1-28, 1964

> <u>see also</u> Inactivity

Bends, <u>see</u> Altitude; Decompression sickness

Benzidrine, <u>see</u> Amphetamine

Beri-beri

> effect of muscular exercise (Hayasaka and Inawashiro) Tohoku J. Exp. Med. <u>12</u>:29-61, 1928

> <u>see also</u> Vitamin B_1

Beta-adrenergic blocking agent

> circulation, effects on in hypertrophic subaortic stenosis (Harrison and others) Circulation, <u>29</u>:84-98, 1964

> haemodynamic effects (Chamberlain and Howard) Brit. Heart J. <u>26</u>:213-217, 1964

> Nethalide (Schröder and Werkö) Clin. Pharmacol. Ther. <u>5</u>:159-166, 1964

> non-esterified-fatty acid and carbohydrate metabolism, effects on at rest and during exercise (Jenkins) Lancet <u>2</u>:1184-1185, 1964; (Muir) Lancet <u>2</u>:930-932, 1964

Bicycle ergometer

> (Sarkar and others) J. Exp. Med. Sci. <u>4</u>:145-154, 1961

> compared with measured step exercise (Tschirdewahn and others) Arch. Kreislaufforsch. <u>42</u>:45-63, 1963

> conversion of treadmill to (Lurie) J. Appl. Physiol. <u>19</u>:152-153, 1964

> muscular work, psychophysical study (Borg and Dahlström) Vetenskapliga Biblioteket, 1960; Nord. Med. <u>62</u>:1383-1386, 1959

> single (Dobeln) J. Appl. Physiol. <u>7</u>:222-224, 1954

> speed and load, effects of (Dickinson) J. Physiol. <u>67</u>:242-255, 1929

> work capacity, children (Cumming G. R. and Cumming P. M.) Canad. Med. Ass. J. <u>88</u>:351-355, 1963; (Cumming and Danzinger) Pediatrics <u>32</u>:202-208, 1963

Bicycle pedalling

> dynamics (Dickinson) Proc. Roy. Soc. <u>103B</u>:225-233, 1928

> efficiency (Hill) J. Physiol. <u>82</u>:207-210, 1934

Bicycle pedalling (Cont.)

    heart-rate, blood-pressure and duration of systole, changes in (Bowen) Amer. J. Physiol. 11:59-77,

        1904

    prolonged, electrocardiogram changes during (Chailley-Bert and others) Arch. Mal. Coeur 49:910-915,

        1956

    use and abuse of, and of medicine, religion and physical exercise (Remondino) Nat. Pop. Rev.,

        Chicago and San Diego 5:59-61, 1894

    see also Cyclists

Bioenergetics

    and growth, efficiency complex in domestic animals (Brody) New York, Reinhold, 1945

Birds

    migrating, homeostasis of nonfat components (Odum and others) Science 143:1037-1039, 1964

Bleeding time

    changes associated with muscular exercise and adrenalin infusion (Egeberg) Scand. J. Clin. Lab.

        Invest. 15:539-549, 1963

Blood

    biochemical constants of serum, value during sport and intensive training (Haralambrie) Acta Biol. Med.

        German. 13:30-39, 1964

    destruction during exercise (Broun) J. Exp. Med. 36:481-500, 1922; 37:113-130, 187-206, 207-220, 1923

    modifications during exercise (Geuens) Acta Belg. Arte Med. Pharm. Milit. 109:155-163, 1956

    morphological changes, after muscular exercise (Hawk) Amer. J. Physiol. 10:384-400, 1904

    plasma viscosity, effect of muscular exercise, correlation with postprandial triglyceridemia (Konttinen

        and Somer) J. Appl. Physiol. 18:991-993, 1963

    reaction, and breathing, after exercise (Barr) J. Biol. Chem. 56:171-182, 1923

    reaction and lung ventilation (Hasselbalch and Lundsgaard) Scand. Arch. Physiol. 27:13-21, 1912

    reaction and muscle work (Arborelius and Liljestrand) Skand. Arch. Physiol. 44:215, 1923,

    and regulation of respiration (Winterstein) Pflüger Arch. ges. Physiol. 138:167-184, 1911

    'reserves', use by exercise, epinephrine, and hemorrhage (Ebert and Stead) Amer. J. Med. Sci. 201:

        655-664, 1941

    serum colloidal osmotic pressure, effect of exercise, rabbit (Kawamoto) Far East Sci. Bull. 1:39, 1941

    in sportsmen (Jokl) Arbeitsphysiol. 4:379-389, 1931

    and sweat reaction to exhausting work (Prokop) Medizinische, pp. 1622-1624, 1952

    and tissue fluid exchange, behaviour in relation to work (Furbetta and others) Folia Med. 42:1299-1312, 1959

    see also Alkali reserve; Oxygen content, blood; Protein, serum

Blood, acids

    effect of physical activity on behaviour of (Julich and Eisfeld) Zeits. klin. Med. 156:222-235, 1960

Blood cells

constituents during training (Thürner) Arbeitsphysiol. 2:116-128, 1930

corpuscles, distribution of in blood stream, effect of exercise (Isaacs and Gordon) Amer. J. Physiol.
71:106-111, 1924

erythrocyte count, consecutive, changes, in muscular training (Rougier and Dupuy) Arch. Mal. Prof.
20:176-177, 1959

erythrocyte and hemoglobin increase, blood, during and after exercise (Schneider and Crampton) Amer.
J. Physiol. 112:202-206, 1935

erythrocyte number, and percentage of hemoglobin, effect of work (Boothby and Berry) Amer. J. Physiol.
37:378-382, 1915

erythrocyte and plasma volume after prolonged severe exercise (Åstrand and Saltin) J. Appl. Physiol.
19:829-832, 1964

erythrocytes, effect of exercise (Smith and Kumpf) Amer. J. Med. Sci. 184:537-546, 1932

erythrocytes, increased, conditioned reflex before exertion (Láng) Kiserl. Orvostud. 15:375-380,
1963

erythrocytes, pentose cycle, activity (Sonka and others) Endokrinologie 45:174-186, 1963

erythrocytes, resistance to laking, relation to exertion (Heath) Amer. J. Physiol. 139:569-573, 1943

erythrocytes, sedimentation rate, effect of exercise (Black and Karpovich) Amer. J. Physiol. 144:
224-226, 1945

erythrocytes, size, before and after exercise (Dryerre and others) Quart. J. Exp. Physiol. 16:69-86, 1926

erythroleucocyte picture, changes, trained and untrained subjects (Lazzari) Gazz. Int. Med. Chir.
68:2527-2531, 1963

exercise, effect of repeated light, on rats (Moorhouse) Amer. J. Hyg. 21:214-223, 1935

exercise, effect on blood count (Babbitt) Amer. Phys. Educat. Rev. 6:240-245, 1901

leukocyte changes, muscular work (Wachholder) Int. Zeits. angew. Physiol. 16:356-360, 1957

leucocyte count, effect of exercises of graded intensity (Tuttle) Res. Quart. Amer. Phys. Educ. Ass.
6(Suppl.):37-45, 1935

leucocytes, differential and total count, effect of hard laboratory exercise (Meyer and Pella) Res.
Quart. 18:271-278, 1947

leucocytes and histamine in blood during muscular work (Dunér and Pernow) Scand. J. Clin. Lab.
Invest. 10:394-396, 1958

leucocytes, motility, influence of stress conditions (Charva and others) Int. Rec. Med. 170:672-677, 1957

leucocytes, and muscle work (Rohde and Wachholder) Arbeitsphysiol. 15:165-174, 1953

leucocytes, respiration, effect of muscular activity prior to venepuncture (Bisset and Alexander) Nature
181:909-910, 1958

leucocytes, response to brief severe exercise (Andersen) J. Appl. Physiol. 7:671-674, May, 1955

muscular work, immediate effects on blood count (Auvergnat) Comptes Rend. Soc. Biol. 152:176-181,
1958

Blood cells (Cont.)

    reticulocyte count, changes in fatigue, muscular work (Rosenblum and Mendjuk) Arbeitsphysiol. 2: 395-408, 1930

Blood changes

    associated with exercise (Ikkala) Duodecim 80:115-117, 1964; (Ikkala and others) Nature 199: 459-461, 1963; (Dill) J. Lancet 56:313-315, 1931

    chemical components after rest and effort (Geuens) Acta Belg. Arte Med. Pharm. Milit. 110: 601-610, 1957

    chemical, during recovery from exhaustive exercise (Selye) Canad. J. Res. 17(Sect. D):109-112, 1939

    evaluation and respiratory function (MacCagno and Pellegrino) Lotta Tuberc. 24:930-938, 1954

    after muscular activity and during training (Schneider and Havens) Amer. J. Physiol. 36:239-259, 1915; (Schneider) Amer. Phys. Educ. Rev. 32:178, 250, 1927

    during muscular activity and recovery (De Lanne and others) J. Appl. Physiol. 15:31-36, 1960

    in muscular activity, especially fitness for work (Pezzeri and others) Rass. Med. Industr. 32: 390-394, 1963

    muscular work, influence of (Hannisdahl) Arbeitsphysiol. 11:165-174, 1940; (Willebrand) Scand. Arch. Physiol. 14:176-187, 1903

    in sportsmen (Hartmann and Jokl) Arbeitsphysiol. 2:452-460, 1930

    see also Oxygen content, blood; Carbon dioxide

Blood circulation, see Circulation, blood

Blood clotting, see Bleeding time; Coagulation

Blood destruction

    during exercise (Broun) J. Exp. Med. part I, 36:481-500, 1922; part II 37:113-130, 1923; part III, 37:187-206; part IV, 37:207-220, 1923

Blood distribution

    (Tigerstedt) Scand. Arch. Physiol. 3:145-243, 1892

    blood depots (Venrath and others) Zeits. Kreislaufforsch. 46:612-615, 1957

    and blood volume regulation (Sjöstrand) Klin. Wschr. 34:561-569, 1956

    and blood volume, significance in regulating circulation (Sjöstrand) Physiol. Rev. 33:202-228, 1953

    and circulation during physical work (Asmussen and Christensen) Scand. Arch. Physiol. 82:185-192, 1939

    and circulation, physiology of (Müller and Veiel) Sammlung klin. Vorträge inn. Med. No. 194-196: 641-724, 1910.

    importance to lungs (Sjöstrand) Acta Physiol. Scand. 2:231-248, 1941

Blood donation

and work capacity (Balke and others) J. Appl. Physiol. 7:231-238, 1954

work capacity of athletes, influence on (Ostyn and Styns) Arch. Belg. Med. Soc. 17:375-387, 1959

Blood flow

aortic, during treadmill exercise, dogs (Franklin and others) J. Appl. Physiol. 14:809-812, 1959

in arm during supine leg exercise (Bishop and others) J. Physiol. 137:294-308, 1957

in arm (resting), during supine leg exercise (Muth and others) Clin. Sci. 17:603-610, 1958

arterial stenosis and sympathectomy, influence of, ergogram (Van de Berg and others) Ann. Surg. 159:623-635, 1964

in arteries: superior mesenteric, renal and common iliac (Herrick and others) Amer. J. Physiol. 128:338-344, 1940

artery, reversed vertebral, effects of limb exercise and hypertensive agents (Sammartino and Toole) Arch. Neurol. 10:590-594, 1964

blood debt repayment following rhythmic exercise of forearm muscles, effect of continuous infusions of ATP, histamine and acetylcholine (Patterson and Shepherd) Clin. Sci. 13:85-91, 1954

caffeine, effect of in normal subjects (Means and Newburgh) J. Pharmacol. Exp. Ther. 7:449-465, 1915

in calf of leg after running (Livingstone) Amer. Heart J. 61:219-224, 1961

in calf (leg), after prolonged walking (Halliday) Amer. Heart J. 60:110-115, 1960

calf (leg), requirements, after walking and running (Black) Clin. Sci. 18:89-93, 1959

calf (leg), at rest, after occlusion and after exercise, normal and in intermittent claudication (Strandell and Wahren) Acta Med. Scand. 173:99-105, 1963

circulatory debt, law of constancy, in function of cardiac power (Pachon and Fabre) Comptes Rend. Soc. Biol. 105:30-31, 31-32, 1930

coronary, effects of exercise, denervated and partly denervated trained dogs (Essex and others) Amer. J. Physiol. 138:687-697, 1943

coronary, influence of exercise, dog (Essex and others) Amer. J. Physiol. 125:614-623, 1939

coronary, in intact conscious dog, studies with miniature electromagnetic flow transducers (Hepps and others) J. Thorac. Cardiov. Surg. 46:783-794, 1963

coronary, myocardial oxygen consumption and cardiac efficiency, effect of exercise (Lombardo and others) Circulation 7:71-78, 1953

iliac vein (external), and oxygen consumption, effect of exercise in normal, and occlusive arterial disease (Pentecost) Clin. Sci. 27:437-445, 1964

forearm, changes during physical training (Rohter and others) J. Appl. Physiol. 18:789-793, 1963

forearm, during intra-arterial infusions of adrenaline (Glover and Shanks) J. Physiol. 167:268-279, 1963

in forearm muscles during sustained hand-grip contractions (Humphreys and Lind) J. Physiol. 163: 13P-19P, 1962

Blood flow (Cont.)

in forearm veins, during rhythmic exercise, origin (Idbohrn and Wahren) Acta Physiol. Scand. 61:
301-313, 1964

hepatic blood debt, variation during physical exercise (Baschieri and others) Cardiologia 29:229-237,
1956

hepatic, estimated, and indocyanine green clearance, during exercise (Rowell and others) J. Clin.
Invest. 43:1677-1690, 1964

leg, during leg exercise in relation to cardiac output response (Donald and others) Clin. Sci. 16:
567-591, 1957

local, muscular work (Borgatti and others) Boll. Soc. Ital. Biol. Sper. 39:269-273, 1963

low physical working capacity due to inadequate adjustment of peripheral blood flow (Holmgren and
others) Acta Med. Scand. 158:413-436, 1957

through lower extremities in obliterative arterial diseases, analysis (Pernow) Scand. J. Clin. Lab.
Invest. 15(Suppl. 76):57-60, 1963

through lungs, measurements (Krogh and Lindhard) Scand. Arch. Physiol. 27:100-125, 1912

lungs, measurement during exercise, using nitrous oxide (Becklake and others) J. App. Physiol. 17:
579-586, 1962

metabolism, and exudation in organs, and functional activity (Barcroft and Kato) Proc. Roy. Soc.
88B:541-543, 1915

muscle, following exercise and circulatory arrest (Dornhorst and Whelan) Clin. Sci. 12:33-40, 1953

muscle, during sustained contraction (Barcroft and Millen) J. Physiol. 97:17-31, 1939

muscle, local regulation (Hyman and others) Circ. Res. 12:176-181, 1963

muscle strength and endurance development, effect of (Vanderhoff and others) J. Appl. Physiol. 16:
873-877, 1961

myocardial, local, indicated by disappearance of NaI[131] from heart muscle during rest, exercise,
and following nitrite administration (Hollander and others) J. Pharmacol. Exp. Ther. 139:53-59,
1963

and oxygen debt, repayment in exercising skeletal muscle (Coffman) Amer. J. Physiol. 205:365-369,
1963

peripheral, changes, maximal exercise (Wilmore and Horvath) Amer. Heart J. 66:353-362, 1963

peripheral, in intermittent claudication (Hillestad) I. Postural tests Acta Med. Scand. 172:301-305, 1962; II.
Skin thermometry, Acta Med. Scand. 172:307-314, 1962; III. Oscillometry, Acta Med. Scand.
172:573-583, 1962; IV. Claudication distance, Acta Med. Scand. 173:467-478; V.-VII. Plethysmographic studies, Acta Med. Scand. 174:23-41, 671-685, 687-700, 1963

peripheral, and respiratory exchange, effects of exercise (Foster) Med. Arts & Sci. 10:145-151, 1956

pulmonary capillary volume and diffusing capacity during exercise (Johnson and others) J. Appl. Physiol.
15:893-902, 1960

Blood flow (Cont.)

    pulmonary, zonal distribution, effect of exercise (Read and Fowler) J. Appl. Physiol. 19:672-678, 1964

    rate, and oxygen saturation following contraction of forearm muscles (Love) Clin. Sci. 14:275-283, 1955

    renal, and sodium excretion, effects of exercise, dogs (Carlin and others) J. Appl. Physiol. 3:291-294, 1950

    splanchnic, and splanchnic volume, effect of exercise (Wade and others) Clin. Sci. 15:457-463, 1956

    splanchnic circulation, influence of muscular exercise, dog (Lacroix) Arch. Int. Physiol. 71:108-111, 1913

    sympatholysis, functional, during muscular activity; influence of carotid sinus on oxygen uptake (Remensnyder and others) Circ. Res. 11:370-380, 1962

    uterine, during exercise, in normal and pre-eclamptic pregnancies (Morris and others) Lancet 2:481-484, 1956

    and venous oxygen saturation during sustained contraction of forearm muscles (Barcroft and Whelan) J. Physiol. 168:848-856, 1963

    see also Cardiac output; Cerebral circulation; Circulation, blood

Blood gases, see Gas, blood

Blood loss

    effect on performance in Balke-Ware treadmill test (Howell) Res. Quart. Amer. Ass. Health Phys. Educ. 35:156-165, 1964

Blood pH

    change after physical effort (Styns and Ostyn) Comptes Rend. Soc. Biol. 151:415-416, 1957

    and O_2 and CO_2 tensions in exercised control and emphysematous horses (Gillespie and others) Amer. J. Physiol. 207:1067-1072, 1964

    standard bicarbonate and pCO_2 in deep veins of forearm during and after strong sustained contraction (Barcroft and others) J. Physiol. 169:34P-35P, 1963

    see also Acid-base equilibrium

Blood platelets, see Thrombocytes

Blood pressure

    ankle, venous pressure of, in venous valvular defects; effect of exercise and body position (Pollack and others) J. Clin. Invest. 28:559-563, 1949

    aortic, direct measurement method, dog (Skouby) Acta Physiol. Scand. 10:366-373, 1945

    aortic, variations during exercise, influence by drugs and aortic insufficiency (Skouby) Acta Physiol. Scand. 17(Suppl. 58):3-115, 1948

    arterial, behaviour in different amounts of body loads (Israel) Zeits. ges. inn. Med. 14:432-435, 1959

    arterial, changes, during physical exercise (Rubenstein and others) Acta Physiol. Lat. Amer. 13:130-137, 1963; (Engels and Nieske) Zeits. exp. Med. 110:81-91, 1942

Blood pressure (Cont.)

    arterial, conditions determining volume (Henderson and Barringer) Amer. J. Physiol. 31:288-299,
       1913

    arterial, during march (Soler and Soler) Prensa Méd. Argent. 28:1364-1374, 1941

    arterial, intra, measurement during exercise (Eskildsen and others) Acta Med. Scand. 138(Suppl. 239):
       245-250, 1950

    arterial, pulmonary, mild exercise, supine position, normal subjects (Slonim and others) J. Clin.
       Invest. 33:1022-1030, 1954

    arterial, pulse and leucocyte formation during muscular exercise (Bergman) Rev. Asoc. M. A.,
       Sect. Soc. Biol. 35:289-296, 1922

    arterial, pulse, and respiration changes, children, after physical exercise (Ostrovskaia) Vop. Okhr.
       Materin. Dets. 8:41-46, 1963

    arterial, and pulse rate during effort syndrome (Christensen) Acta Med. Scand. 121:194-216, 1945

    arterial, pulse-rate and oxygen pulse, under low barometric pressure (Schneider and Clarke) Amer. J.
       Physiol. 88:633-649, 1929

    arterial, and pulse rate, statistical study, in recumbency, standing and after standard exercise (Schneider
       and Truesdell) Amer. J. Physiol. 61:429-474, 1922

    arterial, systemic, during exercise in pulmonary hypertension (Jonsson and Lukianski) Acta Med. Scand.
       173:73-81, 1963

    capillary, current strength, relation, in skeletal muscle vessels (Schroeder) Zeits. Kreislaufforsch.
       53:47-53, 1964

    and cardiac output, instantaneous increase at onset of muscular activity (Guyton and others)
       Circ. Res. 11:431-441, 1962

    children and young men during physical activity and rest (Rutenfranx and others) Zeits. Kinderheilk.
       85:317-342, 1961; 89:227-244, 1964

    exercise, effects on denervated and partly-denervated trained dogs (Essex and others) Amer. J. Physiol.
       138:687-697, 1943

    exercise, influence on, dog (Essex and others) Amer. J. Physiol. 125:614-623, 1939

    exercise, variations during, and myocardial efficiency (Robertson) Med. J. & Rec. 122:213-219, 1925

    in exercised extremities (Gambill and Hines) Amer. Heart J. 28:782-785, 1944

    fluctuations during working period (Renker and Adam) Zeits. Aertzl. Fortbild. 54:903-905, 1960

    heart measurement (right) and spirometry (Lukiánski and others) Gruzlica 31:907-912, 1963

    and heart rate, during and after muscular exercise (Brouha and Harrington) J. Lancet 77:79-80,
       1957

    and heart rate, effects of muscular exertion and verbal stimuli (Astrup and Gantt) Recent Advances
       Biol. Psychiat. 4:39-42, 1961

Blood pressure (Cont.)

and heart-rate changes, and duration of systole, resulting from bicycling (Bowen) Amer. J. Physiol.
11:59-77, 1904

hexamethonium, effect during exercise (Fowler and Guz) Brit. Heart J. 16:1-7, 1954

hypotensive drugs, effect of (Weidmann and Klepzig) Zeits. Kreislaufforsch, 49:723-731, 1960

measurements, simultaneous direct and indirect, at rest and work (Henschel and others) J. Appl.
Physiol. 6:506-508, 1954

muscular work, influence on (Tangl and Zuntz) Pflüger Arch, ges. Physiol. 70:544-558, 1898

normal, during and after exercise (Korner) Aust. J. Exp. Biol. Med. Sci. 30:375-384, 1952

ocular, blood pressure and body weight in extreme prolonged physical work (Kern) Ophthalmologica
147:82-92, 1964

oscillation frequency products, and heart minute volume (Schoenewald) Zeits. ges. exp. Med. 79:
620-634, 1931

and physical exertion, relation between (Adler) Med. Press 205:181-183, 1941; (Yo) Far East Sci.
Bull. 2:89, 1942

physical work, during and after difficult (Christensen) Arbeitsphysiol. 4:128-153, 1931

post exercise, in maximum exertion tests, various relationships (Cureton) J. Lancet 77:81-82,
1957

post-exercise, reflex regulation (Korner) Aust. J. Exp. Biol. Med. Sci. 30:385-394, 1952

pressor reactions, acute, and hypertension, haemodynamic basis (Brod) Brit. Heart J. 25:227-245,
1963

pulmonary artery, and total pulmonary resistance, response of untrained convalescent man to prolonged
mild steady state exercise (Sancetta and Rakita) J. Clin. Invest. 36:1138-1149, 1957

and pulse, during regulated work and gymnastics (Budnick) Kallmünz, M. Lassleben, 1934

and pulse, influence of exercise (Pembrey and Todd) J. Physiol. 37:lxvii-lxviii, 1908

and pulse rate during and after physical work (Mechelke and Nusser) Deutsch. Arch. klin. Med.
202:599-633, 1955

and pulse rate, normal values, various age groups, during rest, orthostatism, and light exertion (Gubser
and others) Schweiz. Zeits. Sportmed. 11:17-31, 1963

and pulse rate, relative influence of mental and muscular work (Gillespie) J. Physiol. 58:425-432,
1924; (Gillespie and others) Heart 12:1-22, 1925

regulation, reference to muscular work (Euler and Liljestrand) Acta Physiol. Scand. 12:279-300, 1946

'Saluetikum-Reserpin,' influence of (Strasburger and Klepzig) Med. Welt 41:2079-2083, 1963

sucking and tilting in newborn premature infant, response to (Hanninen and others) Ann. Paediat. Fenn.
10:92-98, 1964

systolic, diastolic, and pulse, and pulse rate, effects of exercise (Lowsley) Amer. J. Physiol. 27:446-466,
1911

systolic, following exercise; remarks on cardiac capacity (Rapport) Arch. Int. Med. 19:981-989,
1917

Blood pressure (Cont.)

> venous, ambulatory, measurement, lower extremity (Lofgren) Surg. Forum 5:163-168, (1954)
> 1955
>
> venous, central, in relation to cardiac 'competence', blood volume and exercise (Landis and others)
> J. Clin. Invest. 25:237-255, 1946
>
> venous, effect of exercise (Hooker) Amer. J. Physiol. 28:235-248, 1911; (McCloy) Physical Training
> 14:300-309, 1917; (Szekely) Amer. Heart J. 22:360-366, 1941
>
> venous, changes, effect of heart glycosides (Zöllner and König) Zeits. Kreislaufforsch. 47:31-39,
> 1958
>
> venous, changes, exercise normal, elderly (González Cruz) Med. espãn. 32:124-149, 1954
>
> venous, increased, mechanism, with exercise, congestive heart failure (Wood) J. Clin. Invest. 41:
> 2020-2024, 1962
>
> venous, influence on heart rate (Sassa and Miyazaki) J. Physiol. 54:203-212, 1920
>
> venous, measurement, new method, under load (Tepper and Effert) Zeits. klin. Med. 146:509-515, 1950
>
> venous, and onset and disappearance of dyspnea in acute left ventricular heart failure (Mauck and others)
> Amer. J. Cardiol. 13:301-309, 1964
>
> venous, peripheral, suppression during and after manual work (König and Zöllner) Deutsche. Arch.
> klin. Med. 204:107-122, 1957
>
> venous, and regulation of circulation (Jørgensen) Copenhagen, Danish Science Press, 1954; (Basevi
> and others) Folia Cardiol. 14:37-51, 1955
>
> venous, in saphenous vein at ankle during exercise and changes in posture (Pollack and Wood) J. Appl.
> Physiol. 1:649-662, 1949
>
> venous pressure in saphenous vein at ankle, during exercise and changes in posture (Pollack and Wood) J.
> Appl. Physiol. 1:649-662, 1949
>
> venous, relation to cardiac efficiency (Henderson and Barringer) Amer. J. Physiol. 31:352-369, 1913
>
> see also Hypertension; Hypotension

Blood, venous

> antecubital, relationship between level of physical condition and pH (Heusner and Bernauer) J. Appl.
> Physiol. 9:171-175, 1956
>
> femoral venous blood oxygen, normal and abnormal subjects, rest and exercise (Wilson) S. Afr. J. Med.
> Sci. 15:115-119, 1950; 19:161-164, 1954
>
> variations during muscular activity (De Lanne) Bruxelles, Presses academiques europennes, 1957
>
> see also Venous return

Blood vessels

> carbon dioxide, action of on (Bayliss) J. Physiol. 26:xxxii-xxxiii, 1901
>
> and exercise (Brown and others) J. Geront. 11:292-297, 1956

Blood volume (Cont.)

variations, effect on pulse rate, supine and upright position and during exercise (Gullbring and others)
Acta Physiol. Scand. 50:62-71, 1960

see also Blood distribution

Blood volume, heart

anthropometric data, relation to, in old and young men (Strandell) Acta Med. Scand. 176:205-218,
1964

body weight, physical capacity and blood volume, relation between (Musshoff and others) Acta
Radiol. 57:377-400, 1962

measuring, different methods (Bornstein) Pflüger Arch. ges. Physiol. 132:307-318, 1910

and physical performance, relations between (Schmidt and others) Zeits. Kreislaufforsch. 51:
165-176, 1962

and respiration, in sport (Albrecht and others) Zeits. ges. exp. Med. 122:356-368, 1953

rest and during exercise, changes during (Ruosteenoja and others) Acta Med. Scand. 162:263-275,
1958

separate measurement present in 2 ventricles (Durand and others) Arch. Sci. Physiol. 15:55-78, 1961;
J. Physiologie 52:88-90, 1960

and skeletal muscle, changes during and after activity (Fischer) Amer. J. Physiol. 113:42-43, 1935

stroke volume, arterio-venous difference, cardiac output, and physical working capacity, relation to
(Musshoff and others) Acta Cardiol. 14:427-452, 1959

and stroke volume, relation between, recumbent and erect positions (Mylin) Scand. Arch. Physiol.
69:237-246, 1934

supine and sitting position, at rest and during muscular work (Holmgren and Ovenfors) Acta Med.
Scand. 167:267-277, 1960

systolic and diastolic, variations, during and after effort (Plas and Pallardy) Presse Méd. 71:2436-2438, 1963

total hemoglobin and physical working capacity in former athletes, relationship with (Holmgren and
Strandell) Acta Med. Scand. 163:149-160, 1959

training, effect of (Holmgren and others) Acta Physiol. Scand. 50:72-83, 1960

ventricles, curve, significance to heart-beat and filling (Henderson) Amer. J. Physiol. 16:325-367,
1906

ventricular, during blood pooling and exercise, effect on performance animals (Gauer) Physiol. Rev.
35:143-155, 1955

ventricular, measurement (Fick) Sitzungsb. physik. med. Ges. Wurzburg, 1870, p. 16

ventricular, regulation, isolated heart, adjustable load (Röckemann) Arch. Kreislaufforsch. 44:274-287, 1964

ventricular, rest and physical exercise in hepatic cirrhosis (Bini and others) Cuore Circ. 48:67-81, 1964.

Blood volume, plasma

changes, and anaerobic metabolism, correlation following exercise (Iseri and others) Ann. Intern. Med.
59:788-797, 1963

changes, error in measurement (Ebert and Stead) Proc. Soc. Exp. Biol. Med. 46:139-141, 1941

in heart failure, effect of exercise (Gilbert and Lewis) Circulation 2:402-408, 1950

and red cell volume after prolonged severe exercise (Åstrand and Saltin) J. Appl. Physiol. 19:829-832,
1964

Blood volume, pulmonary

in acquired heart disease, effect of exercise (Schreiner and others) Circulation 27:559-564, 1963

blood depot, importance of (Sjöstrand) Acta Physiol. Scand. 2:231-248, 1941

capillary, flow and diffusing capacity during exercise (Johnson and others) J. Appl. Physiol. 15:893-902,
1960

capillary, and pulmonary membrane diffusing capacity, measurement, effects of exercise and position
(Lewis and others) J. Clin. Invest. 37:1061-1070, 1958

contained in lungs (Grehant and Quiquaud) Comptes Rend. Soc. Biol. Eighth series 3:159-160, 1886

exercise, effect of (Chaffee and others) Amer. Heart J. 66:657-663, 1963

expiratory reserve, volume during muscular exercise, in health (Petit and others) Arch. Int. Physiol.
67:350-357, 1959

measurement during muscular work (Paulet and Van Den Driessche) Comptes Rend. Soc. Biol. 154:
2314-2316, 1960

and pulmonary circulation time and cardiac output (Stewart) Amer. J. Physiol. 58:20-44, 1921

study by quantitative radiocardiography (Giuntini and others) J. Clin. Invest. 42:1589-1605, 1963

Blood volume, splanchnic

and blood flow, effect of exercise (Wade and others) Clin. Sci. 15:457-463, 1956

Body composition

gross, studies by direct dissection (Pitts) Ann. N. Y. Acad. Sci. 110:11-22, 1963

impact of diet, age, and exercise (Parízková) Ann. N. Y. Acad. Sci. 110:661-674, 1963

influence of previous exercise, rat (Horst and others) J. Nutr. 7:251-275, 1935

and weight gain, effect on performance, dog (Young) J. Appl. Physiol. 15:493-495, 1960

Body constitution

and physical capacities of ground national defence force personnel (Sugiura and others) Nat. Def.
Med. J. 10:562-568, 1963; 11:57-60, 1964

Body efficiency

influence of physical culture (Allen) J. Psych. Med. (London) new series 2:156-160, 1876

of young men, at various times (Schwarz) Zbl. Arbeitsmed. 13:186-192, 1963

Body size

maximal oxygen intake, and total hemoglobin, normal man (Döbeln) Acta Physiol. Scand. 38:193-
199, 1956

C

Calcium

    40- and 47-, metabolism, effect of exercise (Ragan and Briscoe) J. Clin. Endocr. 24:385-392, 1964

    and magnesium, excretion with thermal sweat (Bara) Pol. Arch. Med. Wewnet, 33:1125-1132, 1963

    and phosphorus balance, effect of exercise (Konishi) Army Med. Nutrition Lab. Report 211, pp. 1-17,
       1957

    serum, changes during hyperventilation (George and others) New Eng. J. Med. 270:726-728, 1964

    serum concentration, total, effect of venous stasis and muscular exercise (Radcliff and others) Lancet 2:
       1249-1251, 1962

    therapy, increased performance during physical exercise (Full) Zeits. ges. phys. Ther. 41:98-104, 1931

Caloric requirements

    under adverse environmental conditions (Johnson) Fed. Proc. 22:1439-1446, 1963

    calorigenic action of methylene blue during muscular exercise (Guild and Rapport) Proc. Soc. Exper.
       Biol. 34:459-461, 1936

    nutrient ratios in applied nutrition (Crampton) J. Nutr. 82:353-365, 1964

    see also Energy expenditure

Cancer

    and exercise (Rigan) J. Amer. Osteopath. Asso. 62:596-599, 1963

Capacity, aerobic

    (Andersen) T. Norsk. Laegeforen. 80:1087-1091, 1960

    and anaerobic changes in seal muscles, during diving (Scholander and others) J. Biol. Chem. 142:431-440,
       1942

    and anaerobic work capacity after dehydration (Saltin) J. Appl. Physiol. 19:1114-1118, 1964

    and circulation at exercise, prolonged exercise and/or heat exposure (Saltin) Acta Physiol. Scand. Suppl.
       230:1-52, 1964

    Eskimos (Andersen & Hart) J. Appl. Physiol. 18:764-768, July, 1963

    maximal work, ergometry (Garimoldi and others) Gior. Ital. Tuberc. 18:226-242, 1964

    nomogram for calculation from pulse rate during submaximal work (Åstrand and Rhyming) J. Appl. Physiol.
       7:218-221, 1954

    rapid determination (Binkhorst and van Leeuwen) Int. Zeits. angew. Physiol. 19:459-467, 1963

    see also Oxygen; Respiration; Work, muscular

Capacity, cardiac

    and systolic blood pressure following exercise (Rapport) Arch. Intern. Med. 19:981-989, 1917

Capacity, physical working

    analysis of the effect of previous muscular efforts, on rested muscles (Muravov and Tkachev) Fiziol. Zh.
       10:163-169, 1964

    bicycle ergometer, children (Cumming, G. R. and Cumming, P. M.) Canad. Med. Ass. J. 88:351-355,
       1963

Carbon dioxide (Cont.)

  and oxygen tensions, alveolar air and arterial blood, at rest and after exercise (Galdston and Wollack)
    Amer. J. Physiol. 151:276-281, 1947

  and oxygen tensions, alveolar, influence of muscular activity (Hough) Amer. J. Physiol. 30:18-36, 1912

  and oxygen tensions, arterial blood, during heavy and exhaustive exercise (Holmgren and Linderholm)
    Acta Physiol. Scand. 44:203-215, 1958

  physical-chemical system of blood in respiration and circulation: carbon dioxide inhalation and hyperpnea
    (Hochrin and others) Naunyn Schmiedeberg Arch. exp. Path. 143:170-183, 1929

  quantity expired during 24 hours (Scharling) Ann. Chem. Pharm. 45:214-242, 1843

  and pulmonary ventilation in muscular exercise (Kao and others) J. Appl. Physiol. 19:1075-1080, 1964

  reduction due to muscular exercise (Andersen & Bugge-Asperheim) Acta Physiol. Scand. 47:91-96, 1959

  respiration, effect on, using new method of administration (Fenn and Craig) 18:1023-1024, 1963

  respiratory and cardiovascular centers, effect on: perfusion of mammalian medulla (Hooker and others)
    Amer. J. Physiol. 43:351-361, 1917

  respiratory response, and alveolar oxygen pressure, relation between (Lloyd and others) Quart. J. Exp.
    Physiol. 43:214-227, 1958

  respiratory response to noradrenaline, effect on (Barcroft and others) J. Physiol. 137:365-373, 1957

  ventilation stimuli relation to neurogenic ventilation stimuli (Lefrançois and Dejours) Rev. Franc. Etud.
    Clin. Biol. 9:498-505, 1964

  ventilatory response to, during work at normal and at low oxygen tensions (Asmussen and Nielsen) Acta
    Physiol. Scand. 39:27-35, 1957

  see also Alkali reserve

Carbon monoxide

  diffusing capacity during exercise (Hanson and Tabakin) J. Appl. Physiol. 15:402-404, 1960

  diffusion, in athletes and non-athletes, effect of exercise, body and lung size (Newman and others) J.
    Appl. Physiol. 17:649-655, 1962

  oxygen tension of arterial blood, method of investigation on (Douglas and Haldane) Skand. Arch. Physiol.
    25:169-182, 1911

  uptake and pulmonary diffusing capacity, at rest and during exercise (Filley and others) J. Clin. Invest.
    33:530-539, 1954

Cardiac disease, see Heart disease

Cardiac failure, see Heart failure

Cardiac insufficiency, see Insufficiency, cardiac

Cardiac output

  (Christensen) Ergebn. Physiol. 39:348-407, 1937; (Gross and Mittermaier) Arch. ges. Physiol. 212:136-149,
    1926

Cardiac output (Cont.)

and anerobic metabolism and exercise (Thomas and others) J. Appl. Physiol. 19:839-848, 1964

arterial pressoreceptors during muscular exercise, role of (Leusen and Lacroix) Arch. Int. Pharmacodyn.
130:470-472, 1961

arterio-venous difference, and oxygen absorption and output (Musshoff and others) Zeits. Kreislaufforsch.
48:255-277, 1959

and arteriovenous oxygen difference, exercise and resting (Thomas and others) J. Appl. Physiol. 17:
922-926, 1962

atrial, right, (Stead and others) J. Clin. Invest. 24:326-331, 1945

and blood pressure, oscillation frequency products (Schoenewald) Zeits. ges. exp. Med. 79:620-634,
1931

during carbon dioxide inhalation during exercise (Forssander) J. Appl. Physiol. 8:509-512, 1956

and central blood volume, rest and exercise, dye method (Nowy and others) Zeits. Kreislaufforsch. 46:
382-393, 1957

and central blood volumes, measurement, in physical work (Noder) Zeits. Kreislaufforsch. 52:1206-1210,
1963

circulation time (Stewart) Amer. J. Physiol. 58:20-44, 1921; J. Physiol. 22:159-183, 1897

and circulation time, during body loading, healthy young men (Rothlin and Alsleben) Schweiz. Zeits.
Sportmed. 12:73-79, 1964

coal miners during work (Peretti and Granati) Arch. Sci. Biol. 26:149-153, 1940

dependence on body surface (Noder) Arch. Kreislaufforsch. 45:19-28, 1964

determination, and function of circulation (Bansi and Groscurth) Klin. Wschr. 41:1902-1907, 1930

determination, acetylene (Grollman) Amer. J. Physiol. 88:432-443, 1929

determination, direct Fick method, effects of posture, venous pressure change, atropine, and adrenaline
(McMichael and Sharpey-Schafer) Brit. Heart J. 6:33-40, 1944

determinations, simultaneous and rapidly repeated, by dye-dilution method (Hanson and Tabakin) J. Appl.
Physiol. 19:275-278, 1964

determination, thermodilution method, exertion, dog (Cerretelli and others) Boll. Soc. Ital. Biol. Sper.
39:2038-2040, 1963

determined from blood pressure (Blasius) Zeits. Kreislaufforsch. 33:201-208, 1941

determined with ethyl iodide (Lehmann) Arbeitsphysiol. 1:114-129, 1928; 1:595-599, 1929

determined by indirect physical test, silicosis (Borney) Minerva Cardioangiol. 11:707-710, 1963

determined by right atrial catheterization (Stead and others) J. Clin. Invest. 24:326-331, 1945

determined simultaneously by acetylene and dye injection methods, rest and work (Asmussen and Nielsen)
Acta Physiol. Scand. 27:230, 1953

digitalis, effect of on cardiac output in normal heart, rest and exercise (Rodman and others) Ann. Intern. Med.
55:620-631, 1961

Cardiac output (Cont.)

in difficult physical work (Christensen) Arbeitsphysiol. 4:470-502, 1931

dye-dilution technique during exercise (Levy and others) Brit. Heart J. 23:425-432, 1961

estimation, clinical reliability of acetyl method (Baumann and Grollman) Zeits. klin. Med. 115:
41-53, 1930

estimation, gas analysis in rest and during difficult muscle work (Christensen) Arbeitsphysiol. 4:
175-202, 1931

ethyl iodide method, for measuring (Kaup and Grosse) Arbeitsphysiol. 1:357-376, 1929

ethyl iodide and nitrous oxide method, rest and work (Kaup and Grosse) Zeits. Kreislaufforsch. 21:44-48,
1929

in exercise (Asmussen and Nielsen) Ann. Vol. Physiol. Exp. Med. Sci. India 2:21-26, 1958-1959; (Bailie
and others) J. Appl. Physiol. 16:107-111, 1961; (Donald and others) Clin. Sci. 14:37-73, 1955; (Meek
and Eyster) Amer. J. Physiol. 63:400-401, 1922; (Grollman) Amer. J. Physiol. 96:8-15, 1931

during exercise (Collett and Liljestrand) Scand. Arch. Physiol. 45:29-42, 1924

during exercise, prolonged, serial determination (Grimby and others) Scand. J. Clin. Lab. Invest. 15(Suppl. 76):
52, 1963

and gas metabolism (Odaira) Tohoku J. Exp. Med. 6:325-366, 1925

in health and disease (Grollman) Springfield, Charles C. Thomas, 1932

in heart disease, compensated, during rest and exercise (Nielsen) Acta Med. Scand. 91:223-266, 1937

in heart disease, and normal, during exercise (Morbelli and Mascaretti) Cardiologia 43:317-336, 1963

heart minute volume, oxygen consumption, and arterial and venous blood gases, in volunteers, rest and exercise
(Ulmer and Berta) Pflüger Arch. ges. Physiol. 280:281-296, 1964

heart rate, and arteriovenous oxygen difference, rest and exercise (Nitter-Hauge) T. Norsk. Laegeforen. 83:
1310-1316, 1963; in heart and lung disease (Nitter-Hauge) T. Norsk. Laegeforen. 83:1316-1322, 1963

impedance plethysmographic determination (Kinnen and others) Tech. Docum. Rep. No. SAM-TDR-64-15,
U.S. Air Force Sch. Aerospace Med. 1-8, 1964

and instantaneous increase at onset of muscular activity (Guyton and others) Circ. Res. 11:431-441, 1962

measurement, acetylene method, normal and diseased men (Grollman and others) Naunyn Schmiedeberg Arch.
exp. Path. 162:463-471, 1931

and output investigations, oxygen consumption, and arterial and venous blood gases, in volunteers, rest and
exercise (Ulmer and Berta) Pflüger Arch. ges. Physiol. 280:281-296, 1964

oxygen consumption, and arterial saturation during work of increasing intensity (Morbelli and others)
Atti. Soc. Ital. Cardiol. 22:323-324, 1962

posture and atropine, effects of (Weissler and others) J. Clin. Invest. 36:1656-1622, 1957

posture, effect of (Lindhard) Skand. Arch. Physiol. 30:395-408, 1913; (McGregor and others) Circ. Res.
9:1089-1092, 1961; (Grollman) Amer. J. Physiol. 86:285-301, 1928

Cardiopulmonary (Cont.)

function in young smokers (Krumholz and others) Ann. Intern. Med. 60:603-610, 1964

hemodynamics during exercise, in pulmonary emphysema, rest and exercise (Williams and Behnke)
Ann. Intern. Med. 60:824-842, 1964

and metabolic aspects of muscular work (Bergamaschi and others) Minerva Ginec. 16:831-838, 1964

performance, maximal oxygen intake as objective measure (Taylor and others) J. Appl. Physiol. 8:73-80,
1955

performance, under unusual stress during exercise (Bruce and others) Arch. Industr. Hyg. Occup. Med. 6:
105-112, 1952

physiological responses to heavy exercise, in anemia (Sproule and others) J. Clin. Intern. 39:378-388,
1960

system during adolescence (Birčák and Niks) Bratisl. Lek. Listy 2:701-709, 1963; (Birčák and others) Bratisl.
Lek. Listy 2:541-558, 637-648, 1963

Cardiovascular

adaptations to prolonged physical effort (Beckner and Winsor)' Circulation 9:835-846, 1954

disease and exercise, review (Taylor and Stamler) Nat. Conf. Cardiov. Dis. 2:358-360, 1964

disease, effect of exercise on cardiac output and pulmonary arterial pressure (Hickam and Cargill) J.
Clin. Invest. 27:10-23, 1948

disease, functional, dispensary observations, children (Filippova and Zernov) Vop. Okhr. Materin. Dets.
8:55-59, 1963

diseases, sinoauricular block in effort electrocardiogram (Solti and Goldesy) Zeits. ges. inn. Med. 17:
930-933, 1962

exercise, cardiovascular response to graded (Fries) Arch. Phys. Ther. 25:540-545, 1944

exercise, cardiovascular response to graded in sympathectomized-vagotomized dog (Ashkar and Hamilton)
Amer. J. Physiol. 204:291-296, 1963

exercise, cardiovascular response to, techniques for determination, unanesthetized monkeys (Smith and others)
J. Appl. Physiol. 17:718-721, 1962

exercise and diencephalic stimulation, cardiovascular response to (Smith and others) Amer. J. Physiol. 198:
1139-1142, 1960

effects of exercise, duration (Boigey) Bull. Acad. Med., 3rd series 91:220-224, 1924

effects of exercise, normal and cardiac (Lowenthal and others) Brit. J. Phys. Med. 17:13-15, 1954

exercise, sedentary men and athletes, cardiovascular response to (Wang and others) Physiologist 3:173,
1960

fitness in children, exercise tests (Kramer and Lurie) Amer. J. Dis. Child. 108:283-297, 1964

function, assessment (McIlroy and Naimark) Biochem. Clin. 1:161-168, 1963

function, effect of physical conditioning, ballistocardiography (Holloszy and others) Amer. J. Cardiol.
14:761-770, 1964

function, index, formulae based on concept of humoral regulation of respiration (Vacca and Vacca) Riv.
Med. Aero. 26:223-235, 1963

Cardiovascular (Cont.)

    health and physical activity (Fox and Skinner) Amer. J. Cardiol. 14:731-746, 1964

    physical exercise, cardiovascular reactions to (Briol) Bordeaux, Delmas, 1937

    responses of pre-adolescent boys to muscular activity (Schneider and Crampton) Amer. J. Physiol.

        114:473-482, 1936

    step test and hand cranking test, response of patients to indicate exercise tolerance (Michael and Wolffe)

        Arch. Phys. Med. 44:327-331, 1963

    system, effects of muscular work and heat (Brouha) Industr. Med. Surg. 29:114-120, 1960

    system, reflexogenic areas (Heymans and Neil) Churchill, 1958

    test variable, factor analysis (Cureton & Sterling) J. Sport Med. 4:1-24, 1964

    tests, relation to measurements of motor performance and skills (Fowler and Gardner) Pediatrics 32(Suppl.):

        778-789, 1963

    training for underwater swimming, cardiovascular responses to (Michael) J. Sport Med. 3:218-220, 1963

Carotene

    effects of exercise on blood plasma concentration (Hillman and Rosner) J. Nutr. 64:605-613, 1958

Carotid body

    reflexes, and chemical regulation of respiration, dog (Comroe & Schmidt) Amer. J. Physiol. 121:75-97,

        1938

Carotid sinus

    and cardio-aortic homologous zone (Heymans and Regniers) Paris, G. Doin et Cie, 1933

    function (McDowall) Arch. Int. Pharmacodynam. 140:168-172, 1962

    influence on oxygen uptake, functional sympatholysis during muscular activity (Remensnyder and others)

        Circ. Res. 11:370-380, 1962

    sensitivity to chemical stimulus and blood output of femoral artery (Heymans) Comptes Rend. Soc.

        Biol. 119:542-545, 1935

Catalase

    blood, activity rest and muscular work (Rougier and Babin) J. Physiologie 56:436-437, 1964

    and secondary anoxia in work carried out in anaerobiosis (Ghiringdelli and Molina) Med. Lavoro 43:

        463-467, 1952

Catecholamines

    and atropine, effect on cardiovascular response to exercise, dog (Keck and others) Circ. Res. 9:566-570,

        1961

    content, brain and heart, hedgehog (Erinaceus Europaeus) hibernation, and active (Uuspää) Ann. Med.

        Exp. Fenn. 41:340-348, 1963

    excretion, urinary, relation to waking/sleeping rhythm and work (Pelosse and Soulairac) Ann. Endocr.

        25:661-669, 1964

    see also Epinephrine; Norepinephrine

Cerebral circulation

   exercise at various atmospheres, control during (Lambertsen and others) J. Appl. Physiol. $\underline{14}$:966-982, 1959

   fatigue, influence on (Horiuchi) Arbeitsphysiol. $\underline{1}$:75-84, 1928

   and metabolism, effects of vigorous physical exercise (Scheinberg and others) Amer. J. Med. $\underline{16}$:549-554, 1954

   and metabolism, in pulmonary emphysema and fibrosis, effects of mild exercise (Scheinberg and others) J. Clin. Invest. $\underline{32}$:720-728, 1953

   muscular exercise, behaviour during (Hedlund and others) Acta Physiol. Scand. $\underline{54}$:316-324, 1962

   physical activity, changes (Lazzari) Gazz. Int. Med. Chir. $\underline{69}$:1340-1345, 1964

   physiological effort, adaptation to (Remky) Ann. Ocul. $\underline{188}$:849-858, 1955

   in regulation of respiration (Defares and others) Acta Physiol. Pharmacol. Neerl. $\underline{9}$:327-360, 1960

Cerebral cortex, see Cortex, cerebral

Cerebrospinal fluid

   hydrogen ion concentration and CO_2 pressure in, influence on respiration (Loeschcke) Klin. Wschr. $\underline{38}$: 366-376, 1960

   influence of pH on respiration (Leusen) Experientia $\underline{6}$:272, 1950

Chemoreceptors

   aortic, location and function (Comroe) Amer. J. Physiol. $\underline{127}$:176-191, 1939.

Chemosensitivity

   intracranial, interaction with peripheral afferents to respiratory centers (Loeschcke and others) Ann. N.Y. Acad. Sci. $\underline{109}$:651-660, 1963

   of regions on surface of medulla, respiratory responses mediated by (Mitchell and others) J. Appl. Physiol. $\underline{18}$:523-533, 1963; Ann. N.Y. Acad. Sci. $\underline{109}$:661-681, 1963

Chest

   expansion, electrical gymnastic device (Vaust) Bull. Soc. Sci. Med. Nat. Bruxelles pp. 56-58, 1864

   pain, differential diagnosis, and silent coronary heart disease detected by exercise test (Master and Rosenfeld) J.A.M.A. $\underline{190}$:494-500, 1964

   pain, exercise electrocardiogram (Gubner) J. Occup. Med. $\underline{3}$:110-120, 1961

   see also Lungs; Pulmonary

Chloride

   blood, urine, and sweat content, in muscular activity (Koriakina and others) Arbeitsphysiol. $\underline{2}$:461-473, 1930

   concentration during exercise, dog (Schlutz and Morse) Amer. J. Physiol. $\underline{121}$:293-309, 1938

   metabolism during hot work (Lehmann and Szakáll) Arbeitsphysiol. $\underline{10}$:608-646, 1939

   serum, kidney excretion during exercise, dog (Morse and Schultz) J. Biol..Chem. $\underline{119}$:lxxi-lxxii, 1937

   and sodium, elevated in sweat, in adult without cystic fibrosis (Gup and Briggs) Arch. Intern. Med. $\underline{112}$: 699-701, 1963

Chlorothiazide

> effects on working capacity (Danzinger and Cummings) J. Appl. Physiol. 19:636-638, 1964

Cholesterol metabolism

> arteriosclerosis and physical activity (Karvonen) Schweiz. Zeits. Sportmed. 9:90-100, 1961

> effect of physical activity on synthesis in rat liver (Aleksandrow and others) J. Atheroscler. Res. 4: 351-355, July-Aug., 1964

Cholesterol, blood

> concentration, relationship of physical activity to (Naughton) J. Okla. Med. Ass. 57:540-541, 1964

> dietary cholesterol, dietary fat, and exercise, effects of, mouse (Peltonen and Karvonen) Ann. Med. Exp. Fenn. 34:246-252, 1956

> exercise, acute, and training, response to in medical personnel (Naughton and Balke) Amer. J. Med. Sci. 247:286-292, 1964

> exercise effects in middle-aged men (Montoye and others) Amer. J. Clin. Nutr. 7:139-145, 1959

> exercise, lack of effect of, in two types of experimental obesity (Mayer and others) Experientia 13: 250-251, 1957

> and glucose, serum, concentration changes after prolonged physical effort (Preisler and Pankowska) Bull. Soc. Amis. Sci. Poznan (Med.) 12:61-70, 1963

> level, changes middle-aged and aged during exercise (Babarin and others) Sovet. Med. 26:109-111, 1963

> level during physical activity (Chailley-Bert and others) Presse Méd. 63:415-416, 1955

> level, influence of physical stress, seafarers (Ejsmont) Bull. Inst. Mar. Med. Gdansk. 15:199-205, 1964

> lipid metabolism and pantothenic acid with low cholesterol diet, rats (Lazzari) Gazz. Int. Med. Chir. 69:1151-1154, 1964

> and lipids, liver, effects of exercise and food restriction (Jones and others) Amer. J. Physiol. 207:460-466, 1964

> and lipids, other, and physical activity (Taylor and others) Proc. Soc. Exp. Biol. Med. 95:383-386, 1957

> non-esterified fatty acids, triglycerides, and phospholipids, arteriovenous relationships, in exercise (Konttinen and others) Ann. Med. Exp. Fenn. 40:250-256, 1962

> and physical activity (Lumia and Giarnieri) Gior. Geront. 8:615-618, 1960

> physical activity and diet in populations differing in (Keys and others) J. Clin. Invest. 35:1173-1181, 1956

Cholesterol synthesis

> in rat liver, effect of physical activity (Aleksandrow and others) J. Atheroscler. Res. 4:351-355, July-Aug., 1964

Cholinesterase

> activity, blood, influence of physical work (Billewicz-Stankiewicz and Tyburczyk) Int. Zeits. angew. Physiol. 18:361-375, 1960

Cholinesterase (Cont.)

    activity of serum, brain, and muscle in normal and adrenalectomised rats (Overbeek) Arch. Int.

        Pharmacodyn. 79:314-322, 1949

    blood, effect of work in hot environment on (Liska and others) Prac. Lek. 15:291-293, 1963

    and muscular activity (Croft and Richter) J. Physiol. 102:155-169, 1943

    serum, changes, violent muscular exercise and hypoglycaemia shock (Huidobro and others) Rev.

        Med. Aliment. 6:38-40, 1943-1944

    serum, effect of muscular exercise, myasthemia gravis (Stoner and Wilson) J. Physiol. 102:1-4, 1943

Cinematometer

    Zhukovs'kii, evaluation (Ashmarin) Fiziol. Zh. 9:479-484, 1963

Circulation, blood

    and aerobic work capacity at exercise, prolonged exercise and/or heat exposure (Saltin) Acta Physiol.

        Scand. Suppl. 230:1-52, 1964

    altitudes, high; pulse-rate, arterial and venous pressures, effects of exertion (Schneider and others) Amer. J.

        Physiol. 40:380-417, 1916

    arterial and central venous pressures in systemic circulation, during muscular work (Holmgren) Scand. J.

        Clin. Lab. Invest. 8(Suppl. 24):1-97, 1956

    athletics and exercise, effect on (Pyorala) Duodecim 80:101-109, 1964

    autonomic nervous system inhibition, effect on circulatory response to muscular exercise (Kahler and others)

        J. Clin. Invest. 41:1981-1987, 1962

    bed rest for two weeks, effect on circulatory functions (Miller and others) Aerospace Med. 35:931-939, 1964

    beta adrenergic blockage in hypertrophic subaortic stenosis, effects of (Harrison and others) Circulation 29:

        84-98, 1964

    blood distribution during physical exercise, influence of (Asmussen and Christensen) Scand. Arch. Physiol.

        82:185-192, 1939

    body position, at rest and during exercise, effect of (Bevegård and others) Acta Physiol. Scand. 49:279-298,

        1960

    cardiac, changes, in rest and effort, influence of doping agents (Segers and others) Actualites Cardiol. Angeiol.

        Int. 12:195-204, 1963

    cardioacceleration by methyl scopolamine nitrate, at rest and during exercise, effect of (Bevegård) Acta

        Physiol. Scand. 57:61-80, 1963

    children, reactions, after exercise (Wilson) Arch. Pediat. 37:368-371, 1920

    circulating capacity, total, importance of training factors on, old people (Landen) Deutsch. med. Wschr. 68:

        168, 1942

    coronary collateral, effect of exercise and coronary artery narrowing on (Eckstein) Circ. Res. 5:230-235,

        1957

    coronary, response to exercise, to drugs, and to anoxic stresses (Essex) J. Aviation Med. 21:456-460, 1950

Circulation, blood (Cont.)

after dehydration, response to submaximal and m aximal exercise (Saltin) J. Appl. Physiol. 19:1125-1132, 1964

and distribution during work (Kaufman) Cardiologia 30:102-114, 1957

dye dilution methods during training with physical load (Schneider and others) Verh. deutsch. Ges. inn. Med. 70:140-144, 1964

dynamics, effect of exercise (Dexter and others) J. Appl. Physiol. 3:439-453, 1951

dynamics at rest and on exercise, hyperkinetic states (Bishop and others) Clin. Sci. 14:329-360, 1955

effort, great physical, reaction to (Baldes and others) München. med. Wschr. 53:1865-1866, 1906

effort, reaction to (Fabre and Fabre) J. Physiologie 44:645-654, 1952

effort, repercussions of, dog (Fabre and Rougier) J. Physiologie 44:655-661, 1952

estimation during rest and work (Hochrein and others) Naunyn Schmiedeberg Arch. exp. Path. 143:147-160, 1929

exercise, changes associated with (Starling) J. Roy. Army Med. Corps 34:258-272, 1920; (Akzhigton) Ter. Arkh. 36:90-97, 1964; (Donald and others) Clin. Sci. 14:37-73, 1955; (Gordon) Northwest Med. 25: 376-379, 1926; (MacPhail) Brit. Med. J. 2:637-638, 1915; (Marshall and Shepherd) Circulation 27: 323-327, 1963; (Piédallu) J. Méd. Paris 46:32, 1927

during exercise, dogs, normal and with valvular lesions (Barger and others) Amer. J. Physiol. 201:480-484, 1961

exercise, prolonged severe; response to (Saltin and Stenberg) J. Appl. Physiol. 19:833-838, 1964

exercise, regulation of circulation during; cardiac output: direct Fick and metabolic adjustments, dog (Barger and others) Amer. J. Physiol. 184:613-623, 1956

exercise, resistance, effect of (Brunton and Tunnicliffe) Brit. Med. J. 2:1073-1075, 1897

exercise, supine, changes during (Reeves and others) J. Appl. Physiol. 16:279-282, 1961

exercising dogs (Cerretelli and others) J. Appl. Physiol. 19:29-32, 1964

fatigue and exercise, changes after 2-ethyl-amino-3-phenyl-norcamphan (Weidmann and Klepzig) Zeits. Kreislaufforsch. 49:1103-1108, 1960

and heart action, in young workers (Zuntz) Deutsch. Zeits. Thiermed. 18:261-277, 1892

in heart disease and health, rest and exercise (Loewy and Lewandowsky) Zeits. ges. exp. Med. 5: 321-348, 1917

and heart, effect of exercise (Larrabee) Boston Med. & Surg. J. 147:318-323, 328-330, 1902

and heart, immediate and remote effects, athletics (Stengel) Amer. J. Med. Sci. 118:544-553, 1899

heart impulse, relation between production and conduction, before and after exercise, health and disease (Sato) Acta Sch. Med. Univ. Imp. Kioto 11:457-517, 1929

and heart in athletes (Reindell and others) Med. Welt. 31:1557-1563, 1960

and heart, possible injury by physical strain (Hollmann) Aerztl. Wschr. 14:605-609, 1959

Circulation, blood (Cont.)

hemodynamics, cerebral and general, effect of mild steady state exercise, untrained subjects (Kleinerman and
Sancetta) J. Clin. Invest. 34:945-946, 1955

hyperventilation and exercise, responses of (Thompson and others) Amer. Heart J. 63:106-114, 1962

hyperventilation, effect of (Lüthy and others) Cardiologia 30:139-144, 1957

impulse conduction time and ventricular contraction, change in; effect of exercise (Saito and others) Acta
Sch. Med. Univ. Imp. Kiot 14:353-364, 1932

and kidney function, influence of effort, in cardiac disease (Himbert and others) Sem. Hôp. Paris 32:415-423, 1956

lesser, effect of repeated exercise (Widimsky and others) J. Appl. Physiol. 18:983-986, 1963

in malnutrition, rest and exercise (Frade Fernández) Medicina (Madrid) (Part 2) 11:1-16, 1943

men, old, healthy, rest and exercise (Granath and others) Acta Med. Scand. 176:425-446, 1964; (Granath and Strandell)
176:447-466, 1964; Acta Med. Scand. 169:125-126, 1961

mental effort and exercise, effects of, relation to industry (McDowall) J. Industr. Hyg. 10:94-100, 1928

metabolic effects, different types of inactivity (Birkhead and others) Amer. J. Med. Sci. 247:243, 1964

and metabolic reactions to work in heat (Williams and others) J. Appl. Physiol. 17:625-638, 1962

in mitral stenosis, based on gas exchange data (Beliaeva) Ter. Arkh. 35:60-65, 1963; (Eliasch) Circulation
5:271-278, 1952

in muscle work after eating and fluid intake (Jarisch and Liljestrand) Skand. Arch. Physiol. 51:235-248, 1927

in muscular work (Leusen) Belg. T. Geneesk. 15:930-939, 1959

muscular work, prolonged, effect of (Mahomed) Brit. Med. J. 1:359-361, 1876

normal relation and gross function; dependence of heart minute volume on body surface (Noder) Arch.
Kreislaufforsch. 45:19-28, 1964

in occupation and sport, influence of muscular work (Stadler) Samml. klin. Vorträge, Leipzig, n.F.,
No. 688 (Inn. Med. No. 224):673-692, 1913

occupation, effect on, and extent of pressure variations (Henri) Arch. Mal. Prof. 23:161-163, 1962

peripheral, local regulation, during muscular work (Grandpierre) Acta Belg. Arte Med. Pharm. Milit. 110
(Part 2):337-344, 1957

peripheral, in valvular heart disease, effect of muscular exercise (Abramson and others) J. Clin. Invest.
21:747-750, 1942

physical training, effect of on (Frick and others) Amer. J. Cardiol. 12:142-147, 1963

physical working capacity, old men (Strandell) Acta Med. Scand. Suppl. 414:1-44, 1964

physiological modifications during prolonged effort (Ulmeanau and Mestes) Minerva Med. 48:1319-1323,
1957

positive pressure breathing, influence of (Werkö) Acta Med. Scand. (Suppl. 193):3-125, 1947

Circulation, blood (Cont.)

pressure mean circulatory, and cardiac output, instantaneous increase at onset of muscular activity
(Guyton and others) Circ. Res. 11:431-441, 1962

pulmonary, changes in pH and pCO_2 during CO_2 breathing and exercise (Froeb and Kim) Med. Thorac. 19:
306-316, 1962

pulmonary circulation time, blood volume in lungs, cardiac output (Stewart) Amer. J. Physiol. 58:
20-44, 1921

pulmonary circulatory changes during exercise (Shepherd) Pediatrics 32 (Suppl.):683-690, 1963

pulmonary, effects of acute hypoxia and exercise on (Fishman and others) Circulation 22:204-215, 1960

pulmonary and peripheral, orthostatic changes (Lagerlöf and others) Scand. J. Clin. Lab. Invest. 3:
85-91, 1951

pulmonary, effects of work, in mitral stenosis (Eliasch and others) Circulation 5:271-278, 1952

and pulmonary emphysema, during treadmill exercise (Blount and Reeves) Amer. Rev. Resp. Dis. 80:
128-130, 1959

pulmonary, response to infusion of norepinephrine and isoproterenol (Aramendía and others) Acta Physiol.
Lat. Amer. 13:20-25, 1963

rate, determination at rest and work (Boothby) Amer. J. Physiol. 37:383-417, 1915

rate, method for estimating (Meakins and Davies) Heart 9:191-198, 1922

rate, regulation (Douglas and Haldane) J. Physiol. 56:69-100, 1922

regional, in association with exercise and heart disease (Donald) Brit. Med. J. 1:985-994, 1959

regulation, to right heart (Krogh) Scand. Arch. f. Physiol. 27:227-248, 1912

regulation, significance of blood volume and distribution (Sjöstrand) Physiol. Rev. 33:202-228, 1953

regulation, with special reference to stroke volume, muscular work, body position and heart rate (Bevegård)
Acta Physiol. Scand. 57 (Suppl. 200):1-36, 1962

and respiration, adaptation during long-term, non-steady state exercise, and sitting (Ekelund and Holmgren)
Acta Physiol. Scand. 62:240-255, 1964

and respiration, adaptation to serve muscular work (Åstrand and others) Acta Physiol. Scand. 50:254-258,
1960

and respiration changes in response to muscular exercise (Paterson) J. Physiol. 66:323-345, 1928

and respiration, effect of excess of carbon dioxide and of want of oxygen (Hill and Flack) J. Physiol. 37:
77-111, 1908

and respiration, influence of exercise (Boigey) J. Méd. Franc. 16:298-304, 1927

and respiration, influence of muscular work, dog (Leusen and others) Acta Cardiol. 13:153-172, 1958

and respiration, influence of work and training, clinical and physiological observations (Hollmann)
Dormstadt, Steinkopf, 1959

Circulation, blood (Cont.)

   and respiration, mechanism (Bourdon) Baillière, 1820

   and respiration, nervous factors controlling, during exercise employing blocking of blood flow (Asmussen and
          Nielsen) Acta Physiol. Scand. 60:103-111, 1964

      and respiration, regulation during muscular work, initial stages (Krogh and Lindhard) J. Physiol. 47:112-136, 1913

      and respiration, regulation through oxygen pressure in mixed venous blood (Hilpert and others) Pflüger Arch. ges.
          Physiol. 279:1-16, 1964

      and respiratory responses of anesthetized dogs to induced muscular work (Kao and Ray) Amer. J. Physiol.
          179:249-254, 1954

      in rest and work on Mount Evans (4,300m.) (Asmussen and Consolazio) Amer. J. Physiol. 132:555-563,
          1941

      rowing, effect of, sphygmograph (Fraser) J. Anat. & Physiol. 3:127-130, 1868-1869

      through skeletal muscle (Hyman) Pediatrics 32(Suppl.):671-679, 1963

      smoking, effect of (Steinman and Voegeli) Deutsch. Arch. klin. Med. 189:319-325, 1942

      speed, in rest and exercise, 100 healthy subjects (Mosco) Endocr. Pat. Costit. 15:3-29, 1940

      and sport (Prokop and Slapak) Wien. Moudrich, 1958

      strain, effect of (Fothergill) Brit. Med. J. 1:281, 1873

      stroke volume in normal subjects at rest and during exercise, recumbent position (Holmgren and others)
          Acta Physiol. Scand. 49:343-363, 1960

      studies (Loewy and Schrötter) Zeits. exp. Path. Ther. 1:197-310, 1905; (Akzhigton) Ter. Arkh. 36:
          90-97, 1964

      and tension development, comparison in biceps and triceps (Gersten and others) Amer. J. Phys. Med. 42:
          156-165, 1963

      time and heart minute volume, during body loading, healthy young men (Rothlin and Alsleben) Schweiz.
          Zeits. Sportmed. 12:73-79, 1964

      time, required to circulate blood once in body (Smith) Trans. Coll. Physicians Phila.; third series
          7:133-152, 1884

      upper limb, changes during static loading (Titievskaia) Fiziol. Zh. SSSR Sechenov. 50:1129-1135, 1964

      and ventilation, reaction by aged subjects during static effort, normal air and oxygen inhalation (Binet and
          Bochet) Rev. Franc. Geront. 10:7-19, 1964

      ventricular rate, effect of varying, with artificial pacemakers, at rest and during exercise (Bevegård)
          Acta Med. Scand. 172:615-622, 1962

      volumes, comparison of (Noder) Zeits. Kreislaufforsch. 52:1157-1159, 1963

      in voluntary muscle (Grant) Clin. Sci. 3:157-173, 1938

      Mr. Weston's 500-mile walk, observation on (Mahomed) Lancet 1:432, 1876

      see also Blood; Capillaries; Cardiovascular; Cerebral circulation; Renal

Circulatory organs

  effect of strain on (Fothergill) Brit. Med. J. 1:281, 1873

Cirrhosis, liver

  circulatory changes during exercise and rest (Bayley and others) Clin. Sci. 26:227-235, 1964

  clot lysis in, effect of exercise on (Jang and others) Clin. Sci. 27:9-13, 1964

  ventricle blood volume, rest and physical exercise (Bini and others) Cuore Circ. 48:67-81, 1964

Citric acid

  and oxalic acid, muscle content, changes in various functional conditions (Chagovets) Ukr. Biokhim. Zh.
    36:499-505, 1964

Claudication

  circulation in calf after arterial occlusion, and after exercise (Strandell and Wahren) Acta Med. Scand.
    173:99-105, 1963

  of hemodynamic response, evaluation of (Strandness and Bell) Surg. Gynec. Obstet. 119:1237-1242, 1964

  peripheral blood flow (Hillestad) I. Postural tests, Acta Med. Scand. 172:301-305, 1962; II. Skin
    thermometry, Acta Med. Scand. 172:307-314, 1962; III. Oscillometry, Acta Med. Scand. 172:
    573-583, 1962; IV. Claudication distance, Acta Med. Scand. 173:467-478, 1963; V.-VI.
    Plethysmographic studies, Acta Med. Scand. 174:23-41, 671-685, 687-700, 1963

Climate see Environment

Climbing

  mountain, medical and physiologic notes (Mason) Anesth. Analg. 43:125-132, 1964

Coagulation, blood

  changes immediately after mental irritation and physical exercise (Vuori) Ann. Med. Int. Fenn. 37:
    167-181, 1948; Acta Med. Scand. 138(Suppl. 239):296-300, 1950

  changes in warm and cold influences, and during physical work (Schimpf) Deutsch. Arch. klin. Med.
    204:472-478, 1957

  exercise, effect of (Keeney and Laramie) Circ. Res. 10:691-695, 1962; (Kesseler and others) Klin.
    Wschr. 35:1088-1089, 1957; (Cioffi and Imbimbo) Boll. Soc. Ital. Biol. Sper. 37:813-817, 1961

  and fibrinolysis, effect of physical exercise (Iatridis and Ferguson) J. Appl. Physiol. 18:337-344, 1963

  hemostatic changes associated with exercise (Ikkala and others) Nature 199:459-461, 1963

  and lipid, relation to diet and physical activity (Fidanza and others) Minerva Med. 51:1183-1188, 1960

  and muscular work (Casula and others) Gior. Clin. Med. 42:619-638, 1961

Coal miners see Miners, coal

Coarctation of aorta

  haemodynamic observations (Dahlbäck and others) Scand. J. Clin. Lab. Invest. 16:339-346, 1964

Coitus

  physiologic responses during (Bartlett) J. Appl. Physiol. 9:469-472, 1956

Colon

  motility, modification induced by exercise (De Young and others) Amer. J. Physiol. 99:52-63, 1931

  and spleen, effect of exercise on vascular conditions (Barcroft and Florey) J. Physiol. 68:181-189, 1929

Coronary arteries

exercise, effect on size, rat (Stevenson and others) Circ. Res. 15:265-269, 1964

small animals, effect of exercise and anemia, corrosion-cast technique (Tepperman and Pearlman) Circ. Res. 9:576-584, 1961

see also Coronary disease; Insufficiency, coronary

Coronary disease

background (Keys and Blackburn) Progr. Cardiov. Dis. 6:14-44, 1963

civilized pattern of human activity and (Minc) Med. J. Aust. 2:87-91, 1960

coronary artery narrowing and exercise, effect on coronary collateral circulation (Eckstein) Circ. Res. 5:230-235, 1957

diet and exercise (Mann) Illinois Med. J. 116:20-21, 1959

effort, relation to (Somerville) Med. Sci. Law 3:172-179, 1963

epidemiology, national differences and role of physical activity (Holloszy) J. Amer. Geriat. Soc. 11:718-725, 1963

exercise, effect of on cardiac performance (Messer and others) Circulation 28:404-414, 1963

with hypertension, ballistocardiographic changes (Huang and others) Chin. Med. J. 82:202-207, 1963

individual characteristics (Taylor and others) Cuore Circ. 47:277-292, 1963

ischemic heart disease and arterial hypertension, electrocardiogram T/U strokes and U waves (Torreggiani and others) Folia Cardiol. 22:461-471, 1963

latent, detected by electrocardiogram before and after exercise (Rumball and Acheson) Brit. Med. J. 1:423-428, 1963

latent, determination by exercise electrocardiogram (Robb and Marks) Amer. J. Cardiol. 13:603-618, 1964

mortality, relationship to physical activity of work (Kahn) Amer. J. Public Health 53:1058-1067, 1963

in physically active and sedentary populations (Taylor) J. Sport Med. 2:73-82, 1962

silent, and differential diagnosis of chest pain, detected by exercise test (Master and Rosenfeld) J.A.M.A. 190:494-500, 1964

syncope on exertion, relation to (Engelhardt and Sodeman) Ann. Intern. Med. 22:225-233, 1945

see also Angina pectoris; Insufficiency, coronary

Coronary occlusion

acute, heavy work causing (Sigler) Amer. J. Cardiol. 7:305-306, 1961

acute, relation of effort and trauma to (Master and others) Industr. Med. 9:359-364, 1940; Med. Ann. District of Columbia 10:79-86, 1941

physical effort and emotion in acute coronary thrombosis (Friedberg) Circulation 27:855-857, 1963

Cortex, cerebral

changes of electrical activity in different sections, during muscular work (Ivanhova) Zh. Vyssh. Nerv. Deiat. Pavlov. 13:972-979, 1963

cortical stimulation, influence of muscular activity on (Cardot and others) Comptes rend. Soc. Biol. 97:698-701, 1927

Corticoids see Adrenocorticosteroids

Creatine, blood

    muscular exercise, influence of (Planet and Cardoso) Comptes Rend. Soc. Biol. 112:1509-1510, 1933

    muscular exercise, strenuous (Gemmill and Riberio) Sunti Congr. Internaz. Fisiol. 14 Congr. 1932,

        p. 98

    serum and muscle, in exercising ageing rats (Gsell and others) Gerontologia 9:42-51, 1964

    training, intense, variations in (Backman and others) Scand. Arch. Physiol. 78:304-312, 1938

Creatine phosphokinase

    and adenosine triphosphatase activity in muscles of exercised rats (Rawlinson and Gould) Biochem. J.

        73:44-48, 1959

    and other enzyme activity after controlled exercise (Swaiman and Awad) Neurology 14:977-980, 1964

    serum, variations in activity in normal (Pearce and others) J. Neurol. Neurosurg. Psychiat. 27:1-4,

        1964

Cyanosis

    and arterial pulmonary hypertension (Oñata and Ramos) Rev. Esp. Tuberc. 32:557-562, 1963

    see also Hypoxia; Oxygen content, blood

Cyclists

    retardation of decline in intellect in (Clement) Rev. Franc. Geront. 7:379-412, 1961

Cytochrome C

    intravenous, effect on capacity for effort without pain in angina of effort (Bakst and Rinzler) Proc. Soc.

        Exp. Biol. Med. 67:531-533, 1948

Cytotoxic factor

    in sudden death during exercise (Forssman and Bergman) Acta Allerg. 18:471-473, 1963

D

Dead space

    and alveolar gas pressures at rest and during muscular exercise (Asmussen and Nielsen) Acta Physiol. Scand.

        38:1-21, 1956

    at rest and during exercise (Young) J. Appl. Physiol. 8:91-94, 1955

Death, sudden

    during exercise, cytotoxic factor (Forssman and Bergman) Acta Allerg. 18:471-473, 1963

    non-traumatic, acute fatal collapse, associated with physical exertion (Jokl and Suzman) Amer. Heart J.

        23:761-765, 1942

    non-traumatic, associated with physical exertion in identical twins (Jokl and Wolffe) Acta Genet. Med.

        3:245-246, 1954

Decompression

  altitude pain, role of exercise (aviator's bends) (Henry) Amer. J. Physiol. 145:279-284, 1946

  at sea level from high barometric pressures, bubble formation in animals relation of exercise (Harris and

    others) J. Gen. Physiol. 28:241-251, 1945

  sickness, comparison of altitude and exercise (Cook and others) War Med. 6:182-187, 1944

  sickness, during exercise at simulated low altitudes after exposure to compressed air, rats (Philp and

    Gowdey) Aerospace Med. 33:1433-1437, 1962

  sickness, effects of altitude and exercise (Gray and Masland) J. Aviation Med. 17:483-485, 1946

  sickness, factors affecting incidence of bends at altitude (Burkhardt and others) J.A.M.A. 133:373-377,

    1947

  sickness, symptoms during and after artificial decompression to 38,000 feet for 90 minutes with exercise

    during exposure (Bridge and others) J. Aviation Med. 15:316-327, 1944

Deer hunting

  and the heart (Kerkhof and Kolars) Minnesota Med. 46:1092; 1126; 1189, 1963

Dehydration

  aerobic and anaerobic work capacity after (Saltin) J. Appl. Physiol. 19:1114-1118, 1964

  and physical performance (Döbeln) Acta Physiol. Scand. 25(Suppl. 89):16, 1951

  thermal, circulatory response, submaximal and maximal exercise after thermal dehydration (Saltin)

    J. Appl. Physiol. 19:1125-1132, 1964

Denervation, cardiac

  cardiovascular adjustment, initial, dogs (Donald and Shepherd) Amer. J. Physiol. 207:1325-1329,

    1964

  denervated heart, effects on of stimulating nerves of liver (Cannon and Uridil) Amer. J. Physiol.

    58:353-364, 1921

  exercise, response to (Donald and Shepherd) Amer. J. Physiol. 205:393-400, 1963

  heart rate, changes in with intravenous infusion in dogs with chronic cardiac denervation (Donald and

    Shepherd) Proc. Soc. Exp. Biol. Med. 113:315-317, 1963

  maximal capacity, effect on, racing greyhound (Donald and others) J. Appl. Physiol. 19:849-852,

    1964

  preparation of denervated heart for detecting internal secretion (Cannon and others) Amer. J. Physiol. 77:

    326-352, 1926

  sustained capacity for exercise, dogs (Donald and Shepherd) Amer. J. Cardiol. 14:853-859, 1964

Deprivation, perceptual

  prolonged, counteracting effects of physical exercises (Zubek) Science 142:504-506, 1963

Dextrose

  ingestion, muscular work, and development of hypoglycemia (Bøje) Scand. Arch. Physiol. 83:308-312,

    1940

Diabetes

adolescent, functional adaption to vigorous training (Larsson and others) J. Appl. Physiol. 19:
629-635, 1964

childhood, acetone bodies in blood after exercise (Akerblom and Maijala) Ann. Paediat. Fenn. 10:
36-41, 1964

and exercise (Errebo-Knudsen) Thesis, Copenhagen, 1948

hyperlabile, metabolism, effects of exercise and multiple-dose insulin regimes (Molnar and others)
Metabolism 12:157-163, 1963

juvenile, effect of exercise on blood-lipids (Larsson and others) Lancet 1:350-355, 1964

lipids and polysaccharides, work (Rao) Folia Med. 37:496-499, 1954

metabolism during and after muscular exercise (Hetzel and Long) Proc. Roy. Soc. 99B:279-306, 1926

phenformin on blood lactic acid during exercise, influence of (Glittler and others) Diabetes 12:420-423, 1963

physical work capacity, schoolchildren (Sterky) Acta Paediat. 52:1-10, 1963

serum phosphatase, during work (Zambrano) Folia Med. 35:143-151, 1952

see also Ketonemia; Ketosis

Diarrhea

chronic, muscle electrolytes (Bergström) Scand. J. Clin. Lab. Invest. 14(Suppl. 68):1-110, 1962

Dibazol

effect, and adaptation to muscular work and cold cn animals with Ehrlich tumor (Rusin) Vop. Onkol.
9:60-66, 1963

Diet

activity and body-weight, women (Taggart) Brit. J. Nutr. 16:223-235, 1962

and body condition, and the energy production during mechanical work interrelation between, dog
(Anderson and Lusk) Proc. Nat. Acad. Sci. 3:386-389, 1917

and discipline, effect on prisoners (Smith and Milner) Part 1 Rep. 31st Meeting British Ass. Adv. Sci.
(Manchester) pp. 44-81, 1861; also; London, Taylor and Francis, 1862

exercise, and coronary disease (Mann) Illinois Med. J. 116:20-21, 1959

high-fat, effect of exercise on serum and hepatic lipids, rats (Lewis and others) Amer. J. Physiol.
201:4-8, 1961

reduced, effect on random and voluntary activity, rats (Olewine and others) J. Geront. 19:230-233, 1964

varying conditions of, influence of muscle work on metabolism (Cathcart and Burnett) Proc. Roy.
Soc. 99B:405-426, 1926

work metabolism, effect of (Issekutz and others) J. Nutr. 79:109-115, 1963

see also Food; Nutrition; Weight, body

Digestion

exercise, influence of (Campbell and others) Guy's Hosp. Rep. 78:279-293, 1928

Diuretics

>effect on pulse rate, blood pressure, and electrocardiogram during exercise (Christensson and others) Acta Med. Scand. 175:727-734, 1964

Doping agents

>and cardiac circulation, rest and effort (Segers and Delille) Actualites Cardiol. Angeiol. Int. 12: 195-204, 1963

Drugs

>analeptic, tranquilising and vasodilating, effects on physical work capacity and orthostatic tolerance (Ganslen and others) Aerospace Med. 35:630-633, 1964

>centrally acting, effect on muscular exercise, rats (Jasmin and Bois) Canad. J. Biochem. Physiol. 37: 417-423, 1959

>and exercise, effect on normal electrocardiogram and particularly T wave changes (Hartwell and others) J. Clin. Invest. 21:409-417, 1942

>to increase performance efficiency (Spengler) Schweiz. Zeits. Sportmed. 5:97-124, 1957

>injection and acetylene methods to determine cardiac output (Asmussen and Nielsen) Acta Physiol. Scand. 27:230, 1953

>relaxant, influence of exercise on neuromuscular activity (Foldes and others) Canad. Anaesth. Soc. J. 8:118-127, 1961

>see also names of specific drugs

Dye dilution methods

>cardiac output, use in determination of (Hanson and Tabakin) J. Appl. Physiol. 19:275-278, 1964

>for circulation studies during training (Schneider and others) Verh. deutsch. Ges. inn. Med. 70:140-144, 1964

>curve analysis during body loading, haemodynamic study (Rost and Schneider) Verh. deutsch. Ges. inn. Med. 70:144-148, 1964

>curve, during work of increasing intensity (Mascaretti and Morbelli) Folia Cardiol. 23:137-163; (Mascaretti and others) Folia Cardiol. 23:395-422, 1964; (Morbelli and Mascaretti) Folia Cardiol. 23:327-353, 1964

>curves, arterial, of T-1824, during rest and exercise (Mankin and Swan) Fed. Proc. 12:93, 1953

Dyspnea

>cardiac, ventilatory response to muscular exercise in (Fodstad) Scand. J. Clin. Lab. Invest. 8:104-107, 1956

>on exertion in congestive heart failure (Harrison and others) Arch. Intern. Med. 50:695-720, 1932

>exertion, exercise test for measuring (Hugh-Jones) Brit. Med. J. 1:65-71, 1952

>exertional, syncope associated with (Golden) Amer. Heart J. 28:689-698, 1944

>induced by combinations of respiratory stimuli (Kontos and others) Amer. J. Med. 37:374-385, 1964

>relation of respiratory work and pressure during exercise to (Nisell) Acta Med. Scand. 166:113-119, 1960

>shortness of breath (Stuart-Harris) Brit. Med. J. 1:1203-1209, 1964

Da Costa's syndrome

   effect of physical training (Holmgren and others) Acta Med. Scand. 165:89-103, 1959

   see also Neurocirculatory asthenia

                                        E

Ear

   oximetry (Jeyasingham) Ceylon Med. J. 7:23-31, 1962

Edema

   late, after muscular exercise (Brendstrup) Arch. Phys. Med. 43:401-405, 1962

Effort

   attractiveness, and the anticipation of reward: reply to Lott's critique (Aronson) J. Abnorm. Soc.
      Psychol. 67:522-526, 1963

   dietetics (Delfosse) Acta Belg. Arte Med. Pharm. Milit. 110:589-596, 1957; (Soetens and others)
      Acta Belg. Arte Med. Pharm. Milit. 110:597-599, 1957

   experimental and critical contribution to study (Puyou) Bordeaux, Delmas, 1938

   headache of (Chavany) Presse Méd. 58:645, 1945

   intolerance, effect of exercise on soldiers with (Jones and Scarisbrick) Lancet 2:331-332, 1943

   and secondary reinforcement (Lott) J. Abnorm. Soc. Psychol. 67:520-522, 1963

   syndrome, I. Capacity for work and variations in arterial pressures and pulse rate (Christensen) Acta Med.
      Scand. 121:194-216, 1945; II. Large arteries during muscular work (Christensen) Acta Med. Scand.
      121:319-332, 1945

   test, determination and appraisal (Vuylsteek) Bruxelles Med. 43:641-654, 1963

   tests, average duration (Fleisch) Poumon Coeur 15:883-889, 1959

   see also Neurocirculatory asthenia

Electrocardiogram

   in adolescents, effect of exercise on (Urschel) J. Indiana Med. Ass. 37:561-563, 1944; (Jouve and others)
      Presse Méd. 65:1387-1389, 1957

   age, relation of to response to standardized exercise (Silver and Landowne) Circulation 8:510-520, 1953

   anoxia and exercise, effects of on (Baum and others) J. Aviation Med. 16:422-428, 1945

   cardiac aging, study of, rest and after exercise (Mazer and Reisinger) Ann. Intern. Med. 21:645-652, 1944

   consecutive, modifications in intense muscular activity followed by exhaustion (Fabre and others) J.
      Physiologie 56:345-346, 1964

   cycling, prolonged, changes during (Chailley-Bert and others) Arch. Mal. Coeur 49:910-915, 1956

   duration of phases, during and after dynamic and static work, lying and standing (Boeckh and Haebisch)
      Zeits. Kreislaufforsch. 50:425-436, 1961

   during loading, under direct control by visualization (Fleisch) Cardiologia 40:235-244, 1962

   dynamic and postexercise, evaluation in diagnosing coronary insufficiency (Abarquez and others) Amer. J.
      Cardiol. 13:310-319, 1954

   exercise, abnormalities in ischemia and chest pain (Gubner) J. Occup. Med. 3:110-120, 1961

Electrocardiogram (Cont.)

exercise, changes after (Dalderup and others) Lancet 2:1345, 1964; (Dimond) Dis. Chest 39:
  225, 1961; (Freiman and others) Amer. J. Cardiol. 5:506-515, 1960; (Lloyd-Thomas) Brit. Heart J.
  23:260-270, 1961; (Lozada and Tempone) Acta Cardiol. 13:464-485, 1958; (Mercier) Cah. Med.
  Interprof. 3:24-28, 1963; (Moia and Batile) Rev. Argent. Cardiol. 9:339-351, 1943; (Rumball and
  Acheson) Brit. Heart J. 22:415-425, 1960; (Sandberg) Acta Med. Scand. 169(Suppl. 365):1-117, 1961;
  (Sasamoto) Jap. Circ. J. 28:833-839, 1964; (Segers and Delille) Acta Belge Arte Med. Pharm. 110
  (Part 2):635-644, 1957; (Seghizzi and others) Atti Soc. Ital. Cardiol. 2:86-88, 1962; (Simonson) J.
  Appl. Physiol. 5:584-588, 1953; (Simonson) Amer. Heart J. 66:552-565, 1963

exercise, changes in scaler ECG, and in mean spatial QRS and T vectors (Simonson and Keys) Amer. Heart
  J. 52:83-105, 1956

exercise, chest-head leads, use for recording during (Holmgren and Strandell) Acta Med. Scand. 169:
  57-62, 1961

exercise, comparison, children with adults (Bengtsson) Acta Med. Scand. 154:225-244, 1956

in exercise, continuous, evaluation of pentaerythritol tetranitrate (Krasno and Kidera) Angiology 14:
  417-425, 1963

exercise, detection of latent coronary disease by (Rumball and Acheson) Brit. Med. J. 1:423-428, 1963

exercise, during and after, comparison, old and young men (Strandell) Acta Med. Scand. 174:479-499, 1963

exercise, electrical systole changes (Torreggiani and others) Atti Soc. Ital. Cardiol. 2:97, 1962

exercise, 5-year follow-up (Åstrand) Acta Med. Scand. 173:257-268, 1963

exercise electrocardiogram, determination of latent coronary disease (Robb and Marks) Amer. J. Cardiol.
  13:603-618, 1964

exercise, Master 'two-step' test for cardiac function and coronary insufficiency (Master) Amer. J. Med. Sci.
  207:435-450, 1944

exercise, Master two-step tests, true-positive and false-positive results (Lepeschkin and Surawicz) New
  Eng. J. Med. 258:511-520, 1958

exercise, quantitative interpretation, computer techniques (Smith) Proj. MR 005.13.7004 Subtask 8, Rep.
  No. 3, U.S. Naval Sch. Aviat. Med. 1-20, 1964

exercise, recording intervals (Blackburn and others) Amer. Heart J. 67:186-188, 1964

exercise, ST depression (Takahashi and others) Jap. Heart J. 4:104-117, 1963

exercise, standard, as functional test of the heart (Master and others) Amer. Heart J. 24:777-793, 1942

exercise, T-wave changes, influence of drugs (Walser) Cardiologia 10:231-250, 1946

final stroke, changes in, relation to oxygen consumption, after muscular work (Aresu) Rass. Med.
  Sarda 63:125-146, 1961

lead for exercising subjects (Geddes and others) J. Appl. Physiol. 15:311-312, 1960

lead selection after exercise (Blackburn and Katigbak) Amer. Heart J. 67:184-185, 1964

Master test according to Ford and Hellenstein (Caccuri and others) Cuore Circ. 46:121-135, 1962

Electrocardiogram (Cont.)

modification in aerobic and anaerobic work recovery phase, modification in (Borghetti and others)
Gior. Clin. Med. 42:857-867, 1961

monitoring under dynamic conditions (Carbery and others) Aerospace Med. 31:131-137, 1960

particular aspects (Miraldi and others) Boll. Soc. Ital. Cardiol. 8:206-211, 1963

post-exercise, "false-positive" in digitalized patient (Best) J. Nat. Med. Ass. 55:277-279, 1963

posture and exercise, effects on (Wolf) Res. Quart. 24:475-490, 1953

QRS and T vectors, relations to stroke volume and heart frequency, rest and stress (Blasius and others)
Zeits. Kreislaufforsch. 51:105-117, 1961

QT-duration and pulse rate, relation between, and progress in training period (Heinen and others) Zeits.
Kreislaufforsch. 41:375-379, 1952

recorded by radioelectrocardiography during and after exercise (Bellet and others) Amer. J. Cardiol. 8:
385-400, 1961; Circulation 25:686-694, 1962

simultaneous registration in 3 spatial directions during marching (Cavagna and others) Boll Soc. Ital.
Biol. Sper. 36:1802-1804, 1960

T-U strokes and U waves during work, normals, ischaemic heart disease, and arterial hypertension (Torreggiani
and others) Folia Cardiol. 22:461-471, 1963

vectors, magnitude and direction, during and after dynamic and static work, lying and standing (Boeckh
and Haebisch) Zeits. Kreislaufforsch. 50:477-488, 1961

ventricular repolarization during work and voluntary hyperventilation, normal subjects (Salvetti and others)
Cuore Circ. 48:192-208, 1964

work and apnea test in coronary insufficiency (Roganti and others) Cardiol. Prat. 14:367-375, 1963

during work and prolonged effort (Plas) J. Sport Med. 3:131-136, 1963

during work, clinical significance (Klepzig and others) Zeits. Kreislaufforsch. 45:741-750, 1956

work tests, dangers and limits of (Fleisch) Schweiz. med. Wschr. 92:456-460, 1962

of working heart (Plas and Chailley-Bert) Arch. Mal. Coeur 49:916-918, 1956

see also Exercise; Master step test; Tests

Electroencephalography

radio, influence of physical activity on brain function (Götze and Kofes) Zeits. ges. exp. Med. 126:439-443,
1955

Electrolytes

balance, muscular work (Spinazzola) Rass. Med. Sarda 66:649-664, 1964

blood, and muscular exercise (Thiebault and others) Bull. Soc. Sci. Hyg. Aliment. 51:77-84, 1963

excretion, diurnal variation in, particularly calcium and magnesium (Heaton and Hodgkinson) Clin. Chim.
Acta 8:246-254, 1963

excretion, renal mechanism, effect of exercise (Kattus and others) Bull. Johns Hopkins Hosp. 84:344-368, 1949

Electrolytes (Cont.)

    ion balance, and muscular work, rat (Cier and others) Path. Biol. 8:1147-1154, 1960; Comptes

        Rend. Soc. Biol. 153:96-98, 1959

    ion concentrations and osmotic pressure of plasma, during muscular work and recovery (De Lanne and others)

        J. Appl. Physiol. 14:804-808, 1959

    and lactic acid, after muscular exercise, rat (Sréter and Friedman) Canad. J. Biochem. Physiol. 36:

        1193-1201, 1958

    metabolism, muscle training and stress, effect on, rats (Steingass and others) Zeits. ges. inn. Med. 18:

        292-298, 1963

    muscle, determined by neutron activation analysis on needle biopsy specimens, in normal, kidney disease

        and chronic diarrhoea (Bergström) Scand. J. Clin. Lab. Invest. 14 (Suppl. 68):1-110, 1962

    plasma, determinations, venous stasis and forearm exercise during venipuncture (Broome and Holt)

        Canad. Med. Ass. J. 90:1105-1107, 1964

    serum, and iron, serum, concentration changes, after physical effort (Preisler and Kabza) Bull. Soc. Amis.

        Sci. Poznan (Med.) 13:85-93, 1964

    water, sodium and potassium distribution, relation to work performance of old rats (Sréter and Friedman)

        Gerontologia 7:53-61, 1963

    see also Carbon dioxide; Chloride; Potassium; Sodium

Electromyography

    and energy expenditures of rhythmic and paced lifting work (Karvonen) Ann. Acad. Sci. Fenn. (Med.)

        106(Suppl. 19):1-11, 1964

Emetine

    cardiotoxicity, and physical stress (Marino) Experientia 17:116-117, 1961; (Marino and Russo) Boll.

        Soc. Ital. Biol. Sper. 35:1244-1247, 1959

Emotion

    exercise, and adrenal cortex (Editorial) Brit. Med. J. 2:496-497, 1958

    muscular vasodilatation, metabolic changes in forearm muscle and skin during (Brod and others) Clin.

        Sci. 25:1-10, 1963

    and physical stress, and soldier's heart (Donati) Gior. Med. Milit. 94:345-370, 1947

    tension and physical exertion, contrasting effects on excretion of 17-ketosteroids and 17-ketogenic steroids

        (Connell and others) Acta Endocr. 27:179-194, 1958

Emphysema

    blood pH, O_2 and CO_2 tensions in exercised control and emphysematous horses (Gillespie and others)

        Amer. J. Physiol. 207:1067-1072, 1964

    cardiopulmonary hemodynamics at rest and during exercise, effect upon (Williams and Behnke) Ann.

        Intern. Med. 60:824-842, 1964

Energy expenditure (Cont.)

consumption, arterio-venous difference of oxygen, cardiac output and stroke volume (Brandi and Branbilla)
Int. Zeits. angew. Physiol. 19:130-133, 1961

cost of load carriage (Goldman and Iampietro) J. Appl. Physiol. 17:675-676, 1962

cost of stand-up exercises, normal and hemiplegic subjects (Hirschberg and others) Amer. J. Phys. Med.
43:43-45, 1964

cost of work (Ford) Phys. Ther. Rev. 40:859-862, 1960

degraded in recovery processes of stimulated muscles (Hill) J. Physiol. 46:28-80, 1913

in dumbbell exercise (Full and Lehmann) Pflüger Arch. ges. Physiol. 201:611-619, 1923

electrolyte metabolism, and adrenal responses, during work, dogs (Young and others) J. Appl. Physiol. 17:
669-674, 1962

and electromyographic studies of rhythmic and paced lifting work (Karvonen) Ann. Acad. Sci. Fenn. (Med.)
106(Suppl. 19):1-11, 1964

and energy intake, medical college women (Banerjee and Mahindra) J. Appl. Physiol. 17:971-973, 1962

estimation from expired air (Liddell) J. Appl. Physiol. 18:25-29, 1963

in factory work, two types (Bliss and Graettinger) Arch. Environ. Health 9:201-205, 1964

and food intake, elderly people (Durnin) Geront. Clin. 4:128-133, 1962

foodstuffs oxidation, utilization of 'waste heat', in muscular exercise (Rapport) Amer. J. Physiol. 91:
238-253, 1929

fuel used in muscular exercise, type of (Rapport and Ralli) Proc. Soc. Exp. Biol. Med. 24:964-966,
1927

and gas exchange, treadmill running dogs (Young and others) J. Appl. Physiol. 14:834-838, 1959

hemiplegia, in elderly, effect of bracing and rehabilitation training (Dacso and others) Postgrad. Med. 34:
42-47, 1963

and human maximum power, rowing (Henderson and Haggard) Amer. J. Physiol. 72:264-282, 1925

and lactacidemia during muscular work and thermal shivering (Schmitt and others) Comptes Rend. Soc. Biol.
158:770-773, 1964

mechanical, production, on principle of animal muscular action (Kuhn) Triangle 5:37-44, 1961

of miners (Humphreys and Lind) Brit. J. Industr. Med. 19:264-275, 1962; (Pachner and others) Acta
Med. Leg. Soc. 12:53-55, 1959

muscle, production of energy (Needham) Brit. Med. Bull. 12:194-198, 1956

in muscle work (Abramson) Arbeitsphysiol. 1:480-502, 1929, 2:85-96, 1930

muscles, energy conversion (Meyerhof) Pflüger Arch. ges. Physiol. Part I 182:232-283, 1920; Part II
182:284-317, 1920; Part III 185:11-32, 1920; Part IV 188:114-160; Part V 191:128-183, 1921; Part VI
195:22-74, 1922; Part VII 204:295-331, 1924

Energy expenditure (Cont.)

muscular contraction, regulation of supply of energy (Hartree and Hill) J. Physiol. 55:133-158, 1921

muscular, relative value of fat and carbohydrate as sources of energy (Krogh and Lindhard) Biochem. J. 14:290-363, 1920

in muscular work, dogs (Zuntz) Pflüger Arch. ges. Physiol. 68:191-211, 1897

muscular work grades, ranges (Brown and Crowden) Brit. J. Industr. Med. 20:277-283, 1963

during muscular work, light (Laville and others) Arch. Int. Physiol. 71:431-440, 1963

obese and normal (McKee and Bolinger) J. Appl. Physiol. 15:197-200, 1960

obesity and non-obesity, output in, relation to caloric intake, adolescent boys (Stefanik and others) Amer. J. Clin. Nutr. 7:55-62, 1959

physiological basis for 'optimum' level (Wyndham and others) Nature 195:1210-1212, 1962

physiology of breathing and exercise (Simonson) Pflüger Arch. ges. Physiol. 215:752-767, 1927

physiology of exercise (Simonson and Riesser) Pflüger Arch. ges. Physiol. 215:743-751, 1927

physiology, recovery from physical work (Simonson) Pflüger Arch. ges. Physiol. 215:716-742, 1927

physiology of standing (Simonson) Pflüger Arch. ges. Physiol. 214:403-415, 1926

physiology of work, recovery and breathing (Simonson) Pflüger Arch. ges. Physiol. 214:380-402, 1926

pulse count as measure of (Malhotra and others) J. Appl. Physiol. 18:994-996, 1963

pulse frequency, efficiency and behaviour of, treadmill, dog and man (Stegemann) Zeits. Biol. 113: 369-381, 1963

reserves, of energy, utilization during work, dog (Young and Price) J. Appl. Physiol. 16:351-354, 1961

rickshaw pullers (Banerjee and others) Indian J. Physiol. Pharmacol. 3:147-160, 1959

in running (Cerretelli and others) Boll. Soc. Ital. Biol. Sper. 39:1806-1809, 1963; (Margaria and others) J. Appl. Physiol. 18:367-370, 1963

speed, effect of (Pertuzon) J. Physiologie 56:422, 1964

static and dynamic contractions, comparison between (Monod and others) Comptes Rend. Soc. Biol. 157:2152-2155, 1963

and temperature, environmental (Consolazio and others) J. Appl. Physiol. 18:65-68, 1963

treadmill and floor walking, comparison between (Ralston) J. Appl. Physiol. 15:1156, 1960

treadmill work, prediction in (Iampietro and Goldman) U. S. Civil Aeromed. Res. Inst. 62-5:4P, 1962

in walking, level and grade (Bobbert) J. Appl. Physiol. 15:1015-1021, 1960

walking, during level, and bicycle ergometry, different age groups (Grimby and Söderholm) Scand. J. Clin. Lab. Invest. 14:321-328, 1962

walking, horizontal and grade on motor-driven treadmill (Erickson and others) Amer. J. Physiol. 145:391-401, 1946

walking, related to weight, sex, age, height, speed and gradiant (McDonald) Nutr. Abstr. Rev. 31:739-762, 1961

yield of ventilation, relations between muscular activity and respiratory function, healthy subjects different ages (Berloco and others) Gior. Ital. Tuberc. 16:111-113, 1962

see also Food

Environment, hot (Cont.)

continuous or intermittent work, physiological effect (Lind) J. Appl. Physiol. 18:57-60, 1963

extreme heat, and thermal balance (Robinson and Gerking) Amer. J. Physiol. 149:476-488, 1947

fibrinolytic activity and exercise (Bedrak and others) J. Appl. Physiol. 19:469-471, 1964

heat stress, responses of unacclimatized men (Wyndham and others) J. Appl. Physiol. 6:681-686, 1954;

6:687-690, 1954

heat stroke, mechanism (Gilat and others) J. Trop. Med. Hyg. 66:204-212, 1963

humid, and exercise, effect on pulse rate, blood pressure, body temperature, and blood concentration

(Young and others) Proc. Roy. Soc. 91B:111-126, 1920

intolerable conditions, practical assessment (Lind) Fed. Proc. 22:89-92, 1963

moist, effect of muscular exercise on mepacrine concentrations of blood, plasma and urine (Maegraith

and others) Ann. Trop. Med. Parasit. 40:368-371, 1946

muscular work and ambient temperature, effect on cardiac rate (Schaff and Vogt) Comptes Rend. Soc.

Biol. 155:2036-2039, 1961

muscular work and ambient temperature, effect of on rectal temperature and sweating (Schaff and Vogt)

Comptes Rend. Soc. Biol. 155:1112-1116, 1961; 156:168-172, 1962

and the older worker (Brouha) J. Amer. Geriat. Soc. 10:35-39, 1962

protein requirements during work, influence on (Gontzea and others) Rumanian Med. Rev. 5:162-164,

1961; Int. Zeits. angew. Physiol. 18:248-263, 1960

rectal temperature, cardiac rate and sweating, determined by simultaneous registration of muscular work

and ambiant heat (Schaff and Vogt) J. Physiologie 53:468-469, 1961

severe heat, decline in rates of sweating during work (Gerking and Robinson) Amer. J. Physiol. 147:

370-378, 1946

strenuous exercise (Kronfeld and others) J. Appl. Physiol. 13:425-429, 1958

tolerance coefficient, effect of exposure to sun and exercise in Murrah buffalo calves (Bhatnagar and Chaudhary)

Nature 189:844-845, 1961

and urinary excretion of adrenal steroids during exercise (Robinson and MacFarlane) J. Appl. Physiol. 12:

13-16, 1958

work, attitude to (Zannini) Rass. Med. Industr. 32:409-411, 1963

work, effect of on blood cholinesterase activity (Liska and others) Prac. Lek. 15:291-293, 1963

see also Temperature, environmental

Environment, thermal

of aerospace, human tolerance limits (Kaufman) Aerospace Med. 34:889-896, 1963

limits for everyday work, physiological criterion (Lind) J. Appl. Physiol. 18:51-56, 1963

Enzymes

activity of leucocytic peroxidase in fatigued muscles, normal (Fracchia and Antognetti) Gazz. Int. Med.

Chir. 68(Suppl.):3114-3121, 1963

Enzymes (Cont.)

    histochemistry of rabbit aorta, in spontaneous lesions and after acute exercise (Hashimoto and Kobernick)

        Proc. Soc. Exp. Biol. Med. 115:212-215, 1964

    leucocytic perosidases, and glycopolysaccharides after intense and prolonged muscular work (Mazzella)

        Riv. Med. Aero. 23:117-122, 1960

    muscular, after swimming, rats (Gould and Rawlinson) Biochem. J. 73:41-44, 1959

    see also names of specific enzymes

Enzymes, serum levels

    activity, and alteration in substratum concentration in body loading (Loll and Hilscher) Aerztl. Forsch.

        12:85-86, 1958

    blood, in physical work, and in ambulant patients (Otto and others) Klin. Wschr. 42:75-81, 1964

    changes, in altitude tolerance, rats (Altland and others) Aerospace Med. 35:1034-1039, 1964

    exercise, effects of (Altland and Highman) Amer. J. Physiol. 201:393-395, 1961; (Fowler and others)

        J. Appl. Physiol. 17:943-946, 1962; (Gardner and others) J. Sport Med. 4:103-110, 1964; (Halonen

        and Kcnttinen) Nature 193:942-944, 1962; (Venerando and others) Gazz. Int. Med. Chir. 69:2160-2174,

        1964

    exercise, effects of, rats (Garbus and others) Amer. J. Physiol. 207:467-472, 1964

    and lipids, serum, after high-caloric, high fat intake and vigorous exercise regimen, marines (Calvy and

        others) J.A.M.A. 183:1-4, 1963

    and lipids, serum, effect of strenuous exercise (Calvy and others) Milit. Med. 129:1012-1016, 1964

    in muscle disease (Pearce and others) J. Neurol. Neurosurg. Psychiat. 27:1-4, 1964

    muscular work, behavior of (Baumann and others) Schweiz. Zeits. Sportmed. 10:33-51, 1962

    physical activity, effect of (Venerando and others) Gazz. Int. Med. Chir. 69:2160-2174, 1964

    sports activity, effect of (Mueller and Kuechler) Zeits. aerztl. Fortbild. 55:919-922, 1961

    and tissue changes, effect of exercise and training, rats (Highman and Altland) Amer. J. Physiol.

        205:162-166, 1963; (Altland and Highman) Amer. J. Physiol. 201:393-395, 1961

Eosinophils

    count, peripheral blood changes, after work loads (Borský and Hubač) Prac. Lek. 16:193-197, 1964

    response of exercised rats, effects of training (Keeney) J. Appl. Physiol. 15:1046-1048, 1960

    response to physical exertion (McDonald and others) Psychosom. Med. 23:63-66, 1961; (Wake and others)

        J. Aviation Med. 24:127-130, 1953

    see also Blood cells

Ependyma

    spinal, mitosis, and susceptibility of appearance through physical work (Kulenkampff) Verh. Anat. Ges.

        57:230-235, 1963

Epileptics

    ammonia in blood (Luck and others) Brit. J. Exp. Path. 6:276-279, 1925

Epinephrine

blood, after sport (Kinzius and Kötter) Arbeitsphysiol. 14:363-368, 1951

cardiovascular and metabolic responses to leg exercises, effects on (Marshall and Shepherd) J. Appl.
Physiol. 18:1118-1122, 1963

conjugated, and noradrenaline, presence in blood plasma (Häggendal) Acta Physiol. Scand. 59:255-
260, 1963

fibrinolysis, effect on (Biggs and others) Lancet 1:402-405, 1947

histamine formation, effect on (Graham and others) J. Physiol. 172:174-188, 1964

infusion, and muscular exercise, changes in antihemophilic A factor (F. VIII) and bleeding time associated
with (Egeberg) Scand. J. Clin. Lab. Invest. 15:539-549, 1963

infusion, prolonged, intra-arterial, forearm blood flow, and effects on post-exercise hyperaemia (Glover and
Shanks) J. Physiol. 167:268-279, 1963

liberation during muscular exercise (Hartman and others) Amer. J. Physiol. 62:225-241, 1922

liver, action on (Bainbridge and Trevan) J. Physiol. 51:460-468, 1917

and metabolism of exercise (Ring) Amer. J. Physiol. 97:375-385, 1931

and muscular exercise (Courtice and others) Proc. Roy. Soc. 127B:288-297, 1939

muscular fatigue, effect on (Gruber) Amer. J. Physiol. 33:335-355, 1914; 43:530-544, 1917

and noradrenaline in adrenals and brain, before and after muscular work (Beauvallett and others) Comptes
Rend. Soc. Biol. 156:1258-1260, 1962

and noradrenaline, plasma concentration, muscular work (Gray and Beetham) Proc. Soc. Exper. Biol. Med.
96:636-638, 1957

and noradrenaline, plasma content induced by maximum muscular effort of brief duration (Iannacone and
others) Arch. Fisiol. 60:339-348, 1961

and noradrenaline, urinary excretion (Kärki) Acta Physiol. Scand. 39(Suppl. 132):1-96, 1956; (Kärki and
Vasama) Sotilaslaak. Aikak. 34:59-69, 1959

and noradrenaline, urinary excretion in late normal and toxemic pregnancy (Castren) Acta Pharmacol.
20(Suppl. 2):1-98, 1963

-oxidases, changes in blood plasma during physical work (Billewicz-Stankiewicz and Tyburczyk) Int.
Zeits. angew. Physiol. 18:361-375, 1960

in peripheral blood, during muscle work (Katz) Zeits. klin. Med. 123:154-158, 1934

polyglobinuria, and exercise (Binet) Comptes Rend. Soc. Biol. 100:463-465, 1929

proteosynthesis and proteolysis during work, effect on (Bardino and Quatrini) Boll. Soc. Ital. Biol. Sper.
35:453-456, 1959

Ergometer

acute constant-workrate (Atkins and Nicholson) J. Appl. Physiol. 18:205-208, 1963

foot, for graded muscular exercise (Thulesius) Scand. J. Clin. Lab. Invest. 15:550-552, 1963

three types, physiological comparison (Bobbert) J. Appl. Physiol. 15:1007-1014, 1960

see also Bicycle ergometer

Exercise, muscular (Cont.)

behaviour, discipline and studies, effect of physical exercise on (Hurtel) Vie Méd. 2:1162-1164,

1921

biology (Matthias) Leipzig, Quelle and Meyer, 1931

blood counts, effect on (Babbitt) Amer. Phys. Educat. Rev. 6:240-245, 1901

and blood pressure, relation between (Adler) Med. Press 205:181-183, 1941

bodily, book of (1553) (Mendéz) New Haven, Elizabeth Licht, 1960

body (Editorial) J.A.M.A. 175:801-802, 1961

our body-Handbook of anatomy ... (Schmidt) Leipzig, R. Voigtländer 1899

body organs, effect on (Seguin) Paris, Thesis No. 188 Vol. 203, 1826

children, effect of exercise on (Schlesinger) Klin. Wschr. 8:1481-1484, 1929; (Boigey) Bull. Acad.

Med. 3rd series 94:1026-1030, 1925

chronic effects (Steinhaus) Physiol. Rev. 13:103-147, 1933

confinement and, effect on growth, maze learning and organ weights in rats (Cohen and Serrano) Lab.

Anim. Care 13:689-696, 1963

economy (Dill) Physiol. Rev. 16:263-291, 1936

effects (Cook and Pembrey) J. Physiol. 45:429-446, 1913

evolution of organs, influence on; a sub-Lamarck theory of evolution (Gini) Acta Genet. Med. 10:

312-315, 1961

excessive, dangers (Tomkins) New York Med. J. 52:589-595, 1890

excessive, influence on structure and function of rat organs (Asahina and others) Jap. J. Physiol. 9:

322-326, 1959

excretion of uric acid, influence of (Laval) Rev. Méd. 16:384-392, 1896

fitness and breathing (Briggs) J. Physiol. 54:292-318, 1920; J. Roy. Army Med. Corps 37:278-301, 1921

fitness tests, appraisal (Linde) Pediatrics 32(Suppl.):656-659, 1963

fitness tests, physiology and clinical application, children (Dill) Pediatrics 32(Suppl.):653-655, 1963

fuel of (Editorial) Lancet 2:276-277, 1959

and health (Drysdale) Nurs. Times 60:965-966, 1964; (Dufour) Paris Thesis No. 196, vol. 195, 1825;

(Davies and others) Lancet 2:930-932, 1963; (Farez) Paris, Thesis No. 222, vol. 176, 1822; (Fouré) Paris,

Thesis No. 3, vol. 69, 1808

health and disease, limitations in (Cotes) Brit. Med. Bull. 19:31-36, 1963

heart, effect on (Meylan) J. Med. Soc. New Jersey 2:332-335, 1906

human body, effect on, anatomy and physiology (Dettling) Paris, O. Doin, 1905; 3rd ed. 1931

human organism, influence on, reference to military gymnastics (Rudeloff) Berlin, G. Lange and P. Lange,

1873

Exercise, muscular (Cont.)

human visual analyzers, effect of exercise on excitability of (Navakamikian and others) Fiziol. Zh.
SSSR Sechenov. 49:1036-1043, 1963

hygienic influence, dangers of sedentary life (Boigey) Rev. Hyg. 45:1050-1067, 1923

influence (D'Anaya) Paris, Thesis No. 293, vol. 612, 1858

influence on constitution (Thouvenin) Paris, Thesis No. 85, vol. 624, 1858

instability of 'steady state' during (Lukin) Int. Zeits. angew. Physiol. 20:45-49, 1963

intensive, athletes, comparative clinical, electrocardiographic and biochemical observations before and
and after (Loutsides and others) Rev. Méd. Moyen Orient 19:433-437, 1962

and main functions (Boigey) Arch. Méd Pharm. Milit. 79:411-453, 1923; (Boigey) Biol. Méd. 27:
321-357, 1937

mechanism of exertion (Aubert) Lyon Med. 5:383-391, 1890

metabolism, blood-flow and exudation in organs, effect of (Barcroft and Kato) Proc. Roy. Soc. 88B:
541-543, 1915

on motor-driven treadmill (Snellen) J. Appl. Physiol. 15:759-763, 1960

neglect; results and remedies (Gugger) Oest. med. Wschr. 1846, pp. 1-12

nourishment (Vogel) Deutsch. med. Wschr. 59:1254-1256, 1933

organs and their function in health, influence on (Londe) Paris, Thesis No. 55, vol. 145, 1819

organs, effect on (Speck) Arch. Vereins Gemeinschaftl. Arbeiten Förderung Wissensch. Heilkunde,
Göttingen 6:161-324, 1863

and over-exercise (Brunton) Quart. Med. J. Sheffield 7:107-135, 1898-1899

physiological classification (Romero-Brest) Sem. Méd. 12:1-12, 1905

physiological effects (Boigey) Paris Med. 39:231-235, 1921; Un. Méd. Canada 50:287-295, 1921

physiological effects, control by Health Officer (Boigey) Rev. Hyg. 45:460-468, 1923

physiological necessity (Elliott) New Orleans Med. Surg. J. 10:498-508, 1883

physiological and psychological factors (Karpovich) Arbeitsphysiol. 9:626-629, 1937

physiology (Bainbridge) Longmans Green, 1919; 2nd ed. rev. by Anrep, 1923; 3rd ed. rewritten by
Bock and Dill, 1931; (Bock) New Eng. J. Med. 200:638-642, 1929

physiology of (Byford) Amer. J. Med. Sci, n.s. 30:32-42, 1855; (Goule and Dye) New York, Barnes, 1932;
(Hartwell) Boston Med. & Surg. J. 116:297-302; 321-324, 1887

physiology of, dogs (Steinhaus and others) Amer. J. Physiol. 99:487-502, 503-511, 512-520, 1932;
(Steinhaus and Jenkins) Amer. J. Physiol. 95:202-210, 1930

physiology and pathology of (Boldero) Middlesex Hosp. J. 18:217-228, 1914-1915; (Gaisböck) Zeits.
Hyg. Infektionskr. 112:576-600, 1931

physiology, pathology and therapeutics (Byford) Barnet, 1858; Chicago Med. J., n.s. 15:357-382, 1858

Extremities (Cont.)

reflexes, factor in hyperpnea of muscular exercise (Comroe and Schmidt) Amer. J. Physiol.
138:536-547, 1943

see also Arm; Forearm; Blood flow

F

Factor 8, see Antihemophilic A factor (F. VIII)

Fainting, see Syncope

Fat

digestion, relation to respiratory exchange, and potential directly used in muscular work (Chauveau and
others) Comptes Rend. Acad. Sci. 122:1169-1172, 1896

endogenous, utilization during partial fasting and physical stress (Lokatin) Vop. Pitan. 22:27-34, 1963;
Fed. Proc. 23:945-948, 1964

excess, exercise and body weight (Wells and others) J. Ass. Phys. Ment. Rehab. 16:35-40, 1962

metabolism, in muscular exercise (Stewart and others) Biochem. J. 25:733-748, 1931

oxidation, source in exercising dogs (Issekutz and others) Amer. J. Physiol. 207:583-589, 1964

serum, postprandial, effect of physical activity (Nikkilä and Konttinen) Lancet 1:1151-1154, 1962

see also Obesity; Weight, body

Fatigue

(Bock) Trans. Coll. Physicians Phila. 10:75-81, 1942

adenosinetriphosphate, administration of, to rats submitted to hard physical work (Greco) Gazz. Int.
Med. Chir. 69:795-798, 1964

and adrenals, cholinesterase activity, rats (Overbeek) Arch. Int. Pharmacodyn. 79:314-322, 1949

amphetamine sulphate, effect of (Newman) J. Pharmacol. Exp. Ther. 89:106-108, 1947

and anoxemic and normal skeletal muscle (Anders and others) Naunyn Schmiedberg Arch. exp. Path.
217:406-412, 1953

benzedrine, effect of in soldiers (Somerville) Canad. Med. Ass. J. 55:470-476, 1946

biochemistry (Efimoff and Samitschkina) Arbeitsphysiol. 2:341-346, 1929

CO_2 - output in static muscular work, relation to (Frumerie) Scand. Arch. Physiol. 30:409-440, 1913

cardiac insufficiency and cardiac occlusion, in relation to (Puccini) Minerva Medicoleg. 75:133-140,
1955

in cardiac insufficiency, structure and colloidal state of fibers (Maestrini) Policlinico (sez. prat.)
58:933-945, 1951

cerebral circulation, influence of on (Horiuchi) Arbeitsphysiol. 1:75-84, 1928

colloid-chemical changes in muscles (Schmidt) Arbeitsphysiol. 1:136-153, 1929

disintegration of central autonomic regulation, I. Disintegration, pupillographic studies (Lowenstein and
Loewenfeld) J. Nerv. Ment. Dis. 115:1-21, 1952

disintegration of central autonomic regulation II. Reintegration, pupillographic studies (Lowenstein and
Loewenfeld) J. Nerv. Ment. Dis. 115:121-145, 1952

Fatigue (Cont.)

electrocardiogram changes, muscular activity (Fabre and others) J. Physiologie 56:345-346, 1964

electrophysiology, muscular activity (Stepanov and Burkalow) Fiziol. Zh. SSSR Sechenov. 47:43-47, 1961

excitability in respiratory centers, changes in (Franck and others) Comptes Rend. Soc. Biol. 139:835-836, 1945

and exercise, physiology (Schenck) Marburg, N. G. Elwert, 1911

and exercise and rest (Owen) Canad. Med. Ass. J. 47:41-45, 1942

exercise for efficiency of muscles, importance of (Hedvall) Scand. Arch. Physiol. 32:115-197, 1915

and exhaustion (Hartmann) Deutsch. Med. J. 12:260-264, 1961

exhaustion, death (Schönholzer) Schweiz. Zeits. Sportmed. 5:65-80, 1957

and exhaustion, physiological support with antacids, during physical load (Winter) Med. Klin. 53:2195-2196, 1958

heat, produced by, relation to lactic acid in amphibian muscle (Peters) J. Physiol. 47:243-271, 1913

hypoglycemic (Karlan and Cohn) J.A.M.A. 130:553-555, 1946

impairment and psycho-motor learning (Nunney) Percept. Motor Skills 16:369-375, 1963

influence of regular intervals on, in hard work (Müller and Karrasch) Int. Zeits. angew. Physiol. 16:45-51, 1955

ischaemic necrosis of the anterior tibial muscles, caused by (Hughes) J. Bone Joint Surg. 30B:581-594, 1948

isometric strength, and work decrement (Pierson) Percept. Motor Skills 17:470, 1963

march, inhibitory effects of L-aspartic acid salts against (Fujioka and others) Nat. Def. Med. J. 10:525-528, 1963

mental, influence of physical exercise (Leitão and others) J. Soc. Cienc. Med. Lisboa 127:651-730, 1963

muscle action, striated, parameters of potentials (Mitolo and Cotugno) Boll. Soc. Ital. Biol. Sper. 36: 1766-1770, 1960

muscle, and crystallization of myosin (Belagyi and Felker) Acta Physiol. Acad. Sci. Hung. 22:327-330, 1962

and muscle, modification of osmotic properties (Fletcher) J. Physiol. 30:414-438, 1904

muscles, arm, effect on contraction (Long and others) J. Physiol. 58:334-337, 1924

muscular, afferent system in muscle (Matsev and Kiselkova) Izv. Inst. Fiziol. 6:19-33, 1963

muscular, effect of adrenalin (Gruber) Amer. J. Physiol. 43:530-544, 1917; Amer. J. Physiol. 33:335-355, 1914

muscular, arm, contraction, effect on relation between work and speed (Hill and others) J. Physiol. 58:334-337, 1924

muscular, influence of respiration (Speck) Deutsch. Arch. klin. Med. 45:461-528, 1889

muscular, movement factors governing speed and recovery from (Hill) New York, McGraw-Hill Book Co. Inc. 1927

muscular, physiological (Grandjean) Med. Welt. 31:1587-1590, 1960

Fatigue (Cont.)

   muscular, problems (Merton) Brit. Med. Bull. 12:219-221, 1956

   muscular, recovery (Numajiri) J. Sci. Labour 40:153-161, 1964

   muscular, role (Aubert) Acta Belg. Arte. Med. Pharm. Milit. 110(part 2):513-520, 1957

   muscular, role of, on peroxidase activity of leucocytes, in normal subjects (Fracchia and Antognetti) Gazz.
       Int. Med. Chir. 68(Suppl.):3114-3121, 1963

   muscular, threshold level, and recovery of elbow flexor muscles (Pastor) Arch. Phys. Med. 40:247-252,
       1959

   and muscular training, influence on critical effectiveness of local dynamic work (Bourguignon and Scherrer)
       Comptes Rend. Soc. Biol. 154:921-924, 1960

   and muscular work (Scherrer and Monod) J. Physiologie 52:419-501, 1960

   and muscular work, efferent venous blood of working muscle (Monod and others) J. Physiologie 53:697-717, 1961

   myocardium, effect of physical work, rat (Greco) Gazz. Int. Med. Chir. 69:1163-1166, 1964

   nature (Dill) Personnel 9:113-116, 1933; Geriatrics 10:474-478, 1955

   onset, variations of glucuronic acid content of urine and serum, physical exercise (Tamura and Tsutsumi)
       Folia Pharmacol. Jap. 59:70-77, 1963

   oxygen consumption, relation to, measured by electric flicker, during, and after exercise (Suzuki)
       Tohuku. J. Exp. Med. 52:9-16, 1950

   penicillin, effect of on physical work capacity and experience of fatigue (Furberg and Ringqvist) Svensk.
       Lakartidn. 60:2650-2655, 1963

   physiology (Rothschuh and Rave) Jahresk. aerztl. Fortbild. 33:1-11, 1942

   physiology, and excretion of urea (Haig) Lancet 1:610-615, 1896

   present status of study (Miller) N. Carolina Med. J. 9:580-582, 1948

   psychiatry and physiology (Watkins and others) Arch. Phys. Med. 28:199-206, 1947

   psychological criteria (Bartlett) in Symposium on Fatigue, H. K. Lewis, 1953

   and psycho-motor learning (Nunney) Percept. Motor Skills 16:369-375, 1963

   pyruvic acid, role of (Meyer) New York J. Med. 45:1450-1451, 1945

   stimuli, environmental and intrinsic, influence on work capacity and resistance to fatigue (Missiuro)
       Rumanian Med. Rev. 5:191-200, 1961

   and strength (Merton and Pampiglione) Nature 166:527, 1950

   stress-symptom, general, resulting from secretion of ACTH (Wachholder) Int. Zeits. angew. Physiol.
       16:361-364, 1957

   'toxin' and antitoxin (Weichardt) München. med. Wschr. 51:12-13, 1904; 51:2121-2126, 1904

   war medicine (Dill and others) Clinics 2:1126-1154, 1944

   work and nutrition (Christensen and Hansen) Scand. Arch. Physiol. 81:160-171, 1939

   work decrement, and endurance, repetitive task (Pierson) Brit. J. Med. Psychol. 36:279-282, 1963

Fatigue (Cont.)

    work, optimal body efficiency, estimation and change owing to (Balke) Arbeitsphysiol. 15:311-323, 1954

    work, in reduction of atmospheric pressure (Margaria) Arbeitsphysiol. 2:261-272, 1929

    and work of skeletal muscles, in training for physical exercise, aged subjects (Mitolo and others) Gior. Geront. 12:1313-1320, 1964

    work, study by lung function test (Bühlmann and others) Schweiz. med. Wschr. 91:105-109, 1961

Fatty acids

    arterial and venous plasma concentrations, during exercise (Carlson and Pernow) J. Lab. Clin. Med. 53:833-841, 1959

    arterial plasma concentration, during and after exercise (Carlson and Pernow) J. Lab. Clin. Med. 58:673-681, 1961

    arterial plasma concentration during exercise and in subjects with vasoregulatory asthenia (Carlson and Pernow) J. Lab. Clin. Med. 60:655-661, 1962

    in blood, and duration and intensity of muscular work (Cerretelli and others) Boll. Soc. Ital. Biol. Sper. 37:1660-1662, 1961

    blood level, effects of exercise (Basu and others) Quart. J. Exp. Physiol. 45:312-317, 1960

    and blood sugar, reaction to sport (Wuschech and others) Deutsch. Gesundh. 19:1668-1670, 1964

    and carbohydrate metabolism, effects of beta-sympathetic blockade, rest and exercise (Muir) Lancet 2: 930-932, 1964

    and carbohydrate metabolism, effect of beta-sympathetic blockade at rest and during exercise (Jenkins) Lancet 2:1184-1185, 1964

    and carbohydrates, effects of exercise and isoproterenol, cardiac patients (Bruce and others) Amer. J. Med. Sci. 241:59-67, 1961

    exercise, effect of, pigeon (George and Vallyathan) J. Appl. Physiol. 19:619-622, 1964

    exercise, effect on metabolism, pancreatectomized dogs (Issekutz and others) Amer. J. Physiol. 205: 645-650, 1963

    and free amino acids, arterial concentrations at rest and work (Carlsten and others) Scand. J. Clin. Lab. Invest. 14:185-191, 1962

    metabolism, effect of exercise, dog (Miller and others) Amer. J. Physiol. 205:167-172, 1963

    plasma, and anaerobic metabolism, hemodynamic relationships during exercise, trained and untrained subjects (Cobb and Johnson) J. Clin. Invest. 42:800-810, 1963

    plasma, concentration in obesity (Opie and Walfish) New Eng. J. Med. 268:757-760, 1963

    plasma, during exercise and effect of lactic acid (Issekutz and Miller) Proc. Soc. Exp. Biol. Med. 110: 237-239, 1962

    plasma, effect of nicotinic acid on, during exercise (Carlson and others) Metabolism 12:837-845, 1963

    plasma, effect of supplementary feeding (Mager) Metabolism 13:823-830, 1964

    plasma, in exercise (Rodahl and others) J. Appl. Physiol. 19:489-492, 1964

    plasma, influence of muscular effort (Coster and others) Comptes Rend. Soc. Biol. 106:1937-1939, 1962

Fatty acids (Cont.)

   plasma, metabolism during exercise (Friedberg and others) J. Lipid Res. 4:34-38, 1963

   plasma, in muscular activity (Guarnieri and Bianucci) Riv. Crit. Clin. Med. 64:31-44, 1964

   plasma, turnover and concentration, effect of exercise (Friedberg and others) J. Clin. Invest. 39:
      215-220, 1960

   serum, in children with body loads (Werner and Möhlmann) Zeits. Kinderheilk. 89:160-169, 1964

   triglycerides, cholesterol, and phospholipids, arteriovenous relationship, in exercise (Konttinen) Ann.
      Med. Exp. Fenn. 40:250-256, 1962

   turnover rate and oxidation, blood plasma, continuous infusion of palmitate -1-C^{14} (Havel and others) J.
      Clin. Invest. 42:1054-1063, 1963

   turnover rate and oxidation during exercise (Havel and others) J. Appl. Physiol. 19:613-618, 1964

   in venous blood, experimental conditions (Lorentzen) Aerospace Med. 35:649-652, 1964

Femur

   osteochondroma, associated with popliteal aneurysm (Anastasi and others) Arch. Surg. 87:636-
      639, 1963

Fever

   influence on phosphoric acid content of muscles (Adam) Hoppe-Seyler Zeits. physiol. Chem. 113:281-300, 1921

Fibrillation, atrial

   in asymptomatic young men, effect of exercise, digitalization, atropinization, and restoration of normal rhythm
      (Graybiel) Amer. J. Cardiol. 14:828-836, 1964

   heart rate with exercise in (Knox) Brit. Heart J. 11:119-125, 1949

   occupational activity, relation to (Sessa and others) Atti Soc. Ital. Cardiol. 2:118-119, 1962

   transitory flutter, and atrioventricular dissociation after exertion (Jacono and Juliani) Riforma Med. 76:
      429-431, 1962

   ventricular rate response following exercise during, and after conversion to normal sinus rhythm (Wetherbee
      and others) Amer. J. Med. Sci. 223:667-670, 1952

Fibrinogen

   effect of violent exercise on (Hodgkinson) Henry Ford Hosp. Med. Bull. 6:48-54, 1958

Fibrinolysis

   activity, experimental, produced by exercise or adrenaline (Biggs and others) Lancet 1:402-405, 1947

   and blood clotting, effect of physical exercise (Iatridis and Ferguson) J. Appl. Physiol. 18:337-344, 1963

   equilibrium, coagulation, effects of exercise (Burt and others) J. Sport Med. 4:213-216, 1964

   increased, physiologic and pathologic effect, effects of exercise (Ratnoff and Donaldson) Amer. J. Cardiol.
      6:378-386, 1960

   and muscular exercise in heat (Bedrak and others) J. Appl. Physiol. 19:469-471, 1964

   physical activity, changes produced by (Ogston and Fullerton) Lancet 2:730-733, 1961

   plasma, potential of, effect of muscular work (Camerada and others) Rass. Med. Sarda 62:1037-1041, 1960

Fibrinolysis (Cont.)

of whole blood, determination, special reference to effects of exercise and fat feeding (Billimoria and

others) Lancet 2:471-475, 1959

Fick method

direct, for cardiac output, effects of posture, venous pressure change, atropine, and adrenaline (McMichael

and Sharpey-Schafer) Brit. Heart J. 6:33-40, 1944

direct, regulation of circulation during exercise, dog (Barger and others) Amer. J. Physiol. 184:613-623, 1956

direct, reproducibility of cardiac output determination by (Holmgren and Pernow) Scand. J. Clin. Lab.

Invest. 12:224-227, 1960

Fitness

for adults (Guild) J. Sport Med. 3:101-104, 1963

air force personnel, experimental study (Balke and Ware) U.S. Armed Forces Med. J. 10:675-688, 1959

body condition and diet, and the energy production during mechanical work, inter-relation between, dog

(Anderson and Lusk) Proc. Nat. Acad. Sci. 3:386-389, 1917

middle-aged men, changes in, relation to training, non-training and retraining (Cureton and Phillips)

J. Sport Med. 4:87-93, 1964

physical, correlation of selected laboratory tests with military endurance (Rasch and Wilson) Milit. Med.

129:256-258, 1964

physical, in relation to age, experimental studies (Robinson) Arbeitsphysiol. 10:251-323, 1938

physical, of confined dog: criteria and monitoring of muscular performance (Yoder and others) Amer. J.

Vet. Res. 25:727-738, 1964

sex and age, relation to (Åstrand) Physiol. Rev. 36:307-335, 1956

see also Body efficiency; Training

Flicker fusion

critical fusion, variations during intellectual and physical work (Baron and others) Arch. Mal. Prof. 24:

429-433, 1963

Flight

of locusts, biology and physics, lift and metabolic rate (Weis-Fogh) J. Exp. Biol. 41:257-271, 1964

Food

consumption, military personnel, light activities, hot desert environment (Consolazio and others) Metabolism

9:435-442, 1960

deprivation and temperature regulation, in exercise (Thompson and Stevenson) Canad. J. Biochem. 41:

528-530, 1963

deprivation, effect on treadmill running in dogs (Young) J. Appl. Physiol. 14:1018-1022, 1959

deviant patterns of feeding behaviour, man (Mendelson) Fed. Proc. 23:69-72, 1964

and excretion in turtle dove (Boussingault) Ann. Chim. Phys. Sér. 3. 11:433-456, 1844

ingested, effect of muscular work after (Cantone) Arch. Sci. Biol. 48:277-284, 1964

intake and body weight and exercise, normal rats and genetically obese mice (Mayer and others) Amer.

J. Physiol. 177:544-548, 1954

Food (Cont.)

    intake and energy expenditure, elderly people (Durnin) Geront. Clin. 4:128-133, 1962

    intake, voluntary, effect of exercise, rats (Whalley and others) Permanente Found. Med. Bull. 9:
        114-118, 1951

    oxidisation for energy, utilization of "waste heat" in muscular exercise (Rapport) Amer. J. Physiol. 91:
        238-253, 1929

    requirements according to age, sex, size and occupation (Royal Society: Food (War) Committee) London,
        Harrison, 1919

    requirements in relation to activity (Passmore) Lancet 2:853-854, 1964

    to satiety, offered to young soldiers, to test energy requirements and physical achievements according to body
        composition (Allen and others) U.S. Army Med. Res. Nutr. Lab. Rep. 243:1-30, 1960

    and urea, relation to muscular exercise (Anstie) Practitioner 5:353-357, 1870

    utilization, effect of walking, sheep (Clapperton) Brit. J. Nutr. 18:39-46, 1964

    see also Diet; Energy

Forearm

    arterioles and veins, responses to walking during acclimatization to heat (Wood and Bass) J. Clin. Invest.
        39:825-833, 1960

    blood chemistry, deep forearm veins, during and after contraction (Barcroft and others) J. Physiol. 169:
        34P-35P, 1963

    blood flow changes, during physical training (Rohter and others) J. Appl. Physiol. 18:789-793, 1963

    blood volume, physical effort (Altilla and others) Boll. Soc. Ital. Cardiol. 8:490-493, 1963

    contraction, blood flow and venous oxygen saturation (Barcroft and Whelan) J. Physiol. 168:848-856,
        1963

    lactate and pyruvate formation and oxygen utilization during work of high intensity and varying duration
        (Pernow) Acta Physiol. Scand. 56:267-285, 1962

    muscles, contraction, rate of blood flow and oxygen saturation (Love) Clin. Sci. 14:275-283, 1955

    muscles, effect of continuous infusion of ATP, histamine and acetylcholine on blood debt repayment
        (Patterson and Shepherd) Clin. Sci. 13:85-91, 1954

Fructose

    ingestion, effect of muscular work after (Carpenter and Fox) Arbeitsphysiol. 4:532-569; 570-599, 1931

G

Gas, blood

    and acid-base balance, changes during muscular activity (De Lanne and others) J. Appl. Physiol. 14:328-332,
        1959

    and acid base-balance, changes, in exercise, dog (Wathen and others) J. Appl. Physiol. 17:656-660, 1962

Gas, blood (Cont.)

anoxemia, respiratory response (Haldane and others) J. Physiol. 52:420-432, 1919

arterial, and electrolytes during physical work (Buhlmann and Rossier) Zeits. Biol. 111:235-240, 1959

in arterial and venous (Meakins and Davies) J. Path. Bact. 23:451-461, 1920

arterial and venous, oxygen consumption, cardiac output, stroke volume, in normals, rest and exercise
   (Ulmer and Berta) Pflüger Arch. ges. Physiol. 280:281-296, 1964

arterial, and ventilation, time-courses of changes in, induced by exercise (Matell) Acta Physiol. Scand.
   58(Suppl. 206):1-53, 1963

arterial blood, and pH during exercise, effect of temperature (Holmgren and McIllroy) J. Appl. Physiol.
   19:243-245, 1964

arterial blood gas analysis using Fleish's metabograph; determination of ventilation and acid-base balance on
   heavy work (Abelin and Scherrer) Schweiz. med. Wschr. 90:369-374, 1960

arterial, influence on chemoreceptor action potential in the carotid sinus (Witzleb and others) Pflüger Arch.
   ges. Physiol. 261:211-218, 1955

arterial pO_2, measurement in light and heavy exercise (Asmussen and Nielsen) Acta Physiol. Scand. 42(Suppl.
   145):17, 1957

arterial saturation, complete, in heart disease, physical work (Olmes de Carrasco) Klin. Wschr. 20:95-97, 1941

arterial, tension of (Haldane and Smith) J. Physiol. 20:497-520, 1896

arterial tension, and other blood gas analyses in rest and exercise (Doll) Pflüger Arch. ges. Physiol. 271:283-
   295, 1960

arterial tension, investigation by carbon monoxide method (Douglas and Haldane) Skand. Arch. Physiol. 25:
   169-182, 1911

and blood sugar, changes during exercise (Hartman and Griffith) Proc. Soc. Exp. Biol. Med. 21:561-565,
   1924

changes provoked by light and moderate exercise (Barr and others) Acta Physiol. Scand. 60:1-17, 1964

composition, outdoor living (Petrun) Zdravookhr. Beloruss. 9:57-60, 1963

content of (Magnus) Ann. Chim. Phys. Sér. 2. 65:169-192, 1837

oxygen, partial pressure and carbon dioxide content, arterial blood, in health and disease, after physical
   activity (Julich) Zeits. ges. inn. Med. 18:928-932, 1963

tensions, normal variations during moderate exercise (Suskind and others) J. Appl. Physiol. 3:282-290, 1950

variation of proportion (Mathieu and Urbain) Arch. Physiol. Norm. Pathol. 4:5-26, 190-203, 304-318, 447-469,
   573-587, 710-731, 1872

variations in pO_2 and pCO_2, metabolites in muscular effort, young and old (Tinti and others) Gior. Geront.
   12:1121-1132, 1964

venous, coronary circulation and carbohydrate metabolism of heart, muscular work (Lochner and Nasseri)
   Pflüger Arch. ges. Physiol. 269:407-416, 1959

Gas exchange

circulatory disturbances, influence of (Meakins and Davies) Heart 9:191-198, 1922

and energy expenditure, during treadmill running, dog (Young and others) J. Appl. Physiol. 14:834-838, 1959

and evaluation of cardio-pulmonary function (Refsum) Scand. J. Clin. Lab. Invest. 15(Suppl. 76):44-48, 1963

measurement, physical capacity (Herbst) Deutsch. Arch. klin. Med. 162:33-50, 1928

of muscular exercise, restricted (Furusawa) Proc. Roy. Soc. 99B:155-166, 1926

in muscular work, during and after (Goor and Mosterd) Proc. Kon. Ned. Akad. Wet. (Biol. Med.) 64:96-98, 1961

and respiration, external, limited cyclic rapid exercises, boys (Volkov) Fiziol. Zh. SSSR Sechenov. 49: 1456-1430, 1963

respiratory, during recovery from moderate exercise (Berg) Amer. J. Physiol. 149:597-610, 1947; Mem. Rep. Aero Med. Lab. (MCREXD-696-114), 103-131, 1948

respiratory, effect of ethyl alcohol, during rest and exercise (Hebbelinck) Arch. Int. Pharmacodyn. 126: 214-218, 1960

respiratory, measurements, equilibrial state, muscular exercise (Haab) Rev. méd. Nancy 82:872-879, 1957

respiratory, rest and mountain work (Bürgi) Leipzig, Veit and Co., 1900

see also Ventilation

Gas metabolism

carbon dioxide breathing in disease, health and training, influence of (Herxheimer and Kost) Naunyn Schmiede-berg Arch. exp. Path. 165:101-110, 1932

exercise, influence of (Gruber) Zeits. Biol., n.F. 10:466-491, 1891-1892

gymnastics, influence of (Missiuro and Perlberg) Arbeitsphysiol. 9:514-527, 1937

measurement, physical capability (Herbst) Deutsch. Arch. klin. Med. 162:257-279, 1928

and minute volume (Odaira) Tohoku J. Exp. Med. 6:325-366, 1925

Gastric motility

stomach activity, effect of physical exertion, in gastric complaints (Bugyi) Deutsch. Zeits. Verdauungskr. 16:38-40, 1956

Gas stores

of body and unsteady state (Fahri and Rahn) J. Appl. Physiol. 7:472-484, 1955

Gastric secretion

acid, effect of regular muscular activity, rat (Frenkl and others) Acta Physiol. Acad. Sci. Hungary 22:203-208, 1962

inhibitory effect of muscular exercise (Hammar and Öbrink) Acta Physiol. Scand. 28:152-161, 1953

Gelatin

  effects on limitation of muscle work (Robinson and Harmon) Amer. J. Physiol. 133:161-169, 1941

Globulin

  antihaemophilic, level in blood, effect of exercise (Rizza) J. Physiol. 156:128-135, 1961

  gamma, heterogeneity, in post-exercise urine (Freedman and Connell) Canad. J. Biochem. 42:1065-1097,
      1964

Glucides

  and muscular activity (Babinet and Heraud) Bull. Soc. Sci. Hyg. Aliment. 48:3-10, 1960

Gluconeogenesis

  (Krebs) Proc. Roy. Soc. 159:545-564, 1964

  and muscular exercise (Krebs and Yoshida) Biochem. Zeits. 338:241-244, 1963

Glucose

  assimilation, during muscular effort (Conard and Franckson) Arch. Int. Physiol. 68:374-376, 1960

  assimilation, influence of muscular effort (Conard and Franckson) Comptes Rend. Soc. Biol. 151:2228-2230, 1957

  blood, concentration in intact and pancreatectomized dogs, effect of exercise (Moxness and others) Diabetes 13:
      37-43, 1964

  blood, metabolism, during muscular work (Reichard and others) J. Appl. Physiol. 16:1001-1005, 1961

  consumption and muscular work (Babinet and Heraud) Diabete 10:15-17, 1962

  infusion, intravenous, at various rates during heavy muscular work (Wierzuchowski) Acta Physiol. Pol. 15:
      729-758, 1964

  ingestion, effect of muscular work after (Carpenter and Fox) Arbeitsphysiol. 4:532-569, 578-599, 1931

  metabolism, during exercise in rheumatic heart disease (Harris and others) Clin. Sci. 23:561-569, 1962

  metabolism in experimental potassium depletion, effects of insulin, glucagon, and muscular exercise
      (Sagild and Andersen) Acta Med. Scand. 175:681-685, 1964

  metabolism, myocardial (Carlsten and others) Verh. deutsch. Ges. Kreislaufforsch. 27:195-196, 1961

  peripheral utilization, effect of exercise (Sanders and others) New Eng. J. Med. 271:220-225, 1964

  serum, concentration changes after prolonged physical effort (Preisler and Pankowska) Bull. Soc. Amis.
      Sci. Poznan (Med.) 12:61-70, 1963

  uptake, effect of exercise, rats and man (Christopher and Mayer) J. Appl. Physiol. 13:269-272, 1958

Glucuronic acid

  content of urine and serum, and onset of fatigue, physical exercise (Tamura and Tsutsumi) Folia Pharmacol.
      Jap. 59:70-77, 1963

Glutathione

  reduction, organs, and work output, rats (Télupilová-Krestýnova and Santavý) Pflüger Arch. ges.
      Physiol. 266:473-477, 1958

Glycemia

    in effort, during and after (Martin du Pan) Helv. Med. Acta 9:508-528, 1942

    equilibrium and repeated muscular exercise (Rougier and Babin) Comptes Rend. Soc. Biol. 158:1064-
        1067, 1964

Glyceryl trinitrate

    in angina pectoris, test of efficacy (Russek and Howard) J.A.M.A. 189:108-112, 1964

Glycogen

    cerebral, concentration, changes, in physical activity (Jakoubek and Svorad) Pflüger Arch. ges. Physiol.
        268:444-448, 1959

    -lactic acid breakdown in muscle, free energy (Eurk) Proc. Roy. Soc. 104B:153-170, 1929

    metabolism (Meier and Meyerhof) Biochem. Zeits. 150:233-242, 1924

    mobilization and work in rat heart (Hazelwood and Ullrick) Amer. J. Physiol. 200:999-1003, 1961

    resynthesis in fasted rat (Long and Grant) J. Biol. Chem. 89:553-565, 1930

    tissue, effect of violent exercise, albino mice (Wilber) Life Sci. 8:564-568, 1963

Glycogenosis

    skeletal muscle, in identical twins (Lehoczky and others) Brit. Med. J. 2:802, 1964; Ideggyogy Szemle
        17:65-79, 1964

Glycopolysaccharides

    leucocytal peroxidases, and oxidases after intense and prolonged muscular work (Mazzella) Riv. Med. Aero.
        23:117-122, 1960

Glycosides

    cardiac, hemodynamic effects, rest and exercise (Williams and others) J. Appl. Physiol. 13:417-421,
        1958

    heart, and changes in venous blood pressure (Zöllner and König) Zeits. Kreislaufforsch. 47:31-39, 1958

    theophylline and analeptics, influence on cardiac output in congestive heart failure (Berséus) Acta Med.
        Scand. 113(Suppl. 145):1-76, 1943

    see also Digitalis

Gravity spectrum

    physiology and psychology (Di Giovanni and Chambers) New Eng. J. Med. 270:134-139, 1964

Gray's theory

    of respiratory control, application to hypernea produced by passive movements of the limbs (Otis) J. Appl.
        Physiol. 1:743-751, 1949

Grip

    strength, relation to age (Burke and others) J. Appl. Physiol. 5:628-630, 1953

Growth

    body and organ, alterations following daily exhaustive exercise, x-irradiation, and post-irradiation exercise,
        rats (Kimeldorf and Baum) Growth 18:79-96, 1954

    of organs, effect of exercise, rats (Hatai) Anat. Rec. 9:647-665, 1915

    schistosomiasis, effect upon activity and growth, mice (Hearnshaw and others) Ann. Trop. Med. Parasit.
        57:481-498, 1963

Guanethidine

  influence on blood pressure, normal and under physical load (Sturzenegger and others) Deutsch. med. Wschr. 85:
    1275-1277, 1960

Guanylnucleotides

  effect on work capacity, heart hypertrophy and adrenal glands, rats (Kokas and Miczbán) Zeits. Vitamin
    Hormon Fermentforsch. 11:310-319, 1961

Gymnastics

  anatomical and physiological applications (Roblot) 7th ed. Paris, Lamarre, 1925

  Joinville School of, influence of exercise on muscle power, volume and weight of body, and pulmonary
    capacity (Burcq) Gaz. Med. Paris, 6º série 4:473-475, 1822

                                              H

Harvard step test

  and indirect maximal oxygen consumption (Maggio and others) Rass. Med. Industr. 32:362-363, 1963

  modified, for evaluation and prediction of physical fitness (Patterson and others) Amer. J. Cardiol. 14:
    811-827, 1964

  modified, oxygen consumption, normal subjects (Starke and Bartlett) U.S. Naval Sch. Aviat. Med.
    Res. Rep. 14:71, 1962

Headache

  of effort (Chavany) Presse Méd. 53:645, 1945

  paroxysmal, from exertion (Kriz) Cas. Lek. Cesk. 102:137-142, 1963

Health

  preservation, and physical education (Warren) Boston, W. T. Ticknor and Co., 1846

Heart

  abnormal, response to exercise (Harvey and others) Circulation 26:341-362, 1962

  accidents and excess sporting activity (Fabre) J. Med. Bordeaux 136:244-247, 1959

  action and circulation in young workers (Zuntz) Deutsch. Zeits. Thiermed. 18:261-277, 1892

  activity, and respiration, effect of muscle activity (Johansson) Skand. Arch. Physiol. 5:20-66, 1895

  activity, determined by radioelectrocardiography (Fogel'son and Iazburskis) Kardiologiia 4:67-73,
    1964

  adolescent, development, relàtion of exercise (Foster) Arch. Pediat. 26:814-817, 1909

  aging, electrocardiogram, rest and exercise (Mazer and Reisinger) Ann. Intern. Med. 21:645-652, 1944

  altitude and performance (Balke) Amer. J. Cardiol. 14:796-810, 1964

  of athlete (Wolffe) J. Lancet 77:76-78, 1957; (Sjostrand) Arzt u. Sport 80:963-966, 1955

  in athletes, blood circulation (Reindell and others) Med. Welt 31:1557-1563, 1960

  and athletics, electrocardiography and radiology (Cooper and others) Med. J. Aust. 1:569-579, 1937

Heart (Cont.)

and blood vessels, tonicity (Gaskell) J. Physiol. 3:48-75, 1882

body exercise, lasting influence of (Grober) Wien. med. Wschr. 63:441-449, 1913

and circulation, effects of exercise (Larrabee) Boston Med. & Surg. J. 147:318-323, 328-330, 1902

and circulation, immediate and remote effects of athletics (Stengel) Amer. J. Med. Sci. 118:544-553, 1899

and circulation, possible injury by physical strain (Hollmann) Aerztl. Wschr. 14:605-609, 1959

comparative observations, mongrels and greyhound (Schneider and others) Anat. Rec. 149:173-179, 1964

control, mechanisms in exercise (Rushmer and others) Circ. Res. 7:602-627, 1959; Physiol. Rev. 40(Suppl. 4):27-34, 1960

cycle, determination of duration of phases, athletes, muscular work (Shkhvatsabaia) Kardiologiia 4:62-68, 1964

damage, during carbon monoxide and supplementary physical burden (Groetschel) Arch. Gewerbepath. Gewerbehyg. 10:223-237, 1940

diagnosis, in sportsman, and differential diagnostic estimation of findings in ECG and Kymogramme (Reindell) Deutsch. med. Wschr. 65:1369-1373, 1939

dynamics (Straub) Handbuch. der Norm. Path. Physiol. 7(Teil 1):237, 1926

dynamics, adaptation to work of increasing intensity (Mascaretti and others) Atti Soc. Ital. Cardiol. 22: 325-326, 1962

efficiency, coronary blood flow, and myocardial oxygen consumption, effect of exercise (Lombardo and others) Circulation 7:71-78, 1953

effort, determination of possible outcome (Broustet and others) Arch. Mal. Coeur 57 Suppl.: 56-76, 1964

evaluation by exercise performance (Gilbert and others) Amer. J. Med. 34:452-460, 1963

exercise, response, (Bickelmann and others) Circulation 28:238-250, 1963; (Cumming) Canad. Med. Ass. J. 88:80-85, 1963; (Currie) Guy's Hosp. Gaz. 35:113, 1921; (González Deleito) Rev. Españ. Med. Cir. 10:194-201, 1927; (Lawrence) Delaware Med. J. 36:54-57, 1964; (McKenzie) Amer. J. Med.Sci. 145:69-74, 1913; (Meylan) J. Med. Soc. New Jersey 2:332-335, 1906; (Opdyke) Phys. Ther. Rev. 30:462-468, 1950; (Schmidt) Circ. Res. 7:507-512, 1959; (Williamson) Amer. J. Med. Sci. 149:492-503, 1915; (Wang and others) Circulation 24:1064, 1961

filling and emptying, rest and exercise (Nicolai and Zuntz) Berlin. klin. Wschr. 51:821-824, 1914

function and coronary insufficiency, electrocardiogram and 'two-step' exercise (Master) Amer. J. Med. Sci. 207:435-450, 1944

in industry (Haynes) Med. J. Aust. 2:53-57, 1964

injury and effort, effect of, normal and diseased (Master) New York J. Med. 46:2634-2641, 1946

'irritable', effects of exercise on pulse rate and systolic blood pressure in (Cotton and others) Heart 6: 269-284, 1917

'irritable', pulse rate after exercise test in (Meakins and Gunson) Heart 6:285-292, 1917

loafer's (Raab) Arch. Intern. Med. 101:194-198, 1958

and lung, effect of physical exercise (Zander) Gesundh. in Wort und Bild, Berlin, 1904

Heart (Cont.)

mechanical power, and output, cardiovascular, effects of digitalis and of effort (Mottu) Arch. Mal.
Coeur 49:50-56, 1956

motor acceleration, cause (Mansfeld) Pflüger Arch. ges. Physiol. 134:598-626, 1910

muscle mechanics (Sonnenblick) Fed. Proc. 21:975-990, 1962

muscle, mineral content, influence of training and load (Nöcker and others) Int. Zeits. angew. Physiol.
17:243-251, 1958

nourishment, association with physical work (Zuntz) Deutsch. med. Wschr. 18:109-111, 1892

performance, and obesity (Alexander) Amer. J. Cardiol. 14:860-865, 1964

performance, effect of exercise in minimal heart disease (Gorlin and others) Amer. J. Cardiol. 13:
293-300, 1964

performance, in relation to blood volume (Burch and DePasquale) Amer. J. Cardiol. 14:784-795, 1964

in running and swimming, chronic effects of, electrocardiograms, dogs (Steinhaus and others) Amer. J.
Physiol. 99:503-511, 1932

size, functional reduction of (Moritz) München. Wschr. 55:713-718, 1908

in ski-run-contest (Rautmann) Deutsch. med. Wschr. Sonderausgabe 62:42-44, 1936

and sport, pathology and physiology (Herbst) Aerztl. Wschr. 11:877-880, 1956

strain, development of physiologic concept (Parsonnet and Bernstein) Ann. Intern. Med. 16:1123-1136, 1942

strain, effect on (Fothergill) Brit. Med. J. 1:281, 1873

strained (Plas) Gaz. Med. France 68:1637-1642, 1961

strength and effect of aging (Starr) Amer. J. Cardiol. 14:771-783, 1964

surface, roentgenological measurement, in health and disease, rest and exercise (Drews) Zeits. Kreislaufforsch.
51:622-628, 1962

and work (Acker) J. Tenn. Med. Ass. 56:46-48, 1963; (Dill) Amer. J. Cardiol. 14:729-730, 1964

and work (Rosenbaum) New York, Paul Hoeber, 1959

and work, anticipation and ergonometry (Goldner and Burr) Amer. J. Med. Sci. 246:192-199, 1963

in work, difficult, and high performance sport (Knipping and Valentin) München. med. Wschr. 103:
11-15, 1961

x-ray, porters (Podkaminsky) Arbeitsphysiol. 1:306-356, 1929

see also Atrium; Blood volume, heart; Heart rate; Ventricle

Heart block

effect of heart rate, exercise and nitroglycerin on cardiac dynamics (Benchimol and others) Circulation
28:510-519, 1963

intermittent, well-trained sportsman (Hansen) Nord. Med. 62:1386-1388, 1959

paroxysmal, on exertion (Gough and Galpin) Brit. Med. J. 1:1359, 1964

total, minute volume of heart in (Lundsgaard) Deutsch. Arch, klin. Med. 120:481-496, 1916

treated with implanted pacemaker (Chardack) Prog. Cardiovasc. Dis. 6:507-537, 1964

see also Atrioventricular block; Sinoatrial block

Heart disease

Heart rate (Cont.)

fetal, physical working capacity during pregnancy and effect of tests on (Soiva and others) Ann. Chir. Gynaec. Fenn. 53:187-196, 1964

frequency, during and immediately after difficult physical work (Christensen) Arbeitsphysiol. 4:453-469, 1931

hourly, and respiration, health (Smith) British Med. J. 1:52, 1856; Med. Chir. Soc. Trans. 39:35-58, 1856

increased, during muscular work (Aulo) Skand. Arch. Physiol. 25:347-360, 1911

in 'irritable heart' after test exercise (Meakins and Gunson) Heart 6:285-292, 1917

maximum, and maximum oxygen intake, during strenuous exercise (Wyndham and others) J. Appl. Physiol. 14:927-936, 1959

maximum, and recovery pulse rate and post-exercise blood lactate, inter-relation (Montoye) Res. Quart. 24:453-458, 1953

measurement, in exercise (Austin and Harris) Quart. J. Exp. Physiol. 42:126-129, 1957

monitoring device in an ambulation program, use of (Anderson) Arch. Phys. Med. 45:140-146, 1964

in natural muscular activity (by radiotelemetry) (Rozenblat) Fed. Proc. (Transl. Suppl.) 22:761-766, 1963

and obesity, relationship between, at rest and during work (Buskirk and others) Int. Zeits. angew. Physiol. 16:83-89, 1955

the oesophageal temperature and the oxygen debt during exercise (Harris and Porter) Quart. J. Exp. Physiol. 43:313-319, 1958

and oxygen consumption, discrepancy between, during work in the warmth (Brouha and others) J. Appl. Physiol. 18:1095-1098, 1963

and "oxygen debt", influence of atmospheric conditions after running (Campbell) Proc. Roy. Soc. 96B:43-59, 1924

and oxygen intake during early stages of recovery from severe exercise (Lythgoe and Pereira) Proc. Roy. Soc. 98B:468-479, 1925

and oxygen uptake, maximal, in muscular activity (Åstrand and Saltin) J. Appl. Physiol. 16:977-981, 1961

and oxygen uptake while running (Knuttgen) Acta Physiol. Scand. 52:366-371, 1961

performance-heartbeat, frequency regulation, comparative studies (Koessling) Med. Welt 31:1567-1572, 1960

peripheral pulse, effect of exercise (Edwards and others) New Eng. J. Med. 260:738-741, 1959

physical training and practice, acute infections and exercise distress, effect of (Dawson) Amer. J. Physiol. 50:443-479, 1919

physiological significance (Buchanan) Trans. Oxford Scientific Club No. 34, page 35, 1909

pulse, disappearance after exercise in Leriche syndrome (Williams and De Niord) Virginia Med. Monthly 90:281-282, 1963

pulse-index function as a measure of functional capacity (Müller) Arbeitsphysiol. 14:271-284, 1950

Heart rate (Cont.)

Heart size

Heat, see Environment, hot

Heat, muscle

animal (Dulong) Ann. Chim. Phys. Sér. 3, 1:440-455, 1841

contraction muscle, origin (Meyerhof) Pflüger Arch. ges. Physiol. 195:22-74, 1922; 204:295-331, 1924

development and mechanical work, in connection with muscle activity (Fick) Leipzig, 1882

exchange, and body temperature during treadmill running, dogs (Young and others) J. Appl. Physiol. 14: 839-843, 1959

production, muscle, effects of different salts (Sereni) J. Physiol. 60:1-19, 1925

production in muscles treated with caffein or subjected to prolonged discontinuous stimulation (Hartree and Hill) J. Physiol. 58:441-454, 1924

regulation in muscular work (Zuntz) Berlin. klin. Wschr. 33:709, 1896

specific-dynamic, increased production following maximum muscular exercise, dog (Meyer) Arbeitsphysiol. 2:372-386, 1930

Hemiplegia

bracing and rehabilitation training, effect on energy expenditure (Dacso and others) Postgrad. Med. 34: 42-47, 1963

energy cost of stand-up exercises (Hirschberg and others) Amer. J. Phys. Med. 43:43-45, 1964

energy expenditure during walking (Bard) Arch. Phys. Med. 44:268-270, 1963

Hemoconcentration

effects of short period of strenuous exercise on (Darling and Shea) Arch. Phys. Med. 32:392-396, 1961

Hemoglobin

and albumin serum levels, changes in muscular work and sweating (Cohn) Zeits. Biol. 70:366-370, 1919

blood volume, hemoglobin concentration, rest and exercise, old and young men (Strandell) Acta Med. Scand. 176:219-232, 1964

concentration, during rest and exercise, calculation of oxygen saturation (Merrill and others) Amer. J. Clin. Path. 30:209-210, 1958

dissociation curve (Barcroft and Roberts) J. Physiol. 39:143-148, 1909

and erythrocyte increase, blood, during and after exercise (Schneider and Crampton) Amer. J. Physiol. 112: 202-206, 1935

heart volume and physical training in former athletes, relationship with (Holmgren and Strandell) Acta Med. Scand. 163:149-160, 1959

level, influence of acid base balance, ventilation and O_2-diffusion, during hard work, healthy subjects (Kubicek and Scherrer) Schweiz. Med. Wschr. 92:415-420, 1962

oxygen intake, maximal and body size, normal man (Döbeln) Acta Physiol. Scand. 38:193-199, 1956

percentage, and number of red corpuscles, effect of work (Boothby and Berry) Amer. J. Physiol. 37:378-382, 1915

physical training, increase in connection with (Kjellberg and others) Acta Physiol. Scand. 19:146-151, 1949

Hemoglobin (Cont.)

    and physical working capacity in anemia of pregnancy (Robbe) Acta Obstet. Gynec. Scand. <u>37</u>:
        312-347, 1958

    and physical working capacity in normal pregnancy and puerperium (Gemzell and others) Acta Obstet.
        Gynec. Scand. <u>36</u>:93-136, 1957

    pulse rate and heart volume during work, relation to (Kjellberg and others) Acta Physiol. Scand. <u>19</u>:
        152-169, 1949

    training, effect of (Holmgren and others) Acta Physiol. Scand. <u>50</u>:72-83, 1960

    work capacity, muscular, significance in estimation (Pitteloud and others) Schweiz. med. Wschr. <u>94</u>:
        811-816, 1964

    and work capacity of 40-year-old adult (Gander) Helv. Med. Acta <u>31</u>:669-695, 1964

Hemoglobinuria

    exertional (Davidson) J. Clin. Path. <u>17</u>:536-540, 1964

    march, (Bell) Canad. Med. Ass. J. <u>57</u>:43-46, 1947; (Bryce) Med. J. Aust. <u>2</u>:49-52, 1944; (Fisher and
        Bernstein) Bull. Johns Hopkins Hosp. <u>67</u>:457-461, 1940; (Fleming and Kinsman) Southern Med. J.
        <u>38</u>:739-742, 1945; (Hobbs) Amer. J. Clin. Path. <u>14</u>:485-488, 1944; (Holland) Irish J. Med. Sci. 6th
        series: 183-185, 1955; (Kurz) Brooklyn Hosp. J. <u>6</u>:91-94, 1948; (Lindahl and Fatter) J. Urol. <u>53</u>:
        805-807, 1945; (Lowbury and Blakely) Brit. Med. J. <u>1</u>:12-13, 1948; (Makin) Brit. Med. J. <u>1</u>:844, 1944

    march, amino-aciduria (Pare and Sandler) Lancet <u>1</u>:702-704, 1954

    march, clinical characteristics, blood metabolism and mechanism (Gilligan and Blumgart) Medicine <u>20</u>:
        341-395, 1941

    march, variants (Chaiken and others) Amer. J. Med. Sci. <u>225</u>:514-520, 1953

    march, in a woman (Gilligan and Altschule) New Eng. J. Med. <u>243</u>:944-948, 1950

Hemogram

    modifications in swimmers and gymnasts by physical exercise and sauna-bath (Fornoza) J. Sport Med.
        <u>4</u>:37-42, 1964

Hepatitis

    among troops, reference to alcohol, and physical activity (Gardner and others) Ann. Intern. Med., <u>30</u>:
        1009-1019, 1949

Hepatobiliary metabolism

    and muscular exercise (Parturier and others) Paris Med. <u>26</u>:44-47, 1936

Heroin

    intravenous, effects of addiction on physical activity (Fraser and others) Clin. Pharmacol. Ther. <u>4</u>:
        188-196, 1963

Heteroauxin

    activity in urine after exercise (Kral and others) Med. Welt <u>31</u>:1595-1598, 1960

Hexamethonuim

    effect on blood pressure during exercise (Fowler and Guz) Brit. Heart J. 16:1-7, 1954

Hibernation

    catecholamine content of brain and heart, hedgehog (Erinaceus Europaeus), and in active state

        (Uuspää) Ann. Med. Exp. Fenn. 41:340-348, 1963

Histamine

    blood, influence of physical exertion (Verschure and others) Acta Allerg. 10:136-148, 1956

    formation in physical exercise, anoxia, and under influence of adrenaline (Graham and others) J. Physiol.

        172:174-188, 1964

    and hyperaemia of muscular exercise (Schayer) Nature 201:195, 1964

    and leukocytes in blood during muscular work (Dunér and Pernow) Scand. J. Clin. Lab. Invest. 10:

        394-396, 1958

Homeostasis

    and nonfat components of migrating birds (Odum) Science 143:1037-1039, 1964

Hormones, see ACTH; Adrenocorticosteroids; Epinephrine; Ketosteroids; Steroids; Thyroid Hormones, and names of

    other specific hormones

Housework

    energy expended (Weaver and Elliot) J. Amer. Diet. Ass. 39:205-208, 1961

    use and abuse of muscles (Travell) J. Amer. Med. Wom. Ass. 18:159-162, 1963

Hurdling

    and running, physiology (Jokl) Arbeitsphysiol. 1:296-305, 1929

17-Hydroxycorticosteroids, see Adrenocorticosteroids

Hydralazine

    oral therapy in hypertension, cardiovascular and renal function before and during effect of exercise (Judson

        and others) J. Lab. Clin. Med. 49:672-683, 1957

Hydration

    post-exercise ketosis, and metabolic state interrelations (Johnson and Passmore) Metabolism 9:443-451, 1960

Hydrogen-ion concentration, see Acid-base equilibrium

Hyperemia

    exercise and ischaemia, induced by (Dornhorst) Brit. Med. Bull. 19:137-140, 1963

    of exercise, muscular, and histamine (Schayer) Nature 201:195, 1964

    post-exercise, effects of intra-arterial adrenaline (Glover and Shanks) J. Physiol. 167:268-279, 1963

    potassium ions, role of in exercise (Kjellmer) Med. Exp. 5:56-60, 1961

    reactive, contour of toe pulse, and pulse transmission velocity effect of age, exercise and disease (Simonson

        and others) Amer. Heart J. 50:260-279, 1955

Hyperkinetic states

    circulatory dynamics, rest and exercise (Bishop and others) Clin. Sci. 14:329-360, 1955

Hyperlipemia

alimentary, physical effort and its effect in reducing (Cantone) J. Sport Med. 4:329-360, 1955

Hyperpnea

exercise, peripheral neural mechanism (Iaria and others) J. Physiol. 148:48P-50P, 1959

of muscle exercise, limb reflexes as factor (Comroe and Schmidt) Amer. J. Physiol. 138:536-547, 1943

of muscular exercise (Comroe) Physiol. Rev. 24:319-339, 1944

physical chemical system of blood in respiration and circulation: carbon dioxide inhalation and hyperpnea (Hochrein and others) Naunyn Schmiedeberg Arch. exp. Path. 143:170-183, 1929

respiratory control, application of Gray's theory to (Otis) J. Appl. Physiol. 1:743-751, 1949

see also, Dyspnea

Hyperreflexia

of lower limbs after exercise (Spiller) J.A.M.A. 87:639-640, 1926

Hypertension

arterial, and ischaemic heart disease, electrocardiogram T/U complex and U waves (Torregiani and others) Folia Cardiol. 22:461-471, 1963

cardiovascular and renal function before and during oral hydralazine therapy (Judson and others) J. Lab. Clin. Med. 49:672-683, 1957

and hypertension associated with coronary heart disease, ballistocardiographic changes (Huang and others) Chin. Med. J. 82:202-207, 1963

mechanisms in renoprival man (Merrill and Schupak) Canad. Med. Ass. J. 90:328-332, 1964

and pressor reactions, acute, haemodynamic basis (Brod) Brit. Heart J. 25:227-245, 1963

pulmonary, arterial, and cyanosis (Oñate and Ramos) Rev. Esp. Tuberc. 32:557-562, 1963

pulmonary, on exertion, 10,150 feet (Vogel and others) Med. Thorac. 19:461-477, 1962

pulmonary, systemic arterial pressure during exercise in (Jonsson and Lukianski) Acta Med. Scand. 173:73-81, 1963

renin activity in blood in (Helmer) Canad. Med. Ass. J. 90:221-225, 1964

Hyperthermia

and hypothermia, pituitary-adrenocortical function, the effect of work performed (Yang and Endroczi) Acta Physiol. Acad. Sci. Hung. 18:131-136, 1960

relation to available body water, muscular, high temperature, dogs (Shek) Fiziol. Zh. SSSR Sechenov. 49:542-547, 1963

Hypertrophy

cardiac, experimental, work, rats (Visioli and others) Folia Cardiol. 22:473-481, 1963

compensatory, origin and evaluation of heart, adrenal and hypophysis, animal experiments (Beickert) Arch. Kreislaufforsch. 21:115-126, 1954

muscular, evaluation and production (McMorris and Elkins) Arch. Phys. Med. 35:420-426, 1954

Hypothalamus

appetite and obesity (Brobeck) Physiol. Physicians 1:1-6, 1963

hypothalamo-hypophysial neurosecretion; effect of heavy muscular work, rat (Härkünen and others) Ann.
Med. Exp. Fenn. 42:17-21, 1964

injury, effect on adrenal gland and work performance (Kokas and Kurucz) Schweiz. med. Wschr. 86:1067-1070,
1956

Hypothermia

and hyperthermia, pituitary-adrenocortical function, effect of work performed (Yang and Endroczi) Acta
Physiol. Acad. Sci. Hung. 18:131-136, 1960

Hypoxia

acute, and exercise, effects on pulmonary circulation (Fishman and others) Circulation 22:204-215, 1960

arterial, value and significance, exercise (Salvini and others) Folia Med. 38:777-789, 1955

induced, effect on oxygen uptake during muscular exercise (Cronin and Macintosh) Canad. J. Biochem. Physiol.
40:717-726, 1962

mild, effect on ventilation during exercise (Hornbein and Roos) J. Appl. Physiol. 17:239-242, 1962

oxygen consumption and muscular work (Strumza and Traccan) Comptes Rend. Soc. Biol. 154:1412-1415, 1960

prolonged, respiratory activity (Åstrand) Acta Physiol. Scand. 30:343-368, 1954

test and arterial tension, recovery time (Lazzari) Gazz. Int. Med. Chir. 69:304-308, 1964

test, cardiac rate, trained and untrained (Lazzari) Gazz. Int. Med. Chir. 69:602-606, 1964

test, influence on renal function, untrained subjects in strenuous exercise (Lazzari) Gazz. Int. Med. Chir.
68:2883-2886, 1963

test, trained and untrained massive exertion (Lazzari) Gazz. Int. Med. Chir. 69:179-184, 1964

see also Gas, blood; Oxygen content, blood

I

Immersion

total, at various temperatures, effect on oxygen uptake at rest and during exercise (Goff and others)
J. Appl. Physiol. 9:59-61, 1956

Impedance curves

body, significance, alternating currents of low frequency, influence of muscular activity (Plouvier)
Agressologie 3:761-767, 1962

Inactivity

loafer's heart (Raab) Arch. Intern. Med. 101:194-198, 1958

prolonged, circulatory metabolic effects of different types (Birkhead and others) Amer. J. Med. Sci.
247:243, 1964

see also Bed rest; Disuse

Indocyanine green clearance

    and estimated hepatic blood during exercise (Rowell and others) J. Clin. Invest. 43:1677-1690, 1964

Industrial hygiene

    physiology, effects of exercise and mental effort on circulation (McDowall) J. Industr. Hyg. 10:94-100,
        1928

Insects

    locusts, flight, biology and physics, lift and metabolic rate of flying (Weis-Fogh) J. Exp. Biol. 41:257-271,
        1964

Insufficiency, coronary

    apnea test and electrocardiographic diagnosis (Roganti and others) Cardiol. Prat. 14:367-375, 1963

    and cardiac function test for (Master) Amer. J. Med. Sci. 207:435-450, 1944

    diagnosis during loading, electrocardiogram (Kaltenbach and Klepzig) Zeits. Kreislaufforsch. 52:486-497,
        1963

    diagnosis, evaluation of dynamic and postexercise electrocardiogram (Abarquez and others) Amer. J.
        Cardiol. 13:310-319, 1954

    exercise electrocardiogram test (Gubner) J. Occup. Med. 3:110-120, 1961

    exercise test in diagnosis (Grossman and others) Ann. Intern. Med. 30:387-397, 1949

    physiologic advantage of oxygen during exercise (Pons and Berg) Dis. Chest 39:551-556, 1961

Insulin

    activity and effects on pentose transport into muscle (Sacks and Smith) Amer. J. Physiol. 192:287-289,
        1958

    effects on uptake of hexoses by muscle cells (Huycke and Kruhøffer) Acta Physiol. Scand. 34:232-249,
        1955

    and muscular exercise, effect on isolated hindquarter preparation, cat (Bojesen and Egense) Acta Endocr.
        33:347-369, 1960

    plasma insulin-like activity, effect of training and acute physical exercise (Devlin) Irish J. Med. Sci.
        6th series:423-425, 1963

    and potassium, effect on myasthenia gravis (Frenkel) Arch. Neurol. 9:447-457, 1963

    response, effect of exercise, rabbits (Thorp) Quart. J. Pharm. Pharmacol. 17:75-88, 1944

Intellect

    influence of physical activity on retarding decline, cyclists (Clement) Rev. Franç. Geront. 7:379-412,
        1961

Interval work

    influence on mechanical efficiency (Christensen and others) Acta Physiol. Scand. 48:443-447, 1960

    and interval training (Christensen) Int. Zeits. angew. Physiol. 18:345-356, 1960

Inulin

    and endogenous clearance, rest and exercise (Starlinger and Berghoff) Int. Zeits. angew. Physiol.
        19:194-200, 1962

    and PAH clearance; influence of work in high temperature on, and on electrolytic and
        17-21-dihydroxy-10-ketosteroid excretion in urine (Starlinger and Bandino) Int. Zeits. angew.
        Physiol. 18:285-305, 1960

Iodine

    and lipid levels, in tissues, effect of muscular activity and experimental training, rats (Leshkevich) Ukr.
        Biokhim. Zh. 36:726-734, 1964

Iron

    serum, and electrolytes, concentration changes after physical effort (Preisler and Kabza) Bull. Soc. Amis.
        Sci. Poznan (Med.) 13:85-93, 1964

    serum, influence of exercise (Biörck) Acta Physiol. Scand. 15:193-197, 1948

Ischemic muscle-nerve injury

    of legs in physical exercise (Bekeny and Kraft) Wein. Zeits. Nervenheilk. 20:336-348, 1963

Ischemic work

    responses in forearm (McArdle and Verel) Clin. Sci. 15:305-318, 1956

Isoenzymes

    lactic dehydrogenase, after exercise and training, rats (Garbus and others) Amer. J. Physiol.
        207:467-472, 1964

Isolation

    and adynamia, changes in nervous reactions after long stay conditions (Agadzhanian and others) Zh. Vyssh.
        Nerv. Deiat. Pavlov 13:953-962, 1963

    see also Adynamia

Isometric contraction

    (Smedley) New Physician 13:198-199, 1964

    and agricultural work (Monod and Laville) Concours Med. 86:521-522, 1964

    hemodynamic determinants of rate of change in pressure in left ventricle during (Reeves and others) Amer.
        Heart J. 60:745-761, 1960

Isometric exercise

    arm, maximal, injurious consequences (Pierson and Rasch) J. Amer. Phys. Ther. Ass. 43:582-583, 1963

    immobilized muscle, response of (Hislop) J. Amer. Phys. Therap. Ass. 44:339-347, 1964

    quantitative changes in muscular strength during (Hislop) J. Amer. Phys. Therap. Ass. 43:21-38, 1963

    see also Strength

Isometric tension

    endurance and reaction time, effect of exercise programs (Baer and others) Arch. Phys. Med. $\underline{36}$:495-502,
        1955

    local muscular endurance and load, with occluded blood supply (Start) J. Appl. Physiol. $\underline{19}$:1135-1138,
        1964

Isoproterenol

    and exercise, effects on free fatty acids and carbohydrates, cardiac patients (Bruce and Williams) Amer.
        J. Med. Sci. $\underline{241}$:59-67, 1961

    infusion, producing changes in pulmonary haemodynamics in emphysema (Williams and others)
        Circulation $\underline{28}$:396-403, 1963

    and norepinephrine, infusion, response of pulmonary circulation (Aramendia and others) Acta Physiol.
        Lat. Amer. $\underline{13}$:20-25, 1963

J

Jews

    physical exercise, from olden days to the present (Munter) Wien. Manter, 1926

K

17-Ketogenic steroids

    and 17-ketosteroids, excretion, contrasting effects of emotional tension and physical exertion (Connell
        and others) Acta Endocr. $\underline{27}$:179-194, 1958

Ketonemia

    in muscular training (Mitolo) Arch. E. Maragliano Pat. Clin. $\underline{6}$:239-264, 1951

Ketosis

    post-exercise, hydration, and metabolic state interrelations (Johnson and Passmore) Metabolism
        $\underline{9}$:443-451, 1960

17-Ketosteroids

    and 17-ketogenic steroids, excretion, importance of body characteristics in obesity (Jacobson and others)
        New Eng. J. Med. $\underline{271}$:651-656, 1964

    urinary excretion, in athletes (Saitta) Folia Med. $\underline{37}$:345-352, 1954

Kidney, see Renal

L

Lactic acid

    arterial, heart rate, and oxygen uptake, during exercise, old and young men (Strandell) Acta Physiol.

Lactic acid (Cont.)

Scand. $\underline{60}$:197-216, 1964

in blood, after combinations of exercise and hypoxia (Lorentzen) J. Appl. Physiol. $\underline{17}$:661-664, 1962

in blood and tissue, influenced by muscular exercise (Martin and others) Proc. Soc. Exp. Biol. Med. $\underline{26}$:292-293, 1929

blood content, alterations after light exercise, associated changes in CO_2-combining power and alveolar CO_2 pressure (Owles) J. Physiol. $\underline{69}$:214-237, 1930

blood content, and oxygen consumption during strenuous muscular exercise (Volkov) Fed. Proc. $\underline{22}$:118-122, 1963

blood content during and after work, different diseases, bicycle ergometer test (Jasinski) Helv. Med. Acta $\underline{14}$:117-136, 1947

blood content during recovery from sprint runs (Andersen and others) Acta Physiol. Scand. $\underline{48}$:231-237, Mar. 18, 1960

blood content, regional variations (Burt and Martorano) U.S. Naval Med. Field Res. Lab. $\underline{13}$:1-8, 1963

blood content in relation to absolute and relative work load, in normal, mitral stenosis, atrial septal defect and vaso-regulatory asthenia (Holmgren and Strom) Acta Med. Scand. $\underline{163}$:185-193, 1959

blood content at rest (Long) J. Physiol. $\underline{58}$:455-460, 1924

blood, during and after muscular exercise (Bang) Scand. Arch. Physiol. $\underline{74}$(Suppl. 10):49-82, 1936

in blood during exercise, predicted from pH and pCO_2 determinations (Visser and others) Pflüger Arch. ges. Physiol. $\underline{281}$:300-304, 1964

blood, during muscular work (Bang) Bibliot Laeger $\underline{128}$:106-110, 1936

blood, during muscular work in relation to partial pressure of oxygen of inspired air (Lundin and Ström) Acta Physiol. Scand. $\underline{13}$:253-266, 1947

in blood, kinetics during intensive muscular activity (Volkov) Acta Biol. Med. German. $\underline{13}$:659-673, 1964

blood, post-exercise, and maximum pulse rate, and recovery pulse rate, inter-relation (Montoye) Res. Quart. $\underline{24}$:453-458, 1953

in blood during static work. (Marschak) Arbeitsphysiol. $\underline{4}$:1-19, 1931

chemistry (Embden and Laquer) Hoppe-Seyler Zeits. physiol. Chem. $\underline{113}$:1-9, 1921; (Embden and Zimmerman) Hoppe-Seyler Zeits. physiol. Chem. $\underline{141}$:225-232, 1924

formation and oxygen utilization, legs, normal and arteriosclerosis obliterans (Carlson and Pernow) Acta Med. Scand. $\underline{164}$:39-52, 1959

formation, survival respiration and rigor mortis, mammalian muscle (Fletcher) J. Physiol. $\underline{47}$:361-380, 1913

heat combustion (Meyerhof) Biochem. Zeits. $\underline{129}$:594-604, 1922

lactacidemia and energy expenditure during muscular work, and thermal shivering (Schmitt and others) Comptes Rend. Soc. Biol. $\underline{158}$:770-773, 1964

Liver (Cont.)

pyruvic acid, physical work, rat (Cairella and others) Ann. Med. Nav. 69:557-562, 1964

see also Blood flow; Cirrhosis, liver

Loafer's heart, see Inactivity

Longshoremen

evaluation of physical effort in loading with minimum mechanization (Lewalski) Bull. Inst. Mar. Med. Gdansk 14:191-197, 1963

urinary uropepsin level, heavy work load with minimum mechanization (Lewalski) Bull. Inst. Mar. Med. Gdansk 14:199-208, 1963

Lott's critique

reply to: effort attractiveness, and the anticipation of reward (Aronson) J. Abnorm. Soc. Psychol. 67: 522-526, 1963

Lumber-workers

physiological effects of time schedule work (Lundgren) Acta Physiol. Scand. 13(Suppl. 41):1-137, 1946

Lung diseases

chronic, continuous versus intermittent administration of oxygen during exercise (Cotes) Lancet 1:1075-1077, 1963

chronic, effect of breathing oxygen on cardiac output, heart rate, ventilation, systemic and pulmonary blood pressure (Cotes and others) Clin. Sci. 25:305-321, 1963

chronic obstructive, factors influencing prognosis (Mitchell and others) Amer. Rev. Resp. Dis. 89:878-896, 1964

chronic obstructive, ventilatory response to exercise (Gandevia) Amer. Rev. Resp. Dis. 88:406-408, 1963

chronic pneumopathy, acid-base equilibrium and ventilation, rest and effort (Soucy and others) Un. Med. Canada 87:774-786, 1958

chronic, pulmonary circulation in, at rest and during exercise (Riley and others) Amer. J. Physiol. 152: 372-382, 1948

chronic, work capacity (Fogel'son and others) Ter. Arkh. 35:26-33, 1963

and heart, influence of physical exercise (Zander) Gesundh. in Wort und Bild, Berlin, 1904

structural changes induced by training, rat (Minarovjech) Bratisl. Lek. Listy 44:79-90, 1964

see also Hyperventilation; Pulmonary; Ventilation

Lysis

clot, effect of exercise on time, normal subjects and in cirrhosis of liver (Jang and others) Clin. Sci. 27: 9-13, 1964

M

McArdle's syndrome

case with positive family history (Hockaday and others) J. Neurol. Neurosurg. Psychiat. $\underline{27}$:186-197,
1964

hereditary myopathy due to absence of muscle phosphorylase (Rowland and Schotland) Arch. Neurol. $\underline{9}$:
325-342, 1963

Magnesium

and calcium, excretion with thermal sweat (Bara) Pol. Arch. Med. Wewner. $\underline{33}$:1125-1132, 1963

Malnutrition

behaviour of circulation in, rest and exercise (Frade Fernández) Medicina (Madrid) $\underline{11}$:1-16, 1943

Marathon runners

ballistocardiographic study (Brown) J. Lancet $\underline{77}$:89-90, 1957

circulation of a marathoner (Bock) J. Sport Med. $\underline{3}$:80-86, 1963

physiological and pathological effects on circulatory and renal systems (Barach) Arch. Intern. Med.
$\underline{5}$:382-405, 1910

March hemoglobinuria, see Hemoglobinuria

Marching

at various speeds, work against gravity (Cavagna and others) Boll. Soc. Ital. Biol. Sper. $\underline{36}$:1804-1806,
1960

Massage

after muscular exertion, effect on blood, healthy subjects (Lampert) Zeits. ges. phys. Ther. $\underline{39}$:238-253,
1930

influence on metabolism (Dunlop and others) J. Physiol. $\underline{22}$:68-91, 1897

Master step test

according to Ford and Hellerstein (Caccuri) Cuore Circ. $\underline{46}$:121-135, 1962

in coronary heart disease, and in normal (Mason) Heart Bull. $\underline{8}$:67-69, 1959

healthy young men (Catelli and Privitera) Cuore Circ. $\underline{47}$:202-210, 1963

'2-step' exercise test (Master and others) Bibl. Cardiol. (Suppl. to Cardiologia) No. $\underline{9}$:243-254, 1959;
(Thomas) Bull. Johns Hopkins Hosp. $\underline{89}$:181-207, 1951

two-step, recording the electrocardiogram during (Rosenfeld and Master) Circulation $\underline{29}$:212-218, 1964;
(Rosenfeld and others) Circulation $\underline{29}$:204-211, 1964

see also Electrocardiogram

Mechanics

of animals (Perrault) Pairs, 1680

mechanochronometry, automatic, method in physical work (Gumener and others) Gig. Sanit. $\underline{29}$:58-62,
1964

Medulla oblongata

  mammalian, prefusion, effect of carbon dioxide and other substances on respiratory and cardiovascular
    centers (Hooker and others) Amer. J. Physiol. 43:351-361, 1917

  respiratory reactions elicited from, cat (Liljestrand) Acta Physiol. Scand. 29(Suppl. 106):321-393,
    1953

  respiratory responses mediated through superficial chemosensitive areas (Mitchell and others) J. Appl.
    Physiol. 18:523-533, 1963; Ann. N.Y. Acad. Sci. 109:661-681, 1963

Menstruation

  and physical exercise (Areno) Hospital 25:289-293, 1944; (Peregrino and Lourdes-Oliveira) Hospital 25:
    751-759, 1944; (Rougier and Lincuette) Presse Med. 70:1921-1923, 1962

Mental alertness

  in rowers, influence of psychotropic substances (Policreti and others) Ann. Med. Nav. 68:803-808,
    1963

Mental irritation

  changes of blood coagulation time immediately after (Vuori) Ann. Med. Int. Fenn. 37:167-181, 1948;
    Acta Med. Scand. 138(Suppl. 239):296-300, 1950

Mepacrine

  concentrations in blood plasma, and urine, effect of muscular exercise in hot moist environment (Maegraith
    and others) Ann. Trop. Med. Parasit. 40:368-371, 1946

Metabolism

  aerobic and anerobic metabolism, exercising dogs (Cerretelli and others) J. Appl. Physiol. 19:25-28, 1964

  anaerobic, and plasma free fatty acids, haemodynamic relationships during exercise, trained and untrained
    subjects (Cobb and Johnson) J. Clin. Invest. 42:800-810, 1963

  anaerobic, and plasma volume changes following exercise, correlation (Iseri and others) Ann. Intern. Med.
    59:788-797, 1963

  anaerobic, pyruvate and lactate relationships in (Huckabee) Part I J. Clin. Invest. 37:244-254, 1958;
    Part II, J. Clin. Invest. 37:255-263, 1958; Part III, J. Clin. Invest. 37:264-271, 1958

  anaerobic, role in mild muscular work Part II (Huckabee) J. Clin. Invest. 37:1593-1602, 1958; Part III
    (Huckabee and Judson) J. Clin. Invest. 37:1577-1592, 1958

  basal, effect of muscular exercise (Rougier and Osouf) J. Physiologie 52:216-217, 1960

  basal, influence of physical training, animals (Beickert and others) Zeits. ges. exp. Med. 129:60-68,
    1957

  blood-flow and exudation in organs, effect of functional activity (Barcroft and Kato) Proc. Roy. Soc.
    88B:541-543, 1915

  different movements during tiring exertion, influence of (Lehmann) Arch. Ver. gemeinsch. Arb.
    Ford Wissensch. Heilk. 4:484-520, 1860

  exercise, muscular, sweating, and massage, influence of on metabolism (Dunlop and others) J. Physiol.
    22:68-91, 1897

  exercise, previous, influence on metabolism, rat (Horst and others) J. Nutr. 7:251-275, 1935

Methylene blue

    calorigenic action during muscular exercise (Guild and Rapport) Proc. Soc. Exp. Biol. Med. <u>34:</u>
        459-461, 1936

Methyl scopolamine nitrate

    effect of cardioacceleration on circulation at rest and during exercise (Bevegård) Acta Physiol. Scand.
        <u>57</u>:61-80, 1963

Microfilariae

    periodicity, effect of parasympathetic stimulants on distribution (Hawking and others) Trans. Roy. Soc.
        Trop. Med. Hyg. <u>58</u>:178-194, 1964

Middle-age

    capacity and arthropometric measurements (Skinner and others) Amer. J. Cardiol. <u>14</u>:747-752, 1964

    exercise, effects on blood cholesterol (Montoye and others) Amer. J. Clin. Nutr. <u>7</u>:138-145, 1959

    exercise, strenuous muscular, adaptation to (Iakovlev and others) Fiziol. Zh. SSSR Sechenov. <u>49</u>:1067-
        1070, 1963

    normal, and subjects with angina pectoris, hemodynamic response to exercise (Foster and Reeves) J. Clin.
        Invest. <u>43</u>:1758-1763, 1964

    outdoor sport, advocation of (Graham) Med. News <u>61</u>:403-404, 1892

Milk

    intake, protein, and exercise, effect on athletes (Wilcox and others) J. Amer. Diet. Ass. <u>44</u>:95-99,
        1964

Mind-body

    healthy, in healthy body (Schmid) Halae Magdeb., Lit. Hendelianis, 1728

Miners

    cardiac output during work (Peretti and Granati) Arch. Sci. Biol. <u>26</u>:149-153, 1940

    energy expenditure (Humphreys and Lind) Brit. J. Industr. Med. <u>19</u>:264-275, 1962; (Pachner and others)
        Acta Med. Leg. Soc. <u>12</u>:53-55, 1959

    oxygen and carbon dioxide gradients, expiration, rest, muscular exercise and recovery (Siehoff and others)
        Poumon Coeur <u>19</u>(Suppl.):1385-1393, 1963

    respiration, external, influence of exertion (Shevelev) Gig. Tr. Prof. Zabol. <u>7</u>:13-17, 1963

    respiratory physiological studies, reference to silicosis, bronchitis and emphysema, and expiratory-arterial
        oxygen and carbon dioxide pressure differences, rest and exercise (Muysers and others) Int. Arch.
        Gewerbepath. <u>19</u>:589-612, 1962

Mitotic activity

    during muscular exercise (Alov and Abramson) Biull. Eksp. Biol. Med. <u>51</u>:710-714, Nov., 1961

Mitral heart disease

    mechanics of respiration in (Nisell and others) Acta Med. Scand. <u>162</u>:277-285, 1958

    mitral narrowing and respiratory function, spirographic studies (Hatzfeld) Rev. Franç. Etud. Clin. Biol.
        <u>3</u>:345-356, 1958

    stenosis, blood lactate concentration, in absolute and relative work load (Holmgren and Ström) Acta Med.
        Scand. <u>163</u>:185-193, 1959

Mitral heart disease (Cont.)

    stenosis, cardiac output and rhythm, pulmonary vascular pressures and disability, relationships between
        (Bishop and Wade) Clin. Sci. 24:391-404, 1963

    stenosis, circulatory system state based on gas exchange data (Beliaeva) Ter. Arkh. 35:60-65, 1963

    stenosis compensated, alveolar-capillary diffusion of carbon monoxide, progressively increasing muscular
        exercise (Chiavaro and others) Boll. Soc. Ital. Cardiol. 8:634-638, 1963

    stenosis, distensibility of pulmonary arterial vessels, rest and exercise (Lasser and Amram) Amer. Heart
        J. 51:749-760, 1956

    stenosis, distribution of alveolar ventilation, rest and exercise (Raine and Bishop) Clin. Sci. 24:
        63-68, 1963

    stenosis, exercise effect on lung distensibility and respiratory work (Hayward and Knott) Brit. Heart J.
        17:303-311, 1955

    stenosis, exercise effect on mean diastolic left atrial-left ventricular gradient (Litwak and others) J.
        Thorac. Surg. 34:449-468, 1957

    stenosis, exercise phonocardiogram in evaluation of degree (Magri and others) Minerva Med. 49:1258-1263,
        1958

    stenosis, oxygen, carbon dioxide and lactic acid, role of in ventilatory response to exercise (Cotes) Clin. Sci.
        14:317-328, 1955

    stenosis, respiratory function, and blood circulation in, evaluation by physical exercise (Martynov) Ter. Arkh.
        36:97-105, 1964

    stenosis, work, effects on pulmonary circulation (Eliasch and others) Circulation 5:271-278, 1952

Motor

    performance and skills, measurements, relation of cardiovascular tests (Fowler and Gardner) Pediatrics
        32(Suppl.):778-789, 1963

Movement

    animal (Borelli) Lugduni in Batavia, P. vander Aa, 1710

    influence on growing and adult organs (Külbs) Deutsch. med. Wschr. 38:1916-1920, 1912

    joint, range, effect of systematic heavy resistive exercise (Massey and Chaudet) Res. Quart. 27:41-51,
        1956

    local, animal (Fabricius ab Aquapendente) Patavii, J. B. de Martin, 1618

    muscular activity during locomotion (Gray) Brit. Med. Bull. 12:203-209, 1956

    muscular and central nervous sytem (Beevor) London, Adlard 1904

    muscular, effects of speed on mechanical efficiency (Lupton) J. Physiol. 57:337-353, 1923

    muscular, factors governing speed and recovery from fatigue (Hill) New York, McGraw-Hill Book Co. Inc.
        1927

    and rest (Allébé) Schat. d. Gezondh. 3:225;257, 1860

    willed, involuntary patterning associated with, against progressively increasing resistance (Waterland and
        Hellebrandt) Amer. J. Phys. Med. 43:13-30, 1964

    working, rate, physiological factors determining (Kosilov) Fiziol. Zh. SSSR Sechenov. 49:141-148,
        1963

Mucoproteins

   and adrenal corticosteroids, urinary excretion during rest and exercise (Hatch and others) J. Appl. Physiol. 9:465-468, 1956

Multiple sclerosis

   optic neuropathy, and exercise (Goldstein and Cogan) Arch. Ophthal. 72:168-170, 1964

Muscles

   activity (Hill) Baltimore, Williams and Wilkins Company, 1926

   activity and carbohydrate metabolism (Furusawa) Proc. Roy. Soc. 98B:65-76, 1925

   activity and glucides (Babinet and Heraud) Bull. Soc. Sci. Hyg. Aliment. 48:3-10, 1960

   activity, and recovery, various environments, physiological reactions (Brouha and others) J. Appl. Physiol. 16:133-140, 1961

   activity and respiratory function, healthy adults, different ages (Berloco and others) Gior. Ital. Tuberc. 16: 101-104, 105-110, 111-113, 1962

   activity, and strain, physiological effect (Hough) Amer. Phys. Educat. Rev. 14:207-215, 1909

   activity, biophysical values (Davis and Logan) Dubuque, Iowa, W. C. Brown, 1961

   activity, engineering aspect (Hill) Sci. Progr. Twent. Cent. 22:630-640, 1928

   activity, influence of speed on mechanical efficiency (Cathcart and others) J. Physiol. 58:355-361, 1924

   aerobic and anaerobic changes, during diving, seal (Scholander and others) J. Biol. Chem. 142:431-440, 1942

   antagonistic, strength, effect of isometric exercise (Rasch and others) Int. Zeits. angew. Physiol. 19:18-22, 1961

   blood supply, during indirect warming and cooling (Barcroft and others) Pflüger Arch. ges. Physiol. 261: 199-210, 1955

   chemical processes in, and 'heat formation' relation between (Hill) Ergebn. Physiol. 15:340-479, 1916

   dynamic changes during work (Bock and others) J. Physiol. 66:136-161, 1928

   dynamic constants (Hill) Proc. Roy. Soc. 128B:263-274, 1940

   dynamics, and dimensions of animals (Hill) Proc. Roy. Instn. Great Britain 34:450-473, 1950; Sci. Progr. Twent. Cent. 38:209-230, 1950

   efficiency, effect of exercise (Peder) Scand. Arch. Physiol. 27:315-340, 1912

   effort (Bannister) Brit. Med. Bull. 12:222-225, 1956

   elbow flexor recovery, threshold muscular fatigue level (Pastor) Arch. Phys. Med. 40:247-252, 1959

   energy production (Needham) Brit. Med. Bull. 12:194-198, 1956

   exercise (Hill) Proc. Roy. Instn. Great Britain 24:23-38, 1925; Nature 112:77-84, 1923

   exertion and body temperature (Bardswell and Chapman) Brit. Med. J. 1:1106-1110, 1911

   fasciculations in healthy population (Reed and Kurland) Arch. Neurol. 9:363-367, 1963

   force and velocity in muscle, relation between (Wilkie) J. Physiol. 110:249-280, 1949

   forearm, blood chemistry, deep forearm veins during and after contraction (Barcroft and others) J. Physiol. 169:34P-35P, 1963

Muscles (Cont.)

forearm, contraction, blood flow and venous oxygen saturation (Barcroft and Whelan) J. Physiol. 168:
848-856, 1963

forearm, effects of continuous infusions of adenosine triphosphate, histamine, and acetylcholine (Patterson
and Shepherd) Clin. Sci. 13:85-91, 1954

forearm, lactate, and pyruvate formation and oxygen utilization, during work of high intensity and varying
duration (Pernow) Acta Physiol. Scand. 56:267-285, 1962

gas content of active muscle (Mettenleiter) Deutsche. Arch. klin. Med. 117:517-539, 1915

immobilized, response to isometric exercise (Hislop) J. Amer. Phys. Ther. Ass. 44:339-347, 1964

length and tension (Blix) Scand. Arch. Physiol. 4:399-409, 1893; 5:150-172, 173-206, 1895

loading, and endurance (Caldwell) Rep. 486 U.S. Army Med. Res. Lab. 1-11, 1963

metabolism of warm-blooded animals, circulation during tetanic contraction (Kramer and Quensel) Pflüger
Arch. ges. Physiol. 239:620-743, 1937

movement (Canappe) Lyon 1541; Movimento musulorum, Paris, 1546

myofibrils, number per fiber, sartorius muscle, effect of exercise, rat (Holmes and Rasch) Amer. J. Physiol.
195:50-52, 1958

over-use, urinary abnormalities (Arnett and Gardner) Amer. J. Med. Sci. 241:55-58, 1961

power, origin (Fick and Wislicenus) London, Edinburgh & Dublin Philosoph. Mag. Fourth Series (supplement)
31:485-503, 1866; Zurich Vierteljahrsschr. 10:317-348, 1865; Ann. Sci. Nat. (Zool.) 10:257-279,
1868

receptors, metabolism-receptive, localization, and regulation of pulse frequency (Stegemann) Pflüger Arch.
ges. Physiol. 276:511-524, 1963

responses, thermal and mechanical, inseparability (Gasser and Hartree) J. Physiol. 58:396-404, 1924

rested, effect previous muscular efforts, on working capacity (Muravov and Tkachev) Fiziol. Zh. 10:
163-169, 1964

shortening, effect of load on heat (Hill) Proc. Roy. Soc. 159:297-318, 1964

shortening, efficiency of mechanical power development during, and relation to load (Hill) Proc. Roy. Soc.
159:319-324, 1964

shortening or lengthening, thermodynamic phenomena (Azuma) Proc. Roy. Soc. 96B:338, 1924

small, optimal concentration rate (Dolgin) Arbeitsphysiol. 2:205-214, 1929

smooth, molluscan, contraction (Abbott and Lowy) J. Physiol. 141:385-397, 1958

'steady state' and respiratory quotient during work (Bock and others) J. Physiol. 66:162-174, 1928

stimulated, energy degraded in recovery processes (Hill) J. Physiol. 46:28-80, 1913

stretch reflex, triceps surae, effect of exercise (Johnson and others) J. Ass. Phys. Ment. Rehab. 17:
172-176, 1963

striated, action, in training and fatigue, parameters of potentials (Mitolo and Cotugno) Boll. Soc. Ital.
Biol. Sper. 36:1766-1770, 1960

Muscles (Cont.)

 striated, source of activity, and chemistry of contraction (Embden) Klin. Wschr. 6:628-631, 1927

 tension development and circulation, comparison in biceps and triceps (Gersten and others) Amer. J.
  Phys. Med. 42:156-165, 1963

 testing, functional, and isometric strength (Pierson and Rasch) Amer. J. Phys. Med. 42:205-207, 1963

 thermodynamics (Frank) Ergebn. Physiol. 3(Pt. 2):349-514, 1904

 tissue, comparative physiology (Ritchie) Cambridge, University Press, 1928

 tissue, nourishment and respiratory activity, production of mechanical work (Chauveau and Kaufmann)
  Comptes Rend. Acad. Sci. 104:1763-1769, 1887

 training, effects on strength on specific muscle groups (Fries) Arch. Phys. Ther. 25:546-549, 1944

 training, histological and chemical changes in skeletal muscle due to, and to testosterone (Hettinger)
  Aerztl. Forsch. 13:570-574, 1959

 training, physiology (Grandjean) Schweiz. Zeits. Sportmed. 4:1-5, 1956

 voluntarily controlled action, kinetic energy, and frequency of motor discharge (Bergström) Acta Physiol.
  Scand. 47:179-190, 1959

 voluntary, circulatory changes accompanying contraction (Barcroft) Aust. J. Exp. Biol. Med. Sci. 42:
  1-16, 1964

 voluntary, mechanics (Hill) Lancet 2:947-951, 1951

 work, maximum and mechanical efficiency, and most economical speed (Hill) J. Physiol. 56:19-41, 1922

 in work, mechanical, metabolism and respiration (Chauveau and Kaufmann) Comptes Rend. Acad. Sci.
  104:1763-1769, 1887

 in work, muscular and muscular fatigue, afferent system (Mateev and Kiselkova) Izv. Inst. Fiziol. 6:
  19-33, 1963

 see also Contractions, muscles; Fatigue; Movement; Skeletal muscles; Somatic muscle; Soreness, muscular;
  Strong man; and names of specific muscles

Muscular dystrophy

 work and power capacity, measured during stationary swimming, mice (Gey and Kennard) Nature 202:264-
  266, 1964

Myasthenia gravis

 cholinesterase, serum levels, effect of muscular exercise (Stoner and Wilson) J. Physiol. 102:1-4, 1943

 effect of insulin and potassium (Frenkel) Arch. Neurol. 9:447-457, 1963

Myocardial efficiency

 pulse and blood pressure variations during exercise and (Robertson) Med. J. & Rec. 122:213-219, 1925

Myocardial infarction

 effort, importance of in development (Masoni and others) Arch. Pat. Clin. Med. 38:235-240, 1961

 etiology, significance of psychic and socio-economic stress in (Kasanen and others) Ann. Med. Intern. Fenn.
  52(Suppl. 43):1-40, 1963

Myocardial infarction (Cont.)

evaluation and physical conditioning before and after (Naughton and others) Amer. J. Cardiol. 14: 837-843, 1964

experimental, effect of exercise on course and restitution (Shevchuk and Isakova) Pat. Fiziol. Eksp. Ter. 7:42-45, 1963

hemodynamics (Malmcrona) Acta Med. Scand. 176(Suppl. 417):1-54, 1964

hemodynamics during convalescence (Malmcrona and Varnauskas) Acta Med. Scand. 175:19-30, 1964

outcome, and work capacity after, middle-aged and elderly metal workers (Abramova and others) Sovet. Med. 26:22-26, 1963

and physical activity (Editorial) Nutr. Rev. 19:221-222, 1961; (Storstein) Nord. Med. 65:281-283, 1961; (Pernot) Arch. Mal. Prof. 24:555-556, 1963

physical strain as cause (Sigler) Amer. J. Cardiol. 7:458-463, 1961

and physical stress (Teodori and Vlasov) Ter. Arkh. 35:3-10, 1963

Myocarditis

Coxsackie A9, effects of exercise, mice (Tilles and others) Proc. Soc. Exp. Biol. Med. 117:777-782, 1964

Myocardium

continuing effort, action on (Kulczycki) Bull. Int. Acad. Polon. Sci. Lett. Classe Med. 39-60, 1952

contractile function, evaluation (Syvorotkin) Kardiologiia 3:40-46, 1963

and fatigue, effect of physical work, rat (Greco) Gazz. Int. Med. Chir. 69:1163-1166, 1964

hemorrhages and necroses of myocardium in excessive physical exertion (Shul'tsev and Teodori) Arkh. Pat. 25:33-38, 1963

histopathological changes, rabbits, stress and fear (Fanfani) Atti Soc. Ital. Cardiol. 16:232-234, 1954

injury, with premature systoles, produced by exercise test (Salomon) Dis. Chest 43:439-440, 1963

isolated strips, relation of work and oxygen consumption, rat, cat (Whalen) J. Physiol. 157:1-17, 1961

metabolism, in rheumatic heart disease, at rest and during exercise (Harris and others) Clin. Sci. 26: 145-156, 1964

mineral content of, influence of training and load (Nöcker and others) Int. Zeits. angew. Physiol. 17: 243-251, 1958

neurogenic multifocal destruction (Raab) Rev. Canad. Biol. 22:217-239, 1963

protein composition, relation to varying functional activity (Helander) Cardiologia 41:94-100, 1962

Myoglobin

acute paralytic myohemoglobinuria (Bywaters and Dible) J. Path. Bact. 55:7-15, 1943

and its occurrence in man (Biörck) Acta Med. Scand. 133(Suppl. 226):1-216, 1949

concentration in muscle, effect of enforced exercise (Lawrie) Nature 171:1069-1070, 1953

myohemoglobin as oxygen store in man (Åstrand and others) Acta Physiol. Scand. 48:454-460, 1960

Myoglobinuria

   (Rowland and others) Arch. Neurol. 10:537-562, 1964

   after exhaustive muscular effort (Kreisle and others) Texas J. Med. 56: 421-425, 1960

   idiopathic paroxysmal, exertional, defect in skeletal muscle metabolism (Kontos and others) Amer. J.
      Med. 35:283-292, 1963

   idiopathic paroxysmal, with acute renal failure and hypercalcaemia (Tavill and others) New Eng. J.
      Med. 271:283-287, 1964

   primary, and exercise-induced secondary myoglobinuria (Turell) Southern Med. J. 54:442-448, 1961

Myometrium

   and estrus, effect of extreme physical exertion (Kliment and others) Cesk. Gynek. 28:501-503, 1963

Myopathy

   glycogenic, twins (Lehoczky and others) Ideggyogy Szemle 17:65-79, 1964; Brit. Med. J. 2:802, 1964

   hereditary, due to absence of muscle phosphorylase (Rowland and Schotland) Arch. Neurol. 9:325-342,
      1963

Myosin

   crystallization, and muscle fatigue (Belagyi and Felker) Acta Physiol. Acad. Sci. Hung. 22:327-330, 1962

                                             N

Nerves

   endings, adrenergic, in heart, function (Braunwald and others) Circulation 28:958-969, 1963

   neurones, single, differences in utilization of tritiated leucine by, normal and exercised rats, autoradiography
      with microdensitometry (Altman) Nature 199:777-780, 1963

   peripheral, protein metabolism changes during functional activity (Jakoubek and others) Physiol.
      Bohemoslov. 12:553-561, 1963

   to vascular regions, changes in efferent impulsation during muscular exertion (Georgiyev) Fiziol. Zh.
      SSSR Sechenov 47:1517-1524, 1961

Nervous impulse

   voluntarily controlled muscle action and frequency of motor discharge, mechanical work and kinetic energy
      produced by (Bergström) Acta Physiol. Scand. 47:179-190, 191-198, 1959

Nervous system

   1st and 2nd signal systems, relationship between during work (Kosilov) Zh. Vyss. Nerv. Deiat. Pavlov.
      10:481-487, 1960

   influence of great physical effort (Baldes and others) München. med. Wschr. 53:1865-1866, 1906

   influence of movement (Asher) Trans. XV Internat. Congr. Hyg. and Demog. Washington, 1912, 2:
      640-649, 1913

Nethalide

   a beta-adrenergic blocking agent (Schröder and Werkö) Clin. Pharmacol. Ther. 5:159-166, 1964

Neural control

   in effort (Ulmeanau) J. Sport Med. 4:158-164, 1964

Neurocirculatory asthenia

    effect of exercise on soldiers with (Jones and Scarisbrick) Psychosom. Med. 8:188-192, 1946

    soldier's heart and the effort syndrome (Lewis) New York, P. B. Hoeber, 1919

    soldiers with effort intolerance, effect of exercise (Jones and Scarisbrick) Lancet 2:331-332, 1943

    vasoregulatory asthenia, blood lactate concentration in relation to absolute and relative work load (Holmgren and Ström) Acta Med. Scand. 163:185-193, 1959

    vasoregulatory asthenia, effect of physical training (Holmgren and others) Acta Med. Scand. 165:85-103, 1959

    vasoregulatory asthenia, low physical working capacity in suspected heart cases (Holmgren and others) Acta Med. Scand. 158:413-436, 1957

Neuroendocrine

    regulation during physical exertion (Derevenco and Derevenco) Rumanian Med. Rev. 5:141-142, 1961

Neuromuscular

    activity of relaxant drugs, influence of exercise (Foldes and others) Canad. Anaesth. Soc. J. 8:118-127, 1961

    block, partial, influence of increased respiration by muscular work (Ochwadt and others) Pflüger Arch. ges. Physiol. 269:613-621, 1959

Neuropathy

    optic, of multiple sclerosis, and exercise (Goldstein and Cogan) Arch. Ophthal. 72:168-170, 1964

Neurosis

    cardiac, haemodynamics in (Simonyi and others) Cŏr Vasa 6:26-34, 1964

    psychological symptoms and physiological response to exercise (Tanner and Jones) J. Neurol. Neurosurg. Psychiat. 11:61-71, 1948

    response of psychoneurotic patients to brisk submaximal exercise (Franseen and others) Arch. Phys. Med. 30:219-233, 1949

    without heart symptoms, effects of physical training (Holmgren and others) Acta Med. Scand. 165:89-103, 1959

Nicotine

    swimming capacity, and atheromatosis induced by cholesterol feeding in rats, effect on (Grandjean and Abelin) Schweiz. Zeits. Sportmed. 12:132-144, 1964

Nicotinic acid

    effect on plasma free fatty acids during exercise (Carlson and others) Metabolism 12:837-845, 1963

Nitrogen

    absorption and exhalation in respiration (Edwards) Ann. Chim. Phys. 22:35-43, 1823

    balance, influence of effort adaptation (Gontzea and others) Arch. Sci. Physiol. 16:127-138, 1962

    balance, influence of physical exercise, protein requirements (Gontzea and others) Arch. Sci. Physiol. 13:99-108, 1959

    balance, obese subjects, influence of physical exercise (Slabochova and others) Nutr. Dieta 4:251-260, 1962

Nitrogen (Cont.)

elimination by kidneys and intestines during rest and exercise, on a diet without nitrogen (Parkes) Proc.

Roy. Soc. 15:339-355, 1867

elimination, rest and exercise (Parkes) Proc. Roy. Soc. 16:44-59, 1867; Proc. Roy. Soc. 19:349-361,

1870

excretion during respiration in granivores (Eoussingault) Ann. Chim. Phys. Sér. 3 11:433-456, 1844

excretion, effects of severe and protracted muscular exercise (Flint) J. Anat. & Physiol. 11:109-117,

1876-1877

excretion in sweat, relation to nitrogen balance requirements (Consolazio and others) J. Nutr. 79:399-406, 1963

excretion, increased, in urine, influence of muscular exercise (Gontzea and others) Int. Zeits. angew. Physiol.

19:7-17, 1961

excretion, influence of bodily labour on (North) Proc. Roy. Soc. 39:443-503, 1885

loss, with sweat, muscular work (Gontzea and Schutzescu) Int. Zeits. angew. Physiol. 20:90-110, 1963

Nitroglycerin

heart rate, and exercise, effect on cardiac dynamics in complete heart block (Benchimol and others)

Circulation 28:510-519, 1963

Nitrous oxide

use for measurement of pulmonary blood flow during exercise (Becklake and others) J. Appl. Physiol. 17:

579-586, 1962

Noise

effect on physical work (Jansen) Int. Zeits. angew. Physiol. 20:233-239, 1964

Norepinephrine

in adrenals and in brain, before and after muscular work (Beauvallet and others) Comptes Rend. Soc. Biol.

155:2252-2254, 1961; 156:1258-1260, 1962

in brain and effect of forced exercise on toxicity of amphetamine (Beauvallet and Solier) Comptes Rend.

Soc. Biol. 158:2306-2309, 1964

carbon dioxide, effect of on respiratory response (Barcroft and others) J. Physiol. 137:365-373, 1957

cerebral, study (Fugazza) J. Physiologie 55(Suppl. 8):1-76, 1963

and epinephrine, conjugated, in blood plasma (Häggendal) Acta Physiol. Scand. 59:255-260, 1963

and epinephrine plasma concentration, muscular work (Gray and Beetham) Proc. Soc. Exper. Biol. Med.

96:636-638, 1957

and epinephrine, plasma content induced by maximum muscular effort of brief duration (Iannacone and

others) Arch. Fisiol. 60:339-348, 1961

and epinephrine, urinary excretion (Kärki) Acta Physiol. Scand. 39(Suppl. 132):1-96, 1956; (Kärki and

Vasama) Sctilaslaak. Aikak. 34:59-69, 1959

and epinephrine, urinary excretion in late normal and toxemic pregnancy (Castren) Acta Pharmacol. 20(Suppl. 2):

1-98, 1963

and isoproterenol, infusion, response of pulmonary circulation (Aramendía and others) Acta Physiol. Lat. Amer.

13:20-25, 1963

Obesity (Cont.)

 hypothalamus and obesity (Brobeck) Physiol. Physicians 1:1-6, 1963

 inactivity and overeating effect on energy balance, high school girls (Johnson and others) Amer. J.
  Clin. Nutr. 4:37-44, 1956

 nitrogen balance, influence of exercise (Slabochova and others) Nutr. Dieta 4:251-260, 1962

 and oxygen intake, work on bicycle ergometer (Åstrand and others) Acta Physiol. Scand. 50:294-299, 1960

 and physical activity (Chirico and Stunkard) New Eng. J. Med. 263:935-940, 1960; (Dorris and Stunkard)
  Amer. J. Med. Sci. 233:622-628, 1957

 physical activity, girls (Editorial) Nutr. Rev. 21:108-109, 1963; (Stunkard and Pestka) Amer. J. Dis.
  Child. 103:812-817, 1962

 and pulse rate, relationship between, at rest and during work (Buskirk and others) Int. Zeits. angew. Physiol.
  16:83-89, 1955

 and treadmill performance, relationship between, in sedentary and active young men (Dempsey) Res.
  Quart. Amer. Ass. Health Phys. Educ. 35:288-297, 1964

 ventilatory adjustment to exercise (Auchincloss and others) J. Appl. Physiol. 18:19-24, 1963

 weight reduction, effect of on specific gravity and body fat, female adolescents (Goldman and others)
  Ann. N.Y. Acad. Sci. 110:913-917, 1963

Octacosonal

 wheat germ oil, and vitamin E, effect on performance of swimming rats (Consolazio and others) J. Appl.
  Physiol. 19:265-267, 1964

Old age, see Age, old

Organs

 growth, influence of exercise, rats (Hatai) Anat. Rec. 9:647-665, 1915

Oscillograph

 arterial, of the leg, change in volume and size after effort (Ferrero) Cardiologia 30:126-133, 1957

Osmotic pressure, see Pressure

Osmotic properties

 of muscle, modification in fatigue and rigor (Fletcher) J. Physiol. 30:414-438, 1904

Osteochondroma

 femoral, associated with popliteal aneurysm (Anastasi and others) Arch. Surg. 87:636-639, Oct., 1963

Osteoporosis

 etiology and therapy (Bernstein and Guri) Postgrad. Med. 34:407-409, 1963

 management (Devlin) J. Irish Med. Ass. 54:135-140, 1964

Overexertion

 and exercise (Brunton) Quart. Med. J. Sheffield 7:107-135, 1898-1899

 in man (Stark) Edinburgh Med. Surg. J. 74:77-82, 1850

 physical, and effects on health (Knott) Amer. Med. 7:148-150, 1904

Overtraining

morphological changes in muscles and nerves of extremities (Gudz) Arkh. Anat. 45:55-63, 1963

Oxalic acid

and citric acid, muscle content, changes in various functional conditions (Chagovets) Ukr. Biokhim. Zh.
36:499-505, 1964

Oxidases, see Enzymes

Oxigram

clinical value (Serzysko) Pol. Arch. Med. Wewnet. 33:667-674, 1963

minute ventilation, and expired air composition during effort of brief duration (Orlowska and Serzysko)
Pol. Arch. Med. Wewnet. 33:801-805, 1963

Oximetry

ear (Jeyasingham) Ceylon Med. J. 7:23-31, 1962

work test and estimation of work capacity (Bühlmann) Schweiz. med. Wschr. 81:374-376, 1951

Oxygen

absorption, per beat, as a function of stroke volume, of A-V difference of cardiac output and heart volume
(Musshoff and others) Zeits. Kreislaufforsch. 48:255-277, 1959

adding to inspired air, effects of, on respiration and performance during exercise (Bannister and Cunningham)
J. Physiol. 125:118-137, 1954

athletes, effect on (Hill and Flack) J. Physiol. 38:xxviii-xxxvi, 1909; (Hill and others) Brit. Med. J.
2:499-500, 1908

and carbon dioxide content of blood drawn from cubital vein before, after, at different intervals, and various
amounts, and kinds of exercise (Lundsgaard and Möller) J. Biol. Chem. 55:315-321, 477-485, 599-603, 1923

and carbon dioxide, gradients in expiration, miners, rest and exercise, and recovery (Siehoff and others)
Poumon Coeur 19(Suppl.):1385-1393, 1963

and carbon dioxide tensions, alveolar air and arterial blood, at rest and after exercise (Galdston and Wollack)
Amer. J. Physiol. 151:276-281, 1947

and carbon dioxide tensions, arterial blood during heavy and exhaustive exercise (Holmgren and others) Acta
Physiol. Scand. 44:203-215, 1958

and carbon dioxide tensions, alveolar, influence of muscular activity (Hough) Amer. J. Physiol. 30:
18-36, 1912

catabolites, influence on muscle functional capacity (Kudrjawzew) Arbeitsphysiol. 1:203-212, 1929

concentrations, high and low effect of inhalation on respiration, pulse rate, ballistocardiogram and arterial
oxygen saturation (Dripps and Comroe) Amer. J. Physiol. 149:277-291, 1947

continuous versus intermittent administration during exercise in chronic lung disease (Cotes) Lancet 1:1075-1077,
1963

effects of want on respiration (Haldane and Poulton) J. Physiol. 37:390-407, 1908

efferent blood, of working muscle (Monod and others) J. Physiologie 50:417-420, 1958

extraction, myocardial, patterns, during rest and exercise (Messer and others) J. Clin. Invest. 41:725-742, 1962

Oxygen (Cont.)

high, and forced breathing, influence on athletic performances (Vernon and Stolz) Quart. J. Exp. Physiol.
4:243-248, 1911

high, and pulmonary ventilation, in heavy exercise (Asmussen and Nielsen) Acta Physiol. Scand. 43:365-378, 1958

high content in inspired air, effect on excitability of human visual analyzers (Navakamikian and others) Fiziol.
Zh. SSSR Sechenov. 49:1036-1043, 1963

high, effect on cardiac output, heart rate, ventilation, systemic and pulmonary blood pressure in chronic lung
disease (Cotes and others) Clin. Sci. 25:305-321, 1963

high, in supine position, haemodynamic studies (Barratt-Boyes and Wood) J. Appl. Physiol. 11:129-135, 1957

high, role of body temperature in controlling ventilation (Cotes) J. Physiol. 129:554-563, 1955

inhalation and previous forced breathing, effects on distress caused by muscular work (Douglas and Haldane)
J. Physiol. 39:i-iv, 1909

inhalation, influence on muscular work (Hill and Flack) J. Physiol. 40:347-372, 1910; (Hill and Mackenzie)
J. Physiol. 39:xxxiii-xxxv, 1909

muscular activity, and respiratory function, relations, healthy subjects of different ages (Berloco and others)
Gior. Ital. Tuberc. 16:101-104, 1962

and muscular exercise as form of treatment (Hill) Brit. Med. J. 2:967-968, 1908

and muscular exercise, influence on bodily function (Hill) Brit. Med. J. 2:599-606, 1912

muscular exercise, lactic acid and supply and utilization of, parts I-III (Hill and others) Proc. Roy. Soc.
96B:438-475, 1924; parts IV-VI, Proc. Roy. Soc. 97B:84-138, 1924; part VII, Proc. Roy. Soc. 97B:155-167,
1924

portal venous saturation (Hardin and others) Arch. Surg. 87:831-835, 1963

pulse during utilization of 1 watt/kg body weight work (Dransfeld and Mellerowicz) Zeits. Kreislaufforsch.
49:901-906, 1959

pulse, pulse-rate, and arterial blood pressure, under low barometric pressure (Schneider and Clarke) Amer.
J. Physiol. 38:633-649, 1929

refreshing action (Binet and Contamin) Comptes Rend. Acad. Sci. 227:248-251, 1948

respiratory function during inhalation of pure oxygen (Berloco and others) Gior. Ital. Tuberc. 15:185-188,
191-195, 197-199, 1961

revival with (Wenzig) Arbeitsphysiol. 4:503-507, 1931

saturation, arterial blood, during exercise (Rowell and others) J. Appl. Physiol. 19:284-286, 1964

saturation of arterial blood, continued control during spirometry, rest and exercise (Lob and others) Helv.
Med. Acta 17:511-515, 1950

supply and utilization, and muscular exercise and lactic acid (Hill and Long) Ergebn. Physiol. 24:43-51,
1925

survival metabolism of muscle, relation to (Fletcher) J. Physiol. 28:474-498, 1902

survival respiration of muscle, influence on (Fletcher) J. Physiol. 28:354-359, 1902

Oxygen (Cont.)

transport, comparative physiology (Dill) J. Sport Med. 3:191-200, 1963

treadmill walking, cost of (Workman and Armstrong) J. Appl. Physiol. 18:798-803, 1963

utilization and lactic acid formation, legs, normal and with arteriosclerosis obliterans (Carlson and Pernow)
Acta Med. Scand. 164:39-52, 1959

utilization, lactate, and pyruvate formation, forearm muscles, during work of high intensity and varying
duration (Pernow) Acta Physiol. Scand. 56:267-285, 1962

in varicose blood, measurement, effect of walking and confining bandage (Storstein and Gilje) T. Norsk.
Laegeforen. 83:1373-1374, 1963

in venous blood in anemia (Lundsgaard) J. Exp. Med. 30:147-158, 1919

and violent exercise (Hill) Discovery 4:64-69, 1923

Oxygen consumption

administration of 2, amino-6, methyl-6, heptanolochloride, normal men (Eliseo and Grieco) Folia Med.
47:750-759, 1964

atropine, effects of (Robinson and others) J. Appl. Physiol. 5:508-512, 1953

cardiac exertion (Gabagni and others) Minerva Med. 49:1277-1284, 1958

cardiac output, and arterial saturation, during work of increasing intensity (Morbelli and others) Atti Soc.
Ital. Cardiol. 22:323-324, 1962

cardiac output, heart minute volume, and arterial and venous blood gases, in volunteers, rest and exercise
(Ulmer and Berta) Pflüger Arch, ges. Physiol. 280:281-296, 1964

cardiopathic subjects during work (Castelfranco and others) Folia Cardiol. 16:45-70, 1957

carotid sinus, influence, functional sympatholysis during muscular activity (Remensnyder and others)
Circ. Res. 11:370-380, 1962

curves, reflecting circulatory factors in static work (Royce) Int. Zeits. angew. Physiol. 19:222-228,
1962

and debt under low barometric pressures, muscular exercise (Schneider and Clarke) Amer. J. Physiol. 74:
334-353, 1925

different ages (Valentin and others) Zeits. Alternsforsch. 9:291-309, 1955

in exercise in coronary artery insufficiency (Pons and Berg) Dis. Chest 39:551-556, 1961

in exercise, heavy muscular, first minutes of (Åstrand and others) J. Appl. Physiol. 16:971-976, 1961

in exercise, old and young men (Strandell) Acta Physiol. Scand. 60:197-216, 1964

following exercise in anesthetized dogs (Kayne and Alpert) Amer. J. Physiol. 206:51-56, 1964

fatigue, degree of, measured by electric flicker during and after exercise (Suzuki) Tohuku J. Exp. Med.
52:9-16, 1950

and final stroke changes in electrocardiogram, after muscular work (Aresu) Rass. Med. Sarda 63:125-146,
1961

Oxygen consumption (Cont.)

and heart rate, discrepancy between, during work in the warmth (Brouha and others) J. Appl. Physiol. 18:1095-1098, 1963

and hypoxia, muscular work (Strumza and Traccan) Comptes Rend. Soc. Biol. 154:1412-1415, 1960

immersion, total, effect of at various temperatures, at rest and during exercise (Goff and others) J. Appl. Physiol. 9:59-61, 1956

indirect, maximal and Harvard's test (Maggio and others) Rass. Med. Industr. 32:362-363, 1963

and lactic acid content of blood during strenuous muscular exercise (Volkov) Fed. Proc. 22:118-122, 1963

and lactic acid content of muscle, relation between during exercise (Long) Proc. Roy. Soc. 99B:167-172, 1926

limb movements, effects of (Bahnson and others) J. Appl. Physiol. 2:169-173, 1949

maximal, and heart rate in various types of muscular activity (Åstrand and Saltin) J. Appl. Physiol. 16:977-981, 1961

maximal body size, and total hemoglobin, normal man (Döbeln) Acta Physiol. Scand. 38:193-199, 1956

maximal, from different ergometers (Damoiseau) J. Physiologie 55:235-236, 1963

maximal, influence of muscular exercise (Damoiseau and others) Arch. Int. Physiol. 71:275-277, 1963

maximal, objective measure of cardio-respiratory performance (Taylor) J. Appl. Physiol. 8:73-80, 1955

maximal test, physiological meaning (Mitchell and others) J. Clin. Invest. 37:538-547, 1958

maximum, and maximum heart rate during strenuous work (Wyndham and others) J. Appl. Physiol. 14:927-936, 1959

maximum assessment (Newton) J. Sport Med. 3:164-169, 1963

maximum, effect of protracted muscular exercise (Margaria and others) Boll. Soc. Ital. Biol. Sper. 37:1367-1669, 1961

maximum, for work (Wright) Science 112:423-424

maximum, measurement (Maritz and others) Ergonomics 4:97-122, 1961

maximum, simplified measurement (Damoiseau and others) Arch. Int. Physiol. 70:131-132, 1962

of muscles during tetanic contraction (Quensel and Kramer) Pflüger Arch. ges. Physiol. 241:698-716, 1939

and muscular exercise (Milic-Emili and others) Arch. Int. Physiol. 67:10-14, 1959

myocardial, coronary blood flow, and cardiac efficiency, effect of exercise (Lombardo and others) Circulation 7:71-78, 1953

myocardial, during exercise in fasting and lipemic subjects (Regan and others) J. Clin. Invest. 40:624-630, 1961

myocardium, isolated strips of in cat, rat, relation to oxygen consumption (Whalen) J. Physiol. 157:1-17, 1961

obese individuals working on bicycle ergometer (Åstrand and others) Acta Physiol. Scand. 50:294-299, 1960

Oxygen consumption (Cont.)

    peak, treadmill method of determination, healthy young men (Slonim and others) J. Appl. Physiol.
        10:401-404, 1957

    pulmonary ventilation and heart rate, influence of graded exercise (Durnin and Mikulicic) Quart. J. Exp.
        Physiol. 41:442-452, 1956

    and pulmonary ventilation, relation between, after exercise (Barman and others) Amer. J. Physiol. 138:
        16-19, 1942

    and pulse rate during early stages of recovery (Lythgoe and Pereira) Proc. Roy. Soc. 98B:468-479, 1925

    and pulse rate while running (Knuttgen) Acta Physiol. Scand. 52:366-371, 1961

    rate during negative work, effects of force and speed changes (Abbott and Bigland) J. Physiol. 120:319-325,
        1953

    resting, determination, while breathing concentrated oxygen mixtures (Pereira) Proc. Roy. Soc. 98B:480-483, 1925

    in rich oxygen breathing, during exercise (Furusawa) Proc. Roy. Soc. 98B:287-289, 1925

    in running (Hill and Lupton) J. Physiol. 56:xxxii-xxxiii, 1922

    in submaximal exercises (Royce) Int. Zeits. angew. Physiol. 19:218-221, 1962

    after theophylline-ethylenediamine administration in respiratory disease (Sorbini and others) Folia Cardiol.
        22:445-459, 1963

    tread frequency and pedal pressure, effect of, studies with ergometer (Hess and Seusing) Int. Zeits.
        angew. Physiol. 19:468-475, 1963

    in treadmill-walking, normogram for predicting (Workman and Armstrong) J. Appl. Physiol. 19:150-151,
        1964

    at various temperatures and air current velocities (Berdan and others) Rumanian Med. Rev. 5:95-96, 1961

    and work, and sartorius muscle, frog (Whalen and Collins) J. Cell. Comp. Physiol. 61:293-299, 1963

    in work in cardiac disease, acute digitalization (Castelfranco and others) Folia Cardiol. 16:45-70, 1957

    work, measured, relation to requirement during rest (Renner) Int. Zeits. angew. Physiol. 19:56-66, 1961

    see also Hypoxia; Oxygen, partial pressure

Oxygen content, blood

    arterial and venous, comparison after vigorous exercise (Barr and Himwich) J. Biol. Chem. 55:525-537, 1923

    arterial, at critical pressure-altitudes breathing various mixtures of oxygen and nitrogen, effect of exercise
        (Lilienthal and others) Amer. J. Physiol. 145:427-431, 1946

    arterial-hepatic-venous, difference during and after supine leg exercise (Bishop and others) J. Physiol. 137:
        309-317, 1957

    arterial, oxygen tension (Haldane and Smith) J. Physiol. 20:497-520, 1896

    arterio-venous difference, cardiac output and stroke volume in energy consumption (Brandi and Bramvilla)
        Int. Zeits. angew. Physiol. 19:130-133, 1961

Oxygen content, blood (Cont.)

arteriovenous difference, heart rate, and cardiac output, rest and exercise (Nitter-Hauge) T. Norsk. Laegeforenen. 83:1310-1316, 1963; in heart and lung disease (Nitter-Hauge) T. Norsk. Laegeforenen. 83:1316-1322, 1963

arterio-venous difference induced by circulatory changes in muscular work and vasodilators (Kaindl and Pärtan) Wien. Zeits. inn. Med. 38:413-417, 1957

arterio-venous difference, minute to minute changes, and of oxygen uptake and cardiac output, rheumatic heart disease (Donald and others) J. Clin. Invest. 33:1146-1167, 1954

arteriovenous, difference, resting, and exercise cardiac output (Thomas and others) J. Appl. Physiol. 17:922-926, 1962

in axillary venous blood, changes in, in leg exercise (Donald and others) Clin. Sci. 14:531-551, 1955

femoral venous changes, and leg blood flow during leg exercise in relation to cardiac output response (Donald and others) Clin. Sci. 16:567-591, 1957

femoral venous, normal and abnormal subjects, rest and exercise (Wilson) S. Afr. J. Med. Sci. 15:115-119, 1950; 19:161-164, 1954

hepatic venous, during exercise in rheumatic heart disease (Bishop and others) J. Clin. Invest. 34:1114-1125, 1955

jugular and renal arterio-venous, changes during exercise, heart disease (Bishop and others) Clin. Sci. 17:611-619, 1958

variations, influence on reflex excitability of nerves (Heymans and others) Arch. Int. Pharmacodyn. 48:457-487, 1934

see also Gas, blood

Oxygen debt

contracting and paying, role of lactic acid in muscular contraction (Margaria and others) Amer. J. Physiol. 106:689-715, 1933

contraction, aerobic and anaerobic exertion (Castelfranco and others) Folia Cardiol. 17:211-230, 1958

contraction, kinetics (Cerretelli and Brambilla) Boll. Soc. Ital. Biol. Sper. 34:679-682, 1958

contraction, kinetics and mechanism (Margaria and others) J. Appl. Physiol. 18:371-377, 1963

exercise (Dill and Sacktor) J. Sport Med. 2:66-72, 1962

lactate, pyruvate, and excess lactate after muscular work (Knuttgen) J. Appl. Physiol. 17:639-644, 1962

and pulse rate, influence of atmospheric conditions after running (Campbell) Proc. Roy. Soc. 96B:43-59, 1924

and repayment in exercise (Lukin and Ralston) Int. Zeits. angew. Physiol. 19:183-193, 1962

Oxygen, gradient

experimental analysis from alveolar air to arterial blood, sea level and altitude (Lilienthal and others) Amer. J. Physiol. 147:199-216, 1946

Oxygen requirement

    in muscular exercise (Furusawa and others) Proc. Roy. Soc. 97B:167-176, 1924

    in physical activity and altitude (Hall and Wilson) J. Aviation Med. 15:160-166, 1944

    of running and walking (Henry) Res. Quart. 24:169-175, 1953

    and speed in running, relation between (Sargent) Proc. Roy. Soc. 100B:10-22, 1926

    in underwater swimming (Goff and others) J. Appl. Physiol. 9:219-221, 1956

Ozone

    toxicity, effects of exercise and tolerance development (Stokinger and others) Arch. Industr. Health
        14:158-162, 1956

P

Pacemaker, artificial

    cardiac, implanted, hemodynamic studies (Judge) New Eng. J. Med. 270:1391-1395, 1964

    implantable synchronous, clinical and physiological studies (Nathan and others) Progr. Cardiov. Dis. 6:
        538-565, 1964

    implanted, use in heart block (Chardack) Progr. Cardiov. Dis. 6:507-537, 1964

    varying ventricular rate, effect of on circulation at rest and during exercise (Bevegård) Acta Med. Scand.
        172:615-622, 1962

Palmitate-1-C^{14}

    continuous infusion, and turnover rate and oxidation of free fatty acids in blood plasma (Havel and others)
        J. Clin. Invest. 42:1054-1063, 1963

Pantothenic acid

    low cholesterol diet and lipid metabolism, rats (Lazzari) Gazz. Int. Med. Chir. 69:1151-1154, 1964

Paraplegia

    exercise studies (Ruosteenoja and Karvonen) Ann. Med. Exp. Fenn. 34:57-62, 1956

Paralysis

    hyperkalemic (dynamia episodica hereditaria), four cases and clinical studies (Herman and McDowell)
        Amer. J. Med. 35:749-767, 1963

Parasympathetic nervous system, see Autonomic nervous system

Parturition

    induction of labor by exercise (Haufrect) Obstet. Gynec. 7:462-465, 1956

Patterning

    involuntary, associated with willed movement performed against increasing resistance (Waterland and
        Hellbrandt) Amer. J. Phys. Med. 43:13-30, 1964

    involuntary, evoked by exercise stress (Waterland and Munson) J. Amer. Phys. Ther. Ass. 44:91-97,
        1964

Penicillin

    effects of physical activity and site of injection, following administration of 1.2 million units of
        benzathine penicillin G (Lukash and Frank) Amer. J. Med. Sci. 246:429-438, 1963

    effect on physical work capacity and on fatigue (Furberg and Ringqvist) Svensk. Lakartidn. 60:
        2650-2655, 1963

Pentaerythritol tetranitrate

    evaluation of effect by continuous electrocardiogram during exercise (Krasno and Kidera) Angiology
        14:417-425, 1963

Pentose

    transport into muscle, effects of insulin and activity on (Sacks and Smith) Amer. J. Physiol. 192:
        287-289, 1958

Perceptual-motor task

    relation between effort, tension level, skill, and performance efficiency (Eason) Percept. Motor Skills
        16:297-217, 1963

Pericarditis

    chronic constrictive, haemodynamic changes during exercise and histamine infusion (Lindell and others)
        Brit. Heart J. 25:35-41, 1963

Peromyscus maniculatus

    effect of altitude on endurance running (Hock) J. Appl. Physiol 16:435-438, 1961

Pervitin

    effect on physical and psychological efficiency (Alwall) Acta Med. Scand. 114:35-58, 1943

Phenformin

    influence on blood lactic acid in normal and diabetic subjects, during exercise (Cüttler and others)
        Diabetes 12:420-423, 1963

Phlebothrombosis

    in exertion (Correa Castillo) Arch. Soc. Cir. Hosp. 14:551-552, 1944

Phonocardiogram

    changes, muscular activity (Dupuy and Fabre) J. Physiologie 51:456-457, 1959

    exercise, in evaluation of degree of mitral stenosis (Magri and others) Minerva Med. 49:1258-1263, 1958

    modification, following muscular work (Dupuy) J. Physiologie 51:456-457, 1959

Phosphatase

    serum, normal and diabetes, during work (Zambrano) Folia Med. 35:143-151, 1952

Phosphates

    blood, after strenuous exercise (Gemmill and Riberio) Sunti Congr. Internaz. Fisiol. 14 Congr. 1932,
        p. 98

    inorganic, of blood and urine, influence of exercise (Havard and Reay) J. Physiol. 61:35-48, 1926

    serum and red-cell, changes during hyperventilation (George and others) New Eng. J. Med. 270:726-728,
        1964

    supply, and increase of efficiency (Embden and others) Hoppe-Seyler Zeits. physiol. Chem. 113:67-107,
        1921

Phospholipid

metabolism, in a sympathetic ganglion, effects of temperature, calcium and activity (Larrabee and others)
J. Neurochem. 10:549-570, 1963

and non-esterified fatty acids, triglycerides and cholesterol, arterio-venous relationship, in exercise
(Konttinen and others) Ann. Med. Exp. Fenn. 40:250-256, 1962

Phosphoric acid

content, muscular, rabbits (Embden and Adler) Hoppe-Seyler Zeits. physiol. Chem. 113:201-222, 1921

excretion from muscle, influence of work (Embden and Grafe) Hoppe-Seyler Zeits. physiol. Chem. 113:
108-137, 1921

muscle, influence of fever (Adam) Hoppe-Seyler Zeits. physiol. Chem. 113:281-300, 1921

residual, and lactic acid-phosphoric acid content in pigeon and dove muscle (Lyding) Hoppe-Seyler Zeits.
physiol. Chem. 113:223-244, 1921

Phosphorus

blood, influence of muscular exercise (Planet and Cardoso) Comptes Rend. Soc. Biol. 112:1509-1510, 1933

and calcium balance, effect of exercise (Konishi) Army Med. Nutrition Lab. Report 211, pp. 1-17, 1957

distribution in thigh muscles of toad (Panajotakos) Hoppe-Seyler Zeits. physiol. Chem. 113:245-252, 1921

poisoning, influence on lactic acid content of frog muscles (Adler and Isaac) Hoppe-Seyler Zeits. physiol.
Chem. 113:271-280, 1921

poisoning, influence on lactic acid content in rabbit muscles (Embden and Isaac) Hoppe-Seyler Zeits.
physiol. Chem. 113:263-270, 1921

Phosphorylase

muscle, hereditary absence, causing myopathy - McArdle's disease (Rowland and others) Arch. Neurol.
9:325-342, 1963

Physical culture

influence on body (Allen) J. Psych. Med. (London) new series 2:156-160, 1876

Physical education

(Sedgwick) New York, J. D. Torrey, 1860

physiological basis (Brunton) London, Harrison, 1905

and physiology (Baglioni) Gior. Med. Milit. 68:425-440, 1920

Physical handicap

relation between measured muscular force and success in selected tasks (Bender and others) Arch. Phys.
Med. 45:30-40, 1964

Physiology

applied, of exercise (Lipovetz) Minneapolis, Burgess Publishing Co. 1938

of exercise (Goule and Dye) New York, Barnes, 1932; (Hartwell) Boston Med. & Surg. J. 116:
297-302, 1887; (Hutchings) Nat. Hosp. San. Rec. 2:1-6, 1898-1899; (Lagrange) Paris; F. Alcan, 1888;
London, Keegan Paul, Trench and Co., 1889; (McCurdy) Philadelphia, Lea and Febiger, 1924; 2nd ed.
1928; (Melville) J. Roy. San. Inst. 38:373-381, 1912; (Morehouse and Miller) St. Louis, C. V.
Mosby, 1948; (Schenck) J.A.M.A. 22:417-421, 1894; (Schmidt) 3d ed. Leipzig, Voigtländer, 1921;
(Schmidt and Kohlrausch) Philadelphia, F. A. Davis, 1931; (Taylor) Amer. J. Physiol. 135:27-42, 1941

Physiology (Cont.)

    of exercise and fatigue (Schenck) Marburg, N. G. Elwert, 1911

    of exercise and scientific physical education (Piñero) Rev. Soc. Méd. Argent. 12:71-123, 1904

    function, architecture (Barcroft) Cambridge University Press, 1934

    human (Zuntz and Schumberg) Berlin, A. Hirschwald, 1901

    human, textbook (Zuntz and Loewy) 2nd edition, Leipzig, F.C.W. Vogel, 1909

    industrial (Simonson) Ann. Rev. Physiol. 6:543-577, 1944

    medical progress (Hoff) New Eng. J. Med. 229:543-550, 1943

    moderate and strenuous exercise, men and women (Metheny and others) Amer. J. Physiol. 137:318-326, 1942

    pathological and normal, of physical exercise (Knoll and Arnold) Leipzig, J. A. Barth, 1933

    and physical education (Baglioni) Gior. Med. Milit. 68:425-440, 1920; (Lee) Amer. Phys. Educat. Rev. 14:216-223, 1910; (Knoll) Schweiz. med. Wschr. 58:1262-1264, 1928

    physiological action in physical activity (Chailley-Bert) Rev. Prat. 7:2057-2059, 1957

    physiological basis of physical education (Brunton) London, Harrison, 1905

    physiological changes during work performance, porcelain factory, women (Okhrimenko) Gig. Tr. Prof. Zabol. 7:9-13, 1963

    physiological dead space and alveolar gas pressures at rest and during muscular exercise (Asmussen and Nielsen) Acta Physiol. Scand. 38:1-21, 1956

    physiological measurements, variability, rest and during muscular work (Brouha and Savage) Rev. Canad. Biol. 4:131-143, 1945

    physiological parameters, regulation of return to resting values (Ostyn and others) Verh. Kon. Vlaam. Acad. Geneesk. Belg. 25:431-457, 1964

    physiological reactions during muscular activity and recovery in various environments (Brouha and others) J. Appl. Physiol. 16:133-140, 1961

    physiological response to exercise, adolescents (Morse and others) J. Appl. Physiol. 1:683-709, 1949; (Shock) Texas Rep. Biol. Med. 4:368-386, 1946

    physiological work, and its equivalent (Chauveau) Paris, Quantin, 1888; Rev. Scient. 3rd series 15: 129-139, 1888

    simultaneous static and dynamic exercise, effects of (Hellebrandt and others) Amer. J. Phys. Med. 35: 106-117, 1956

    of work (Minard) Arch. Environ. Health 8:427-436, 1964; (Chauderon) Maroc. Med. 42:161-176, 1963

    of work and sport (Kayser) Paris, Hermann, 1947

    of work in health and disease (Luongo) J.A.M.A. 188:27-32, 1964

    work, of physical exercise (Rautmann) Sportmedizin 1:2-4, 1929

    of work, pathological study, parts I and II (Podkaminsky) Arbeitsphysiol. 1:306-356, 577-585, 1929

    of work, premises (Tochilov) Nerv. Sist. 4:176-178, 1963

    of work, principles, and of increase of working capacity (Kosilov) Nerv. Sist. 4:173-175, 1963

Piano playing

   biodynamics (Bernstein and Popowa) Arbeitsphysiol. 1:396-432, 1929

Pituitary-adrenocortical function

   effects on, of work performed in hypothermia and hyperthermia (Yang and Endroczi) Acta Physiol. Acad.

      Sci. Hung. 18:131-136, 1960

Plasma, see Blood; Blood volume, plasma

Plasmocid

   dissociation by forced muscular exercise of cardiotoxic from the myotoxic actions of (Bajusz and others)

      Rev. Canad. Biol. 23:29-36, 1964

Platelets, see Thrombocytes

Pneumonia

   varicella, respiratory function abnormalities (Bocles and others) Ann. Intern. Med. 60:183-195, 1964

Polycythemia

   normovolemic, hemodynamic effects, rest and exercise, dogs (Weisse and others) Amer. J. Physiol. 207:

      1361-1366, 1964

Polyglobulins

   effect of intravenous bicarbonate of soda, muscular exercise (Nitzescu) Comptes Rend. Soc. Biol. 100:

      686-689, 1929

   of exercise, and on adrenalin polyglobulin (Binet) Comptes Rend. Soc. Biol. 100:463-465, 1929

Postoperative walking

   early, influence of exercise on wound healing, rats (Newburger) Surgery 13:692-695, 1943

Posture

   and activity, effects on major fractions of serum protein determined by phosphate turbidity method

      (Aull and McCord) Amer. J. Clin. Path. 27:52-55, 1957

   cardiac output and minute ventilation during exercise, affected by (McGregor and others) Circ. Res. 9:

      1089-1092, 1961

   cardiac output, effected by (Weissler and others) J. Clin. Invest. 36:1656-1662, 1957; (Lindhard) Skand.

      Arch. Physiol. 30:395-408, 1913

   changes, effect of exercise on blood platelet count (Sloan and Allardyce) Quart. J. Exp. Physiol. 40:

      161-167, 1955

   effect on dynamic ventilatory work, during muscular exercise, in health (Petit and others) Arch. Int. Physiol.

      68:437-444, 1960

   left ventricular diameter and exercise (Wilson) Circ. Res. 11:90-95, 1962

   and muscular exercise, effects on electrocardiogram (Wolf) Res. Quart. 24:475-490, 1953

   respiration and pulse rate, influence of (Mark and Neumann) Zeits. ges. exp. Med. 80:150-163, 1931

   variation, effect on cardiac output (Grollman) Amer. J. Physiol. 86:285-301, 1928

Potassium

deficiency and loading, effect on extra and intracellular mineral content of skeletal muscle, untrained
and trained subjects (Schleusing and Noecker) Med. Welt 31:1579-1583, 1960

depletion, experimental, glucose metabolism; effect of insulin, glucagon, and muscular exercise on
(Sagild and Andersen) Acta Med. Scand. 175:681-685, 1964

and insulin, effect in myasthenia gravis (Frenkel) Arch. Neurol. 9:447-457, 1963

ions, role in exercise hyperaemia (Kjellmer) Med. Exp. 5:56-60, 1961

plasma, and sodium, effect of muscular exercise, rat (Sréter and Friedman) Canad. J. Biochem.
Physiol. 36:333-338, 1958

serum, low, effect of exercise on electrocardiograma (Georgopoulos and others) Circulation 23:567-572,
1961

and sodium, concentration in saliva and serum (Salminen and Konttinen) J. Appl. Physiol. 18:812-814,
1963

and sodium ions, influence of muscular work on distribution, rats (Cier and others) Comptes Rend. Soc.
Biol. 153:96-98, 1959

Power

human, maximum, observations on power (Henderson and Haggard) Amer. J. Physiol. 72:264-282, 1925

human, new records (Åstrand) Nature 176:992-993, 1955

see also Strength

Pregnancy

anemia, total haemoglobin and physical working capacity in (Robbe) Acta Obstet. Gynec. Scand. 37:
312-347, 1958

cardio-respiratory aspects and muscular work (Bergamaschi and others) Minerva Ginec. 16:831-838, 1964

early, and cardiac output, in rest and exercise (Schmidt) Geburtsh. Gynak. 90:83-99, 1932

gymnastic exercise on labour pain, influence of (Rütte) Gynaecologia 132:274-276, 1951

normal and pre-eclamptic, effective uterine blood-flow during exercise in (Morris and others) Lancet
2:481-484, 1956

physical working capacity during, effect on fetal heart rate (Soiva and others) Ann. Chir. Gynaec. Fenn.
53:187-196, 1964

and puerperium, normal, total hemoglobin and physical working capacity in (Gemzell and others) Acta
Obstet. Gynec. Scand. 36:93-136, 1957

pulmonary diffusing capacity in rest and exercise (Bedell and Adams) J. Clin. Invest. 41:1908-1914,
1962

renal function, and electrolyte excretion, effect of experience on, healthy and toxemic (Vedra and Horska)
Amer. J. Obstet. Gynec. 90:288-292, 1964

work tests, results, before and after (Dahlstrom and Ihrman) Acta Soc. Med. Upsala 65:305-314, 1960

see also Parturition; Puerperium

Prematurity

    response of blood pressure to sucking and tilting (Hanninen and others) Ann. Paediat. Fenn. <u>10</u>:
        92-98, 1964

Pressure

    osmotic, and ionic concentrations of plasma, changes during muscular work, and recovery (De Lanne
        and others) J. Appl. Physiol. <u>14</u>:804-808, 1959

    retrosternal and precordial, induced by exercise (Pombo) Prensa Méd. Argent. <u>33</u>:355-356, 1946

Pretibial muscles, <u>see</u> Anterior tibial compartment syndrome; Necrosis

Propranolol

    in angina pectoris (Hamer and others) Brit. Med. J. <u>2</u>:720-723, 1964

Protein

    composition in myocardium, relation to varying functional activity (Helander) Cardiologia <u>41</u>:94-100, 1962

    composition of skeletal muscle, influence of exercise and restricted activity (Helander) Biochem. J. <u>78</u>:
        478-482, 1961

    dietary effects of variations on physical well being during manual work (Darling and others) J. Nutr. <u>28</u>:
        273-281, 1944

    metabolism, during prolonged effort (Chailley-Bert and others) Presse Méd. <u>70</u>:705-707, 1962

    metabolism, influence on cortico-adrenal hormones, during work, relation to age (Gattuso and others)
        Sicilia Sanit. <u>1</u>:71-73, 1963

    milk intake, and exercise, effect on athletes (Wilcox and others) J. Amer. Diet. Ass. <u>44</u>:95-99,
        1964

    muscles, sarcoplasmic, content following prolonged muscular activity, and at rest (Krasnova) Ukr.
        Biokhim. Zh. <u>36</u>:209-214, 1964

    requirements during work, influence of hot environment (Gontzea and others) Rumanian Med. Rev.
        <u>5</u>:162-164, 1961; Int. Zeits. angew. Physiol. <u>18</u>:248-263, 1960

    requirements, for work (Gontzea and others) Arch. Sci. Physiol. <u>16</u>:97-120, 1962; Rumanian Med. Rev.
        <u>4</u>:94-96, 1960

    requirements for work, influence of physical exercise on nitrogen balance (Gontzea and others) Arch. Sci.
        Physiol. <u>13</u>:99-108, 1959

    serum, chloride and total fixed base, concentrations, during exercise, dog (Schlutz and Morse) Amer. J.
        Physiol. <u>121</u>:293-309, 1938

    serum, during muscle activity, changes, dogs (Dydenko) Fiziol. Zh. <u>10</u>:55-60, 1964

    serum, effect of physical exercise, elderly persons (Krasnova) Fiziol. Zh. SSSR Sechenov. <u>50</u>:756-761, 1964

    serum, effect of training and competitive swimming (Johnson and Wong) J. Appl. Physiol. <u>16</u>:807-809, 1961

    serum, influence of exhausting graded exercise on, trained athletes (Bojanovský and Filip) Rev. Czech.
        Med. <u>2</u>:339-345, 1956

    serum, influence of mode of life, Madras Indians (Henrotte and others) Acta Trop. <u>20</u>:279-281, 1963

    serum, major fractions, effect of posture and activity, phosphate turbidity method (Aull and McCord) Amer.
        J. Clin. Path. <u>27</u>:52-55, 1957

Proteinuria

    benign, clinical aspects (Kleinschmidt) Deutsche med. Wschr. 88:2283-2288, 1963

    and blood sugar in exercise (Edwards and others) Amer. J. Physiol. 98:352-356, 1931

    determination, comparison of two methods (Poortmans and Van Kerchove) Clin. Chim. Acta 8:485-488,
        1963

    of effort, and diagnosis of congestive heart failure (Brummer) Acta Med. Scand. 124:252-265, 1946

    of effort, physiology and biochemistry (Poortmans and others) Int. Zeits. angew. Physiol. 19:337-354,
        1962

    of effort, quantitative and qualitative changes induced by training (Cerretelli and others) Boll. Soc.
        Ital. Biol. Sper. 36:1276-1278, 1960

    electrophoretic studies, normal and nephropathic subjects, muscular work (Lamperi and Bianchini) Minerva
        Nefrol. 4:17-21, 1957

    exercise and postural, proteins (Rowe and Soothill) Clin. Sci. 21:87-91, 1961

    exercise, characteristics (Taylor) Clin. Sci. 19:209-217, 1960; (Poortmans and Van Kerchove) Clin.
        Chim. Acta 7:229-242, 1962

    exercise, electrophoretic analysis (Nedbal and Seliger) J. Appl. Physiol. 13:244-246, 1958

    following muscular exercise, effect of training (Cantone and Cerretelli) Int. Zeits. angew. Physiol. 18:
        324-329, 1960

    physiological, rest and exercise (Poortmans) Ann. Soc. Roy. Sci. Med. Natur. Brux. 17:89-188, 1964

    and urea clearance during exercise (Light and Warren) Amer. J. Physiol. 117:658-661, 1936

Psychomotor learning

    fatigue, and impairment (Nunney) Percept. Motor Skills 16:369-375, 1963

Psychosis

    and exhaustion syndrome (Shulack) Amer. J. Psychiat. 102:466-475, 1946

Puerperium

    and pregnancy, normal; total hemoglobin and physical working capacity (Gemzell and others) Acta Obstet.
        Gynec. Scand. 36:93-136, 1957

Pulmonary

    insufficiency, spirometric and gas analytic studies, rest and exercise (Larmi) Scand. J. Clin. Lab.
        Invest. (suppl. 12) 6:1-144, 1954

    insufficiency, ventilatory equivalent and oxygen removal (Larmi) Ann. Med. Exp. Fenn. 32:240-247, 1954

Pulmonary artery

    constricted, cardiac performance during exercise, in dogs (Rastelli and others) Circ. Res. 13:410-419, 1963

Pulmonary diffusion

    diffusing capacity and carbon monoxide uptake, at rest and during exercise (Filley and others) J. Clin.
        Invest. 33:530-539, 1954

Pulmonary diffusion (Cont.)

   diffusing capacity and pulmonary capillary blood volume, measurement, effect of exercise and position

      (Lewis and others) J. Clin. Invest. 37:1061-1070, 1958

   diffusing capacity and pulmonary capillary volume and flow during exercise (Johnson and others) J. Appl.

      Physiol. 15:893-902, 1960

   diffusing capacity during rest and exercise, in normal, in atrial septal defect, pregnancy and pulmonary

      disease (Bedell and Adams) J. Clin. Invest. 41:1908-1914, 1962

   diffusing capacity, effect of atropine and reserpine during exercise (Krumholz and Ross) J. Appl. Physiol.

      19:465-468, 1964

   diffusing capacity for carbon monoxide, increased by exercise, mechanism of (Ross and others) J. Clin.

      Invest. 38:916-932, 1959

Pulmonary function

   during effort (Denolin) Acta Belg. Arte. Pharm. Milit. 110:521-572, 1957

Pulmonary resistance

   total, effect of exercise, normal, and in isolated aortic valvular lesions (Sancetta and Kleinerman) Amer.

      Heart J. 53:404-414, 1957

   total, of untrained, convalescent man to prolonged mild steady state exercise (Sancetta and Rakita) J. Clin.

      Invest. 36:1138-1149, 1957

Pulmonic stenosis

   Cardiac performance, with constricted pulmonary artery during exercise, dogs (Rastelli and others) Circ.

      Res. 13:410-419, 1963

   isolated, haemodynamic response to exercise (Lewis and others) Circulation 29:854-861, 1964

Pulse, see Heart rate

Purines

   endogenous, excretion, effects of muscular work (Kennaway) J. Physiol. 38:1-27, 1908

   urinary excretion during muscular exercise (Nasrallah and Al-Khalidi) J. Appl. Physiol. 19:246-248, 1964

Pyruvate

   and lactate formation, and oxygen utilization, forearm muscles, during work of high intensity and varying

      duration (Pernow and Wahren) Acta Physiol. Scand. 56:267-285, 1962

   and lactate, in blood and urine after exercise (Johnson and Edward) J. Biol. Chem. 118:427-432, 1937

   and lactate, relationships in anaerobic metabolism (Huckabee) Parts I-III; J. Clin. Invest. 37:244-254,

      255-263, 264-271, 1958

   oxygen debt, lactate and lactate excess after physical exercise (Knuttgen) J. Appl. Physiol. 17:639-644, 1962

Pyruvic acid

   liver, physical work, rat (Cairella and others) Ann. Med. Nav. 69:557-562, 1964

   role in fatigue (Meyer) New York J. Med. 45:1450-1451, 1945

Q

Quadriceps femoris

strength, effect of brief maximal exercise (Rose and others) Arch. Phys. Med. <u>38</u>:157-164, 1957

R

Radiation

alteration in organ and body growth, effect of exhaustive exercise, x-radiation and post-irradiation exercise,
rat (Kimeldorf and Baum) Growth <u>18</u>:79-96, 1954

dosage, relationship to lethality, exercised animals, exposed to X-rays (Kimeldorf and Jones) Amer. J. Physiol.
<u>167</u>:626-632, 1951

exercise effects on tolerance (Smith and Smith) Amer. J. Physiol. <u>165</u>:662-666, 1951

exhaustive exercise, effect on performance of, rat (Kimeldorf and others) Amer. J. Physiol. <u>174</u>:331-335,
1953

lethality, effect of exercise, rats (Kimeldorf and others) Science <u>112</u>:175-176, 1950

and thyroid, effects on sensitivity to hypoxia, basal rate of O_2 consumption and tolerance to exercise (Smith
and Smith) Amer. J. Physiol. <u>165</u>:651-661, 1951

Radioelectrocardiography

clinical evaluation of exercise test, use in (Furuya) Jap. Heart J. <u>4</u>:81-91, 1963

erythrityl tetranitrate during exercise, effect of (Bellet and others) Amer. J. Cardiol <u>11</u>:600-608, 1963

during exercise (Bellet and others) Amer. J. Cardiol. <u>8</u>:385-400; Circulation <u>25</u>:686-694, 1962

during exertion (Donkerlo) Nederl. T. Geneesk. <u>108</u>:385-387, 1964

quanitative, study of pulmonary blood volume (Giuntini and others) J. Clin. Invest. <u>42</u>:1589-1605, 1963

Radiomicroangiography

investigations during effort (Ulmeanau and others) Rumanian Med. Rev. <u>5</u>:273-274, 1961

Radiotelemetry

determination of heart rate during natural muscular activity (Rozenblat) Fed. Proc. (Trans. Suppl.)
<u>22</u>:761-766, 1963

use in physiological research on work and sport (Rozenblat) Vestn. Akad. Med. Nauk. SSSR <u>19</u>:66-71,
1964

Reaction time

effect of exercise programs (Baer and others) Arch. Phys. Med. <u>36</u>:495-502, 1955

Receptors

chemo- and pressor, arterial and respiration during muscular exercise (Leusen and others) Acta Physiol.
Pharmacol. Neerl. <u>6</u>:43-52, 1957

chemo, aorta, location and function (Comroe) Amer. J. Physiol. <u>127</u>:176-191, 1939

Receptors (Cont.)

    chemosensitive, medullary (Euler and Söderberg) J. Physiol. 118:545-554, 1952

    pressor, arterial, and cardiac debt during muscular exercise (Leusen and others) Arch. Int. Physiol.
        64:564-570, 1956

    pressor, arterial, role in cardiac output during muscular exercise (Leusen and Lacroix) Arch. Int.
        Pharmacodyn. 130:470-472, 1961

    reflexogenic areas of cardiovascular system (Heymans and Neil) London, Churchill, 1958

Recovery

    biochemistry of (Margaria) J. Sport Med. 3:145-156, 1963

    blood changes during, after exhaustive exercise (Selye) Canad. J. Res. 17(Sect. D):109-112, 1939

    following brief severe exercise (Keys) J. Biol. Chem. 105:xlvi, 1934

    and muscular activity, various environments, physiological reactions (Brouha and others) J. Appl.
        Physiol. 16:133-140, 1961

    from muscular fatigue (Numajiri) J. Sci. Labour 40:153-161, 1964

    pause, determination, and theory of, for static work (Rohmert) Int. Zeits. angew. Physiol. 18:123-164,
        191-212, 1960

    from severe exercise, pulse rate and oxygen intake during early stages (Lythgoe and Pereira) Proc. Roy. Soc.
        98B:468-479, 1925

    ventilatory reaction, muscular exercise (Teillac and LeFrançois) J. Physiologie 54:417-418, 1962

    from vigorous exercise of short duration (Sargent) Proc. Roy. Soc. 100B:440-447, 1926

Reflexes

    cardiac (Bainbridge) J. Physiol. 48:332-340, 1914

    controls, theory to explain regulation body temperature at rest and during exercise (Bazett) J. Appl. Physiol.
        4:245-262, 1951

    joint, and regulation of respiration during exercise (Gardner and Jacobs) Amer. J. Physiol. 153:567-579,
        1948

    reflexogenic areas of cardiovascular system (Heymans and Neil) London, Churchill, 1958

    respiratory, man and other mammals (Widdicombe) Clin. Sci. 21:163-170, 1961

    triceps surae, stretch reflex duration, effect of exercise (Johnson and others) J. Ass. Phys. Ment.
        Rehab. 17:172-176, 1963

    ventilatory, effects, stimulation of large afferent fibres, cat (Bessou and others) Comptes Rend. Soc.
        Biol. 153:477-481, 1959

Reinforcement

    secondary, and effort (Lott) J. Abnorm. Soc. Psychol. 67:520-522, 1963

Renal

    circulation and sodium excretion, effect of exercise in recumbent position (Bucht and others) Acta Physiol.
        Scand. 28:95-100, 1953

    circulation, effects of exercise (White and Rolf) Amer. J. Physiol. 152:505-516, 1948

    concentrating mechanism, effect of heavy exercise (Raisz and others) J. Clin. Invest. 38:8-13, 1959

Renal (Cont.)

excretory function and hemodynamics of kidneys in physical activity in heart disease under indifferent
thermal conditions (Kaufmann) Verh. deutsch. ges. Kreislaufforsch. 30:340-345, 1964

function, and circulation, effect of effort, in cardiac disease (Himbert and others) Sem. Hop. Paris
32:415-423, 1956

function during muscular work (Milla and others) Boll. Soc. Ital. Biol. Sper. 23:725-726, 1947

function, effect of exertion, aged (Panno) Boll. Soc. Ital. Biol. Sper. 38:782-784, 1962

function, influence of muscular activity (De Lanne) Acta Belg. Arte Méd. Pharm. Milit. 110:
611-620, 1957

function, reaction to physical activity (Greco) Gazz. Int. Med. Chir. 69:596-601, 1964

hemodynamics and sodium chloride, basal condition and diffuse pulmonary lesions (Basevi and others)
Folia Cardiol. 14:25-35, 1955

hemodynamics, effect of exercise and emotional stress on (Blake) Amer. J. Physiol. 165:149-157,
1951

influence of work in high temperature on inulin and PAH clearance and on electrolytic and 17-21-dihydroxy-
20-ketosteroid excretion, urine (Starlinger and Bandino) Int. Zeits. angew. Physiol. 18:285-305,
1960

manifestations during prolonged muscular exertion (Chevat and others) Lille Med. 6:847-849, 1961

mechanism of electrolyte excretion, effect of exercise (Kattus and others) Bull. Johns Hopkins Hosp.
84:344-368, 1949

muscle electrolytes in kidney disease (Bergström) Scand. J. Clin. Lab. Invest. 14(Suppl. 68):1-110, 1962

plasma flow and filtration rate, effect of exercise, normal and cardiac patients (Merrill and Cargill) J.
Clin. Invest. 27:272-277, 1948

plasma flow, effect of exercise (Chapman and others) J. Clin. Invest. 27:639-644, 1948

response to exercise (Editorial) Brit. Med. J. 2:1281-1282, 1958

responses to exercise, heat and dehydration (Smith and others) J. Appl. Physiol. 4:659-665, 1952

severe physical exercise, effect on the kidneys (Záruba) Med. Exp. 11:233-238, 1964

system, effect of great physical exercise (Baldes and others) München. med. Wschr. 53:1865-1866,
1906

Renin

activity in blood in hypertension (Helmer) Canad. Med. Ass. J. 90:221-225, 1964

Reserpine

and atropine, effect on pulmonary diffusing capacity during exercise
(Krumholz and Ross) J. Appl. Physiol. 19:465-468, 1964

Resistance

non-specific increased, status (Lazarev and Rusin) Nerv. Sist. 4:149-152, 1963

progressively increasing, involuntary patterning associated with willed movement performed against
(Waterland and Hellebrandt) Amer. J. Phys. Med. 43:13-30, 1964

Respiration

(Pembrey) in Text-book of physiology by E. A. Schäfer, Edinburgh and London, Young J. Pentlord, 1898,
v. 1, 698-712; (Allen and Pepys) Phil. Trans. Roy. Soc. 99:404-429, 1809; (Haldane and Priestley)
2nd ed. Oxford, Clarendon Press, 1935; (Pettenkofer) Ann. Chem. Pharm. 2(Suppl.):1-52, 1862-1863

abnormalities in varicella pneumonia (Bocles and others) Ann. Intern. Med. 60:183-195, 1964

following acclimatization, intracontinental regions of Antarctic (Tikhomirov) Biull. Eksp. Biol. Med.
57:20-23, 1964

action of foods on, during the primary processes of digestion (Smith) Phil. Trans. Roy. Soc. 149:
715-742, 1859

of active and passive limb movements, effects (Bahnson and others) J. Appl. Physiol. 2:169-173, 1949

adaptation (Pickfold) Lancet 2:1225-1226, 1954

adaptation during long-term, non-steady state exercise and sitting (Ekelund and Holmgren) Acta Physiol.
Scand. 62:240-255, 1964

adaptation to exercise in anxious patients (Mezey and Coppen) Clin. Sci. 20:171-175, 1961

adaptation to serve muscular work (Åstrand and others) Acta Physiol. Scand. 50:254-258, 1960

adaptations of muscular exercise (Lemarchands) Gaz. Méd. France 67:1093-1104, 1960

air inspired, quantity, day and night, influence of exercise, food, medicine, temperature (Smith)
Proc. Roy. Soc. 8:451-454, 1857

of animals (Seguin and Lavoisier) Hist. Acad. Sci. (1789); 566-584, 1793

of animals, various kinds, chemical researches (Regnault and Reiset) Ann. Chim. Phys. Sér. 3 26:
299-519, 1849

atmospheric pressure, variable, effect of (Speck) Schrifen Ges. Beförderung ges. Naturgewissensch.
Marburg 11:173-256, 1877

blood, function of in work and recovery (Kaup) Arbeitsphysiol. 2:541-574, 1930

and blood reaction after exercise (Barr) J. Biol. Chem. 56:171-182, 1923

body loading, normal and high performance sports, studies of respiration (Kirchhoff) Deutsch. Arch, klin.
Med. 203:423-447, 1956

and breathing apparatus in Physiological Institute of München (Pettenkofer) Sitzungsberichte der Königl.
bayerisch. Acad. Wissensch. München pp. 296-304, 1860

capacity, maximal, effects of inhalation of CO_2 muscular exercise and epinephrine (Lewis and Morton)
J. Appl. Physiol. 7:309-312, 1954

and carbon dioxide (Parker and others) J. Clin. Invest. 42:1362-1372, 1963

carbon dioxide content of expired air on respiratory movement, dependence of (Vierordt) Arch. physiol.
Heilk. 3:536-558, 1845

CO_2, effect of on using new method of administration (Fenn and Craig) J. Appl. Physiol. 18:1023-1024,
1963

Respiration (Cont.)

carbon dioxide, excess and want of oxygen, effect of on (Hill and Flack) J. Physiol. 37:77-111, 1908

CO_2, influence of in cerebral ventricles (Leusen) Amer. J. Physiol. 176:39-44, 1954

and carbon dioxide, relation between (Loeschcke) Anaesthesist 9:38-46, 1960

and cardiac function during muscular exercise and during recovery (Michali) Rev. Franç. Etud. Clin.
Biol. 2:251-261, 1957

and cardiac responses, during prolonged exercise (Michael and others) J. Appl. Physiol. 16:997-1000, 1961

center, effect of direct chemical and electrical stimulation, cat (Comroe) Amer. J. Physiol. 139:490-498, 1943

center, response to carbonic acid, oxygen and hydrogen ion concentration (Campbell and others) J. Physiol. 46:
301-318, 1913

centers, changes in excitability, aviators in state of fatigue (Franck and others) Comptes Rend. Soc. Biol.
139:835-836, 1945

centers, excitability, during muscular work (Lindhard) Arbeitsphysiol. 7:72-82, 1934

centers, interaction of intracranial chemosensitivity with peripheral afferents to (Loeschcke and others)
Ann. N.Y. Acad. Sci. 109:651-660, 1963

centers, slow potentials (Euler and Söderberg) J. Physiol. 118:555-564, 1952

changes in H^+ and total buffer concentrations in cerebral ventricles, influences of (Leusen) Amer. J. Physiol.
176:45-51, 1954

changes, initial, from rest to work and work to rest (Asmussen and Nielsen) Acta Physiol. Scand. 16:
270-285, 1948

changes, transition from work to rest (Krogh and Lindhard) J. Physiol. 53:431-439, 1920

chemical and other phenomena of, modification by physical agencies (Smith) Phil. Trans. Roy. Soc.
149:681-714, 1859

chemical regulation (Gesell) Physiol. Rev. 5:551-595, 1925

chemoreceptor control, arterial (Dejours) Ann. N.Y. Acad. Sci. 109:682-695, 1963

chemoreflexes (Dejours) Physiol. Rev. 42:335-358, 1962

chemoreflex and central components during acid-base displacements in blood (Hesser) Acta Physiol. Scand.
18(Suppl. 64):5-69; appendix, 1949

and circulation, effort test in evaluation (Deloff and Pudelski) Pol. Tyg. Lek. 18:1256-1260, 1963

and circulation in physical work (Hansen) Handbuch der normalen und pathologischen Physiologie, edited
by A. Bethe and others, Berlin, Springer, 1931, vol. 15, part 2

and circulation, influence of work and training, clinical and physiological observations (Hollmann) Dormstadt,
Steinkopf, 1959

control, Gray's theory, application to hypernea produced by passive movements (Otis) J. Appl. Physiol.
1:743-751, 1949

Respiration (Cont.)

difficulty of, cause, also dyspnoea and apnoea (Pflüger) Pflüger Arch. ges. Physiol. $\underline{1}$:61-106,
1868

in exercise, brief (Craig and Cummings) U. S. Army Chem. Warfare Techn. Rep. CWLR 2364:1-22,
1960; J. Appl. Physiol. $\underline{15}$:583-588, 1960

exercise, heavy, factors influencing (Mitchell and others) J. Clin. Invest. $\underline{37}$:1693-1701, 1958

exercise, muscular, response to (Schmidt) Acta Med. Philipp. $\underline{11}$:27-48, 1955

exercise performance, effects of adding oxygen to inspired air (Bannister and Cunningham) J. Physiol. $\underline{125}$:
118-137, 1954

exercise, physical exertion, and fitness (Briggs) J. Physiol. $\underline{54}$:292-318, 1920; J. Roy. Army Med. Corps
$\underline{37}$:278-301, 1920

external, and gas exchange, limited cyclic rapid exercises, boys (Volkov) Fiziol. Zh. SSSR Sechenov.
9:1456-1460, 1963

external, influence of exertion, miners (Shevelev) Gig. Tr. Prof. Zabol. $\underline{7}$:13-17, 1963

external, under controlled physical loading, pulmonary tuberculosis (Vinnik and Filimonov) Probl. Tuberk.
$\underline{42}$:27-34, 1964

forced, and oxygen, influence on athletic performance (Vernon and Stolz) Quart. J. Exp. Physiol. $\underline{4}$:243-248,
1911

forced, previous, and oxygen inhalation, effects on distress caused by muscular work (Douglas and Haldane)
J. Physiol. $\underline{39}$:i-iv, 1909

frequency and volume, under low barometric pressures, muscular exercise (Schneider and Clarke) Amer. J.
Physiol. $\underline{75}$:297-307, 1926

frog muscle (Meyerhof) Pflüger Arch. ges. Physiol. $\underline{175}$:20-87, 1919

and heart activity, effect of muscle activity on (Johansson) Skand. Arch. Physiol. 5:20-66, 1895

and heart beat during exercise, correlation (Wright) Boston Med. & Surg. J. $\underline{162}$:417-424, 1910

and heart minute volume in sport (Albrecht and others) Zeits. ges. exp. Med. $\underline{122}$:356-368, 1953

hemodynamic response to exercise, supine position, while breathing oxygen (Barratt-Boyes and Wood)
J. Appl. Physiol. $\underline{11}$:129-135, 1957

history (Dempster) Detroit Med. J. $\underline{13}$:320-327, 1913

horse, rest and work (Zuntz and Lehmann) J. Physiol. $\underline{11}$:396-398, 1890

and hourly pulsation (Smith) Brit. Med. J. $\underline{1}$:52, 1856; Med. Chir. Soc. Trans. $\underline{39}$:35-58, 1856

hypnotically induced emotion, pain, and exercise, changes associated with (Dudley and others)
Psychosom. Med. $\underline{26}$:46-57, 1964

increased voluntary, effect on speed of recovery after physical work (Simonson) Arbeitsphysiol. $\underline{1}$:
87-101, 1929

lung changes, animal (Lavoisier) Hist. Acad. Sci. pp. 185-194, 1776; (Lavoisier and Seguin) Ann. Chim.
$\underline{91}$:318-334, 1814

mechanical work of, during exercise, trained and untrained subjects (Milic-Emili and others) J. Appl. Physiol.
$\underline{17}$:43-46, 1962

Respiratory regulation (Cont.)

 hypoxia, acute and prolonged (Nielsen and Smith) Acta Physiol. Scand. 24:293-313, 1951

 and joint reflexes, during exercise (Gardner and Jacobs) Amer. J. Physiol. 153:567-579, 1948

 in muscular activity (Kao) Amer. J. Physiol. 185:145-151, 1956

 in muscular exercise (Dejours) in The Regulation of Human Respiration, edited by Cunningham and
     Lloyd, Blackwell, Oxford, 1963

 in muscular work (Euler and Liljestrand) Acta Physiol. Scand. 12:268-278, 1946

 in muscular work, induced in decerebrate dogs (Kao and others) J. Appl. Physiol. 7:379-386,
     1955

 in muscular work, initial stages (Krogh and Lindhard) J. Physiol. 47:112-136, 1913

 in muscular work, studied on perfused isolated head (Heymans and others) Acta Physiol. Scand. 14:
     86-101, 1947

 nervous factors controlling, during exercise employing blocking of the blood flow (Asmussen and Nielsen)
     Acta Physiol. Scand. 60:103-111, 1964

 through oxygen pressure in mixed venous blood (Hilpert and others) Pflüger Arch. ges. Physiol. 279:1-16, 1964

 in work, heavy (Asmussen and Nielsen) Acta Physiol. Scand. 12:171-188, 1946

Respiratory response

 of anesthetized dogs to induced muscular work (Kao and Ray) Amer. J. Physiol. 179:249-254, 1954

 to exercise (McIlroy) Pediatrics 32(Suppl.):680-682, 1963

 to exercise, acute, Eskimoes and white (Erikson) Acta Physiol. Scand. 41:1-11, 1957

 to exercise, acute, in induced metabolic acidosis (Refsum) Acta Physiol. Scand. 52:32-35, 1961

 measurements, underwater swimmers (Goff and others) J. Appl. Physiol. 10:197-202, 1957

 mediated through superficial chemosensitive areas on medulla (Mitchell and others) J. Appl. Physiol.
     18:523-533, 1963; Ann. N.Y. Acad. Sci. 109:661-681, 1963

 muscular exercise, changes in (Paterson) J. Physiol. 66:323-345, 1928

 of pre-adolescent boys to muscular activity (Schneider and Crampton) Amer. J. Physiol. 117:577-586, 1936

 and temperature, in exercise (Morgan and others) Amer. J. Physiol. 183:454-458, 1955

Respiratory system

 influence of muscular exercise (Hough) Trans. XV Int. Congr. Hyg. & Demog., Washington 2:
     651-659, 1913

 static volume-pressure characteristics during maximal effects (Cook and others) J. Appl. Physiol. 19:1016-
     1022, 1964

 water vapor loss from, during outdoor exercise in the cold (Brebbia and others) J. Appl. Physiol. 11:219-222,
     1957; Environ. Protect. Div. QM Res. and Devel. Center, U.S. Army Tech. Rep. EP-57, 1957

Retinal circulation

 used in study of adaptation of cerebral circulation to effort (Remky) Ann. Oculist. 188:849-858, 1955

Rheogram

 pregnancy, normal, rest and exercise (Consiglio and others) Quad. Clin. Ostet. Ginec. 18:1070-1074,
     1963

Rheumatoid arthritis

lactic acid response to muscular exercise in (Kalliomäki and others) Ann. Med. Exp. Fenn. 35:
441-445, 1957

Ribonucleic acid

content of various organs with different forms of protein metabolism, effect of physical training (Lubańska-
Tomaszewska) Acta Physiol. Pol. 15:819-829, 1964

Rickshaw puller

energy expenditure (Banerjee and others) Indian J. Physiol. Pharmacol. 3:147-160, 1959

Rigor

and modification of osmotic properties of muscle (Fletcher) J. Physiol. 30:414-438, 1904

Rigor mortis

lactic acid formation, and survival respiration in mammalian muscle (Fletcher) J. Physiol. 47:361-380,
1913

Rose Bengal test

liver function in rowers (Cairella and others) Ann. Med. Nav. 68:941-946, 1963

Rowing

adrenal cortex reaction to the physical and emotional stress (Renold and others) New Eng. J. Med. 244:754-757,
1951

circulation, effect on, sphygmograph (Fraser) J. Anat. & Physiol. 3:127-130, 1868-1869

human maximum power and its fuel, observations on (Henderson and Haggard) Amer. J. Physiol. 72:264-282,
1925

physical and emotional stress, reaction to (Renold and others) New Eng. J. Med. 244:754-757, 1951

psychotropic substances on mental alertness, influence of (Policreti and others) Ann. Med. Nav. 68:
803-808, 1963

rowers, health (Bradford) Sanitarian 5:529-536, 1877

rowers, liver function, Rose Bengal test (Cairella and others) Ann. Med. Nav. 68:941-946, 1963

Running

air resistance (Hill) Proc. Roy. Soc. 102B:380-385, 1928

blood flow in calf after (Livingstone) Amer. Heart J. 61:219-224, 1961

energy expenditure (Margaria and others) J. Appl. Physiol. 18:367-370, 1963

equation of motion exerting maximal effort (Best and Partridge) Proc. Roy. Soc. 103B:218-225, 1928

heart, chronic effect on, electrocardiogram, dogs (Steinhaus and others) Amer. J. Physiol. 99:503-511, 1932

heart, chronic effect on, roentgenogram, dogs (Steinhaus and others) Amer. J. Physiol. 99:487-502, 1932

and hurdling, physiology (Jokl) Arbeitsphysiol. 1:206-305, 1929

intermittent and continuous (Christensen and others) Acta Physiol. Scand. 50:269-286, 1960

long-distance runners, electrocardiogram (Heim) Schweiz. Zeits. Sportmed. 6:1-72, 1958

mechanical work in (Cavagna and others) J. Appl. Physiol. 19:249-256, 1964

organ weights, effects on, dogs (Steinhaus and others) Amer. J. Physiol. 99:512-520, 1932

oxygen consumption (Hill and Lupton) J. Physiol. 56:xxxii-xxxiii, 1922

positive and negative reinforcer (Hundt and Premack) Science 142:1087-1088, 1963

Running (Cont.)

  pulse rate and 'oxygen debt' after running, influence of atmospheric conditions (Campbell) Proc. Roy.

    Soc. 96B:43-59, 1924

  second wind (Langlois) Médecine 2:915-917, 1921

  speed in, and oxygen requirement, relation between (Sargent) Proc. Roy. Soc. 100B:10-22, 1926

  sprint, blood lactate level during recovery from (Andersen and others) Acta Physiol. Scand. 48:231-237, 1960

  sprint, dynamics (Furusawa and others) Proc. Roy. Soc. 102B:29-42, 1927

  sprint, energy requirement (Furusawa and others) Proc. Roy. Soc. 102B:43-50, 1927

  well-trained runners, energy production, pulmonary ventilation and length of steps, treadmill (Bøje) Acta

    Physiol. Scand. 7:362-375, 1944

Running-wheel

  activity as function of combined food and water deprivation, rat (Moskowitz) J. Comp. Physiol. Psychol. 52:

    621-625, 1959

                                                    S

Salicylates

  elevation of body temperature during exercise, effect on (Downey and Darling) J. Appl. Physiol. 17:323-325,

    1962

  exercise metabolism, effects on (Downey and Darling) J. Appl. Physiol. 17:665-668, 1962

  sodium, effects on physiological responses to work in heart (Jacobson and Base) J. Appl. Physiol. 19:33-36, 1964

Sarcoma

  Yoshida, metastatic spread, effect of muscular stress (Guimaraes and others) Hospital (Rio) 64:967-972, 1963

Sartorius

  comparison between, isolated, energy liberated and work performed, frog (Fenn) J. Physiol. 58:175-203,

    1923

  work and oxygen consumption, frog (Whalen and Collins) J. Cell Comp. Physiol. 61:293-299, 1963

Sauna

  effect on physical performance (Miettinen and Karvinen) J. Sport Med. 3:225-228, 1963

Sewing

  motor, different types, body stress from working (Hubac and others) Int. Zeits. angew. Physiol. 20:

    111-124, 1963

Scar tissue

  anterior tibialis muscle, changes after exertion (Severin) Acta Chir. Scand. 89:426-432, 1943

Schistosomiasis

  effect on activity and growth, mice (Hearnshaw and others) Ann. Trop. Med. Parasit. 57:481-498, 1963

Schizophrenia

motor activity in: effect on plasma factor (Frohman and others) Arch. Gen. Psychiat. 9:83-88, 1963

pupillary abnormalities (May) J. Ment. Sci. 94:89-98, 1948

Scleroderma

involving the heart and respiratory system, pathophysiology (Sackner and others) Ann. Intern. Med. 60:
611-630, 1964

Scoliosis

some ergospirometric indices in adolescents (Orlowska and Jaworska) Pediat. Pol. 39:421-423, 1964

Second wind

(Pembrey and Cook) J. Physiol. 37:lxviii, 1908

second breath of runners (Langlois) Médecine 2:915-917, 1921

Sedimentation rate

during loading, special regard to tuberculosis of the lungs (Wiedemann) Tuberkulosearzt 4:465-470, 1950

in trained and untrained, before and after exertion (Lazzari) Gazz. Int. Med. Chir. 68:2887-2891, 1963

Segontin

effectiveness in angina pectoris: evaluation of O_2 deficiency and exercise load (Kimura and others) J. Ther.
46:162-165, 1964

Sensitivity reaction

through physical exertion (Bartelheimer) Deutsch. med. Wschr. 70:175, 1944

Serotonin

sensitivity, effect of muscular activity, rats (Frenkl and others) Kiserl. Orvostud. 16:391-393, 1964;
Med. Exp. 10:190-194, 1964

Sex and age

and human physical fitness (Åstrand) Physiol. Rev. 36:307-335, 1956

relation to physical working capacity (Åstrand) Copenhagen, Munksgaard, 1952

Shock

exhaustion and restoration during war (Crile and others) Proc. Interstate Postgrad. Med. Ass. N. Amer. 18:
157-160, 1942

fainting and muscular activity (Tomb) Med. J. Aust. 2:274-275, 1944

Shunts

left to right, entering right atrium and great veins, cardiovascular and renal studies during exertion (Schnabel
and others) Acta Med. Scand. 157:241-255, 1957

left-to-right, hemodynamic and ventilatory effects of exercise, upright position (Stephens and others)
Circulation 29:99-106, 1964

left-to-right, pulmonary vascular dynamics in, effect of supine exercise (Swan and others) J. Clin.
Invest. 37:202-213, 1958

Silicosis

> effect of muscular exercise, oxygen inhalation, serpasil and priscol on lesser circulation (Kasalický and
>
> others) Cor Vasa 5:264-272, 1963

Sinoatrial block

> in effort electrocardiogram in cardiovascular diseases (Solti and Foldesy) Zeits. ges. inn. Med. 17:
>
> 930-933, 1962

Sinus rhythm

> and atrial flutter, haemodynamic response to exercise during (Åstrand and others) Acta Med. Scand. 173:
>
> 121-127, 1963
>
> see also Arrhythmia

Skaters

> physical condition during training (Enschedé and Jongbloed) Int. Zeits. angew. Physiol. 20:252-257,
>
> 1964

Skeletal muscles

> anoxemic and normal, relation to fatigue (Anders and others) Naunyn Schmiedberg Arch. exp. Path.
>
> 217:406-412, 1953
>
> capillary permeability during rest and activity (Arturson and Kjellmer) Acta Physiol. Scand. 62:41-45, 1964
>
> exercising, accumulation of fluid (Jacobsson and Kjellmer) Acta Physiol. Scand. 60:286-292, 1964
>
> experimental inactivity, electron microscope findings (Wechsler) Verh. deutsch. Ges. Path. 46:300-305,
>
> 1962
>
> fibers, effects of exercise and reduced food intake on (Goldspink) J. Cell Comp. Physiol. 63:209-216,
>
> 1964
>
> lymph, flow and content of, during rest and exercise (Jacobsson and Kjellmer) Acta Physiol. Scand. 60:
>
> 278-285, 1964
>
> mineral content of, influence of training and load (Nöcker and others) Int. Zeits. angew. Physiol. 17:
>
> 243-251, 1958
>
> passive and active tension length diagrams, normal women, different ages (Botelho and others) J. Appl.
>
> Physiol. 7:93-98, 1954
>
> training, influence of (Hoffmann) Anat. Anz. 96:191-203, 1947
>
> vessels, capillary pressure, current strength, relation (Schroeder) Zeits. Kreislaufforsch. 53:47-53, 1964

Skiers

> electrocardiographic telemetry in, heart rate during competition (Hanson and Tabakin) New Eng. J. Med.
>
> 271:181-185, 1964
>
> heart, in contest (Rautmann) Deutsch. med. Wschr. Sonderausgabe 62:42-44, 1936
>
> long-distance, electrocardiogram (Heim) Schweiz. Zeits. Sportmed. 6:1-72, 1958
>
> physiology of skiing (Christensen and Högberg) Arbeitsphysiol. 14:292-303, 1950

Skin

> loss of water and salts through, physiological adjustments (Hancock and others) Proc. Roy. Soc. 105B:
>
> 43-59, 1930

Stroke volume

cardiac output, regulation by (Warner and Toronto) Circ. Res. <u>8</u>:549-552, 1960

cardiac stroke, force, and exercise (Jokl) J. Ass. Phys. Med. Rehab. <u>18</u>:148-163, 1964

and cardiac work (Müller) Deutsch. Arch. klin. Med. <u>96</u>:127-152, 1909

in graded exercise, dog (Wang and others) Circ. Res. <u>8</u>:558-563, 1960

heart, and capacity of vascular system, relationship (Sjöstrand) Acta Physiol. Scand. <u>42</u>(Suppl. 145):
126-127, 1957

and heart volume, relation between, in recumbent and erect positions (Nylin) Scand. Arch. Physiol.
<u>69</u>:237-246, 1934

leg exercise in supine position, response to, base-line effects (Frick and Somer) J. Appl. Physiol. <u>19</u>:
639-643, 1964

and minute volume after physical exertion of varying intensity (Poruchikov) Fiziol. Zh. SSSR Sechenov.
<u>49</u>:1076-1083, 1963

and minute volume, during heavy work (Christensen) Arbeitsphysiol. <u>4</u>:470-502, 1931

myotonic, atrophy, of Steinert, cardiac stroke (Gfeller and Roux) Cardiologia <u>42</u>:200-205, 1963

and pulse frequency, behaviour after physical stress (Millahn and Sollmann) Int. Zeits. angew. Physiol.
<u>19</u>:143-148, 1962

quantitation of beat-to-beat changes, from aortic pulse contour (Warner and others) J. Appl. Physiol.
<u>5</u>:495-507, 1953

at rest and during exercise (Chapman and others) J. Clin. Invest. <u>39</u>:1208-1213, 1960

spontaneous activity and exercise, baboons, changes (Franklin and Van Citters) Amer. J. Cardiol. <u>12</u>:
816-821, 1963

upright exercise, responses of (Cobb and others) Clin. Res. <u>9</u>:84, 1961

in ventricular responses to exertion, constancy of (Rushmer) Amer. J. Physiol. <u>196</u>:745-750, 1959

in work intensities, different, circulatory data (Holmgren and others) Acta Physiol. Scand. <u>49</u>:343-363, 1960

Strong man

Mr. Maul (Virchow) Berlin. klin. Wschr. <u>29</u>:703, 1892

Subaortic stenosis

hypertrophic subaortic, effects of beta adrenergic blockage on circulation (Harrison and others) Circulation <u>29</u>:
84-98, 1964

Succinic dehydrogenase

activity of heart and skeletal muscle of exercised rats (Hearn and Wainio) Amer. J. Physiol. <u>185</u>:348-350,
1956

and aldolase activities of skeletal muscle of exercised rats (Hearn) J.-Lancet <u>77</u>:80, 1957

Sugar

effect on recovering mental and motor control after exercise (Laird) Med. Rev. of Rev. <u>36</u>:383-386, 1930

metabolism, effect of exercise on (Gordon) Northwest. Med. <u>25</u>:376-379, 1926

<u>see also</u> Dextrose; Fructose; Glucose; Pentose

Sugar, blood

    and blood gases changes during exercise (Hartman and Griffith) Proc. Soc. Exp. Biol. Med. 21:
        561-565, 1924

    and free fatty acids, measured after bicycle ergometry (Wuschech and others) Deutsch. Gesundh. 19:
        1668-1670, 1964

    physical work, during and after (Bøje) Scand. Arch. Physiol. 74(Suppl. 10):1-48, 1936

    regulation after concentrated nourishment connected with muscular work (Glatzel and Rettenmaier) Schweiz.
        Zeits. Sportmed. 11:126-140, 1963

    urine sugar and urine protein in exercise (Edwards and others) Amer. J. Physiol. 98:352-356, 1931

Surgical patients

    activity, observations (Browse) Brit. Med. J. 1:1669-1670, 1964

Sweat

    and blood reaction to exhausting work (Prokop) Medizinisische, pp. 1622-1624, 1952

    electrolyte and lactate content, effect of thermal stress and muscular exercise (Hasan and others) Acta Physiol.
        Scand. 31:131-136, 1954

    electrolytes, and d-aldosterone (McConahay and others) J. Appl. Physiol. 19:575-579, 1964

    elevated, sodium and chloride, in adult without cystic fibrosis (Gup and Bruggs) Arch. Intern. Med. 112:
        699-701, 1963

    and exercise (Kral and others) J. Sport Med. 3:105-113, 1963

    exercise, influence on (Boigey) J. Physiol. Path. Gen. 25:249-253, 1927

    lactate content (Åstrand) Acta Physiol. Scand. 58:359-367, 1963

    loss, effect on body fluids (Kozlowski and Saltin) J. Appl. Physiol. 19:1119-1124, 1964

    magnesium and calcium excretion (Bara) Pol. Arch. Med. Wewnet. 33:1125-1132, 1963

    nitrogen excretion in, and relation to nitrogen balance requirements (Consolazio and others) J. Nutr.
        79:399-406, 1963

    nitrogen loss, muscular work (Gontzea and Schutzescu) Int. Zeits. angew. Physiol. 20:90-110, 1963

    production, effects of atropine, work and heat (Craig) J. Appl. Physiol. 4:826-833, 1952

    serum hemoglobin and albumin, changes in (Cohn) Zeits. Biol. 70:366-370, 1919

    sweating, decline in rates, during work in severe heat (Gerking and Robinson) Amer. J. Physiol. 147:370-378,
        1946

    sweating, influence on metabolism (Dunlop and others) J. Physiol. 22:68-91, 1897

    sweating, rapid response to muscular work (Van Beaumont and Bullard) Science 141:643-646, 1963

    sweating, stimulation by exercise after heat induced 'fatigue' of the sweating mechanism (Ahlman and
        Karvonen) Acta Physiol. Scand. 53:381-386, 1961

    thermal stress and muscular exercise effect on perspiration rate with and without insulin hypoglycaemia (Hasan
        and others) Acta Physiol. Scand. 31:131-136, 1954

Swimming

> aspartic acid salts, effects on performance, rats and dogs (Matoush and others) J. Appl. Physiol. 19:262-264, 1964

> chronic effect on heart, electrocardiogram, and roentgenogram, dogs (Steinhaus and others) Amer. J. Physiol. 99:487-502, 503-511, 1932

> competitive, effect on serum proteins (Johnson and Wong) J. Appl. Physiol. 16:807-809, 1961

> digoxin in guinea pigs, influence (Arienzo) Gior. Med. Milit. 110:575-587, 1960

> of dolphins (Steven) Sci. Progr. Twent. Cent. 38:524-525, 1950

> and eating (Ball) New York J. Med. 63:600-603, 1963

> I^{131} distribution in thyroidectomised, 1-thyroxine maintained rats after injection of I^{131} labelled 1-thyroxine, effects (Escobar Del Rey and Morreale De Escobar) Acta Endocr. 23:393-399, 1958

> muscular enzyme levels after, rats (Gould and Rawlinson) Biochem. J. 73:41-44, 1956

> octacosanol, wheat germ oil, and vitamin E, rats, effect of (Consolazio and others) J. Appl. Physiol. 19:265-267, 1964

> organ weights, dogs, effect of (Steinhaus and others) Amer. J. Physiol. 99:512-520, 1932

> trained swimmers, underwater, elevated end-tidal CO_2 in (Goff and Bartlett) J. Appl. Physiol. 10:203-206, 1957

> 20°C., effect of various pharmacological agents on time of exhaustion, animals (Jacob and Michaud) Arch. Int. Pharmacodyn. 133:101-115, 1961; 135:462-471, 1962; Med. Exp. 2:323-328, 1960

> underwater, oxygen requirements (Goff and others) J. Appl. Physiol. 9:219-221, 1956

> underwater, swimmers, respiratory responses and work efficiency, measurements (Goff and others) J. Appl. Physiol. 10:197-202, 1957

> underwater, training, cardiovascular responses (Michael) J. Sport Med. 3:218-220, 1963

> water temperature on heart rate and rectal temperature, rats, effect on (Baker and Horvath) Amer. J. Physiol. 207:1073-1076, 1964

Sympathectomy

> and arterial stenosis, effect on blood flow and the ergogram (Van de Berg and others) Ann. Surg. 159:623-635, 1964

> denervation and muscular work, effect on histochemically demonstrable acid phosphatase activity in adrenal medulla, rat (Eränkö and Härkönen) Ann. Med. Exp. Fenn. 40:129-133, 1962

> effects on electrocardiogram and effort tolerance in angina pectoris (Apthorp and others) Brit. Heart J. 26:218-226, 1964

> heart rate, in rest and exercise, dog (Brouha and others) J. Physiol. 87:345-359, 1936

> and vagotomy, cardiovascular response to graded exercise, dog (Ashkar and Hamilton) Amer. J. Physiol. 204:291-296, 1963

Sympathetic nervous system, see Autonomic nervous system

Syncope

> associated with exertional dyspnea and angina pectoris (Golden) Amer. Heart J. 28:689-698, 1944

> on exertion, relation to coronary artery disease (Engelhardt and Sodeman) Ann. Intern. Med. 22:225-233, 1945

Temperature, environmental

    and energy expenditures (Consolazio and others) J. Appl. Physiol. 18:65-68, 1963

    high, blood displacement, minute volume, physical work (Marschak) Zeits. ges. exp. Med. 77:
        133-143, 1931

    high, effect on excitibality of human visual analyzers (Navakamikian and others) Fiziol. Zh. SSSR
        Sechenov. 49:1036-1043, 1963

    high, influence of work on urinary excretion of insulin, PAH, electrolytes and 17-21-dihydroxy-20-ketosteroid
        (Starlinger and Bandino) Int. Zeits. angew. Physiol. 18:285-305, 1960

    high, physiological bases of human work in (Lehmann) Concours Méd. 82:2383-2388, 1960

    and humidity, changes, tolerance limits in work and rest (Friedrich) Pflüger Arch. ges. Physiol. 250:
        182-191, 1948

    lactic acid content of frog muscle, influence of on (Adler) Hoppe-Seyler Zeits. physiol. Chem. 113:
        174-186, 193-200, 1921; (Adler and Günzberg) Hoppe-Seyler Zeits. physiol. Chem. 113:187-192, 1921

    second wind, effect on of (Berner and others) Amer. J. Physiol. 76:586-592, 1926

    water, influence on heart rate and rectal temperature, swimming rats (Baker and Horvath) Amer. J. Physiol.
        207:1073-1076, 1964

Testis

    morphology and histochemistry, effect of heavy muscular work rat (Härkönen and others) Acta Endocr. 43:
        311-320, 1963

Testosterone

    causing histological and chemical changes in skeletal muscle (Hettinger) Aertzl. Forsch. 13:570-574, 1959

Tests

    endurance, physiological proof for evaluation of training in physical exercise (Mitolo) Arch. Sci. Biol. 35:
        561-576, 1951

    exercise, children, for cardiovascular fitness (Kramer and Lurie) Amer. J. Dis. Child. 108:283-297, 1964

    exercise, premature systoles with myocardial injury produced by (Salomon) Dis. Chest 43:439-440, 1963

    exercise, studies on electrocardiographic changes during (Sandberg) Acta Med. Scand. 169(Suppl. 365):
        1-117, 1961

    exercise, tolerance (Harris) Lancet 2:409-411, 1958

    exercise, value of longitudinal studies (Sexton) Pediatrics 32(Suppl.):730-736, 1963

    laboratory, selected, of physical fitness, correlation with military endurance (Rasch and Wilson) Milit.
        Med. 129:256-258, 1964

    Step, physiological characteristics (Rovelli and Aghemo) Int. Zeits. angew. Physiol. 20:190-194, 1963

    see also Harvard step test; Master test; and names of other specific tests

Theophylline

    glucosides, and analeptics, influence on cardiac output in congestive heart failure (Berseus) Acta Med.
        Scand. 113(Suppl. 145):1-76, 1943

Thermal conductivity cell

    measurement of evaporative water loss (Adams and others) J. Appl. Physiol. 18:1291-1293, 1963

Thermodilution

    determination of cardiac output, exertion, dog (Cerretelli and others) Boll. Soc. Ital. Biol. Sper. $\underline{39}$:
        2038-2040, 1963

Thermodynamic

    phenomena, exhibited in shortening or lengthening muscle (Azuma) Proc. Roy. Soc. $\underline{96B}$:338, 1924

Thermogenesis

    due to exercise and cold in warm- and cold-acclimated rats (Hart and Janksy) Canad. J. Biochem. $\underline{41}$:
        629-634, 1963

Thermoregulation

    and physical effort (Grandjean) Schweiz. Zeits. Sportmed. $\underline{4}$:65-80, 1956

    see also Temperature, body

Thiamine, see Vitamin B_1

Thoracity cavity

    organs contained in, influence of effort (Cloquet) Paris, Mequignon-Marvis, 1820; Nouv. J. Med. Chir.
        Pharm. (Paris) $\underline{6}$:309-375, 1819

Thorax

    size, influence of physical exercise, systematic (Wolf-Heidegger) Schweiz. med. Wschr. $\underline{83}$:917-919, 1953

Thrombocytes

    adhesiveness, change after physical work (Pfleiderer and Kommerell) Verh. deutsch. Ges. inn. Med. $\underline{70}$:
        220-223, 1964

    count and adhesiveness, effect of physical work (Wachholder and others) Acta Haemat. $\underline{18}$:59-79, 1957

    count, effects of posture changes (Sloan and Allardyce) Quart. J. Exp. Physiol. $\underline{40}$:161-167, 1955

    count, influence of brief periods of strenuous exercise (Gerheim and Miller) Science $\underline{109}$:64-65, 1949

    thrombocytosis, evoked by exercise (Sarajas and others) Nature $\underline{192}$:721-722, 1961

Thrombophlebitis

    axillary vein, exertion (Adrower) Minerva Med. $\underline{54}$:2243-2245, 1963

    upper extremities, exertion (Tlusty and Rehor) Sborn. Ved. Prac. Lek. Fak. Karlov. Univ. $\underline{5(Suppl.)}$:
        313-316, 1962

Thrombosis

    arterial, chronic, Na^{24}-clearance during standard exercise (Tonnesen) Scand. J. Clin. Lab. Invest.
        $\underline{15(Suppl. 76)}$:64-65, 1963

    axillary vein, caused by strain or effort, deep-sea diver (Keener and others) U.S. Naval Med. Bull. $\underline{40}$:
        687-692, 1942

    axillary vein, exertion (Toth and others) Fortschr. Roentgenstr. $\underline{99}$:484-492, 1963

    axillary vein, over-exertion (Velasco-Sanfuentes and others) Rev. Med. Chile $\underline{71}$:779-780, 1943

    of effort (Menges) Nederl. Milit. Geneesk. T. $\underline{16}$:37-44, 1963

    with loads and peripheral obstruction, training problems (Loosen and others) Zeits. gesamt. inn. Med.
        $\underline{7}$:520-523, 1952

    tibial artery, anterior, acute (Albanes) Angiology $\underline{9}$:172-175, 1958

Thrombosis (Cont.)

tibial artery, anterior, isolated, treatment (Leriche) Presse Med. 58:1285, 1950

of Vena cava, inferior, following physical exertion (Foster and others) J.A.M.A. 117:2167-2168, 1941

venous, deep, in leg, following effort or strain (Crane) New Eng. J. Med. 246:529-533, 1952

Thyroid gland

effect of frequent housing changes, and of muscular exercise on, mice (Carrière and Isler) Endocrinology 64:414-418, 1959

hyperthyroid state, peripheral vascular response (Abramson and Fierst) J. Clin. Invest. 20:517-519, 1941

Thyroid hormone

circulatory, effect of muscular exercise (Lashof and others) Proc. Soc. Exp. Biol. Med. 86:233-235, 1954

and radiation, effects on sensitivity to hypoxia, basal rate of O_2 consumption, and tolerance to exercise (Smith and Smith) Amer. J. Physiol. 165:651-661, 1951

running, effect of for 12 hours on I^{131} distribution in thyroidectomized, 1-thyroxine maintained rats after injection of I^{131} labelled 1-throxine (Escobar Del Rey and Morreale de Escobar) Acta Endocr. 23:400-406, 1956

swimming, effect of, for 2 hours in I^{131} distribution in thyroidectomized, 1-thyroxine maintained rats after injection of I^{131} labelled 1-throxine (Escobar Del Rey and Morreale de Escobar) Acta Endocr. 23:393-399, 1956

work metabolism, effect on, dog (Kommerell) Arbeitsphysiol. 1:586-594, 1929

Tibia

fracture, spontaneous, caused by running (Kobayashi) Far East. Sci. Bull. 3:18, 1943

Tibial artery

anterior, acute thrombosis (Albanes) Angiology 9:172-174, 1958

isolated thrombosis of, treatment (Leriche) Presse Méd. 58:1285, 1950

Tissue pressure

estimation, indirect method, during exercise (Kjellmer) Acta Physiol. Scand. 62:31-40, 1964

Tocopherols, see Vitamin E

Tolerance

exercise, measurement (Taylor and Franzen) No. 57, Rep. Div. Res. U.S. Civil Aeronaut. Admin., Washington, 1946

exercise, physiologic variation and measurement of (Taylor) Amer. J. Physiol. 142:200-212, 1944

exertion in the elderly (Schweizer) Schweiz. Zeits. Sportmed. 12:98-104, 1964

limits for changes in room temperature and humidity in rest and work (Friedrich) Pfluger Arch. ges. Physiol. 250:182-191, 1948

limits, human, for some thermal environments of aerospace (Kaufman) Aerospace Med. 34:889-896, 1963

work, age and altitude (Dill and others) J. Appl. Physiol. 19:483-488, 1964; Rep. 63-33, U.S. Civil Aeromed. Res. Inst., 1963

Tone

of heart and blood vessels (Gaskell) J. Physiol. 3:48-75, 1882

Transaminase (Cont.)

    serum, activities in thoroughbred horses in training (Cornelius and others) J. Amer. Vet. Med. Ass. 142: 639-642, 1963

    serum, effect of physical exercise (Schlang) Amer. J. Med. Sci. 242:338-341, 1961

    serum, effects of training, exercise, and tying-up, in horse (Cardinet and others) Amer. J. Vet. Res. 24: 980-984, 1963

    serum levels, effect of strenuous and prolonged physical exercise (Remmers and Kaljot) J.A.M.A. 185: 968-970, 1963

    SGOT levels following physical and emotional exertion, man and monkey (Mandel and others) Aerospace Med. 33:1216-1223, 1962

Transducer

    electromagnetic flow, miniature, to study coronary blood flow in intact conscious dog (Hepps and others) J. Thorac. Cardiov. Surg. 46:783-794, 1963

Treadmill

    Balke-Ware, test, effect of blood loss on performance (Howell) Res. Quart. Amer. Ass. Health Phys. Educ. 35:156-165, 1964

    conversion to cycle ergometer (Lurie) J. Appl. Physiol. 19:152-153, 1964

    exercise, aortic blood flow, dogs (Franklin and others) J. Appl. Physiol. 14:809-812, 1959

    hemodynamic response, normal men (Tabakin and others) J. Appl. Physiol. 19:457-464, 1964

    low cost, for experimental animals (Kouwenhoven and others) J. Appl. Physiol. 7:347-348, 1954

    motor-driven, external work in level and grade walking (Snellen) J. Appl. Physiol. 15:759-763, 1960

    observations (Hutchinson) London Med. & Phys. J. 50:112-118, 1823

    titration schedule (Evans) J. Exp. Anal. Behav. 6:219-221, 1963

    treadwheel, observations (Good) London Med. & Phys. J. 50:205-208, 1823

    treadwheel, remarks on (Hippisley) London Med. & Phys. J. 50:273-274, 1823

    see also Cardiac output; Energy expenditure

Tremor

    magnitude, static neuromuscular, influence of exercises, emotional stress, and age (Mitchem and Tuttle) Res. Quart. 25:65-74, 1954

    neuromuscular, influence of order of exercise bouts (Slater-Hammel) Res. Quart. 26:88-95, 1955

    physiological, analysis, during rest and exhaustion (Vetter and Horvath) J. Appl. Physiol. 16:994-996, 1961

Triglycerides

    non-esterified fatty acids, cholesterol, and phospholipids, arteriovenous relationship (Konttinen and others) Ann. Med. Exp. Fenn. 40:250-256, 1962

    triglyceridemia, postprandial, effect of muscular exercise on plasma viscosity in correlation with (Konttinen and Somer) J. Appl. Physiol. 18:991-993, 1963

Triolein I-131

    resorption, influence of physical work, rats (Simko and others) Med. Exp. 8:156-158, 1963

Tryptophan

    metabolism, during sports activity (Pelikán and others) Cas. Lek. Cesk. 102:967-969, 1963

    metabolites, excretion after physical effort (Schmid) Nature 189:64-65, 1961

    -rich pre-albumin, urinary excretion after strenuous effort (Poortmans) Life Sci. 5:334-336, 1963

Tuberculosis

    experimental, effect of effort on course, guinea pigs (Neciuk-Szczerbinski) Gruzlica 31:889-900,
        1963

    intrapleurally induced, pathogenesis, effects of rest and exercise, guinea pigs (Burke and Mankiewicz) Amer.
        Rev. Resp. Dis. 88:360-375, 1963

    lungs, sedimentation rate during loads (Wiedemann) Tuberkulosearzt 4:465-470, 1950

    pulmonary, external respiration under controlled physical loading in (Vinnik and Filimonov) Probl.
        Tuberk. 42:27-34, 1964

    and rehabilitation, dynamic physical restoration (Chapman and others) Calif. Med. 100:88-91, 1964

    work capacity after lung resection (Baliuk) Probl. Tuberk. 41:40-43, 1963

Tumors

    Ehrlich, effect of dibazol and adaptation to muscular work and cold on animals with (Rusin) Vop. Onkol.
        9:60-66, 1963

    growth, effect of exercise, mouse (Rusch and Kline) Cancer Res. 4:116-118, 1944

    transplanted, influence of exercise on growth, rat (Hoffman and others) Cancer Res. 22:597-599, 1962

    see also Cancer; Sarcoma

Twins

    identical, sudden non-traumatic death associated with physical exertion (Jokl and Wolffe) Acta Genet. Med.
        3:245-246, 1954

U

Ulcer

    gastric, experimental, effect of regular muscular activity on development, rat (Frenkl and others) Acta
        Physiol. Acad. Sci. Hungary 22:203-208, 1962

Ultraviolet irradiation

    and physical working capacity of healthy children (Berven) Acta Paediat. Suppl. 148:1-22, 1963

Urea

    clearance and proteinuria, during exercise (Light and Warren) Amer. J. Physiol. 117:658-661, 1936

    excretion, effect of exercise, and physiology of fatigue (Haig) Lancet 1:610-615, 1896

    and food, relation to muscular exercise (Anstie) Practitioner 5:353-357, 1870

    relation to muscular exercise (Flint) Practitioner 6:250-253, 1871

Uric acid

    excretion, influence of muscular exercise (Nichols and others) J. Appl. Physiol. 3:501-507, 1951

    serum, rise during muscular exercise (Zachu-Christiansen) Scand. J. Clin. Lab. Invest. 11:57-60, 1959

Urine

Valvular

   cardiac performance, with constricted pulmonary artery during exercise, dogs (Rastelli and others) Circ. Res.
      13:410-419, 1963

   defects, venous, effect of exercise and body position on venous pressure at ankle (Pollack and others) J. Clin.
      Invest. 28:559-563, 1949

   heart disease, effect of exercise on venous admixture (Perkins and others) Amer. J. Cardiol. 10:52-56,
      1962

   heart disease, effect of muscular exercise upon peripheral circulation (Abramson and others) J. Clin. Invest.
      21:747-750, 1942

   lesions, cardiac, circulation during exercise, dogs (Barger and others) Amer. J. Physiol. 201:480-484, 1961

   lesions, cardiac, relation to auricular pressure, work tolerance and development of chronic congestive failure,
      dogs (Barger and others) Amer. J. Physiol. 169:384-399, 1952

   see also Aortic valvular lesions; Coarctation of aorta; Rheumatic heart disease

Vanillylmandelic acid

   excretion, in different forms of physical and emotional stress (Schmid) Verh. deutsch. Ges. inn. Med. 70:
      443-445, 1964

   urinary excretion during exercise (Klepping and others) Comptes Rend. Soc. Biol. 158:2007-2009, 1964

Varicose veins, see Veins

Vascular

   bed, skeletal muscle, effect of exercise (Kjellmer) Acta Physiol. Scand. 62:18-30, 1964

   bed, upper extremity, response to exercise, cold, levoarterenol angiotensin, hypertension, heart failure, and
      respiratory tract infection with fever (Kettel and others) J. Clin. Invest. 43:1561-1575, 1964

   disease, vasomotor responses to exercise in the extremities (Redisch and others) Circulation 19:579-582, 1959

   system, capacity, and stroke volume of heart, relation between (Sjöstrand) Acta Physiol. Scand. 42(Suppl. 145):
      126-127, 1957

   see also Blood vessels; Circulation, blood

Vasomotor response

   in arm during leg exercise (Blair and others) Circ. Res. 9:264-274, 1961

   to exercise in extremities in vascular disease (Redisch and others) Circulation 19:579-582, 1959

   in musculocutaneous area during muscular activity (Mitchell and others) Amer. J. Physiol. 205:37-40, 1963

Vasopressin

   and aldosterone, effect on distribution of water, sodium, and potassium, and on work performance, old
      rats (Friedberg and others) Gerontologia 7:65-76, 1963

Veins

   forearm, deep, origin of blood withdrawn from during rhythmic exercise (Idbohrn and Wahren) Acta
      Physiol. Scand. 61:301-313, 1964

   superficial and deep, lower limbs, static and dynamic pressures (Højensgard and Stürup) Acta Physiol. Scand.
      27:49-67, 1952

   varicose, cardiac output during exercise (Grimby and others) Scand. J. Clin. Lab Invest. 16:21-30, 1964

Ventilation (Cont.)

increased, afferent impulses as cause during muscular exercise (Harrison and others) Amer. J. Physiol. 100:68-73, 1932

lactic acid, pulse and electrocardiogram during ergospirometry (De Coster and others) Poumon Coeur 19: 633-639, 1963

maximal, in exhausting work, spirometric indices relation to maximal aerobic work, normal (Ghiringhelli and Bosisio) Riv. Med. Aero. 19:619-637, 1956

mechanism, during muscular exercise (Dejours and others) J. Physiologie 53:318-319, 1961

minute, influence of posture during exercise (McGregor and others) Circ. Res. 9:1089-1092, 1961

minute, oxigram, and expired air composition during effort of brief duration (Orlowska and Serzysko) Pol. Arch. Med. Wewnet. 33:801-805, 1963

muscular activity and respiratory function, relations between, healthy subjects, different ages (Berloco and others) Gior. Ital. Tuberc. 16:105-110, 1962

nervous regulation, components (Torelli and Brandi) J. Sport Med. 4:75-78, 1964; Boll. Soc. Ital. Biol. Sper. 36:1812-1814, 1960; Int. Zeits. angew. Physiol. 19:134-142, 1961; (Torelli and others) Boll. Soc. Ital. Biol. Sper. 39:1747-1750, 1750-1753, 1963

normal, during muscular exercise (Damoiseau and others) Arch. Int. Physiol. 69:310-326, 1961

oxygen breathing in heavy exercise, effect of (Asmussen and Nielsen) Acta Physiol. Scand. 43:365-378, 1958

and oxygen consumption after exercise, relation between (Barman and others) Amer. J. Physiol. 138:16-19, 1942

and pCO_2 of mixed venous blood, during exercise (Storey and Butler) J. Appl. Physiol. 18:345-348, 1963

and perfusion, regional distribution, factors affecting (Bryan and others) J. Appl. Physiol. 19:395-402, 1964

peripheral chemical control (Brassfield) Proc. Soc. Exp. Biol. Med. 26:833, 1929

psychophysiologic studies (Dudley and others) Psychosom. Med. 26:645-660, 1964

and pulmonary gas exchange in prolonged muscular exercise (Andrieu) Montpellier, Mari-Lavit, 1937

regulation (Haldane and Priestley) J. Physiol. 32:225-266, 1905; (Gray) Springfield, Charles C. Thomas, 1950; (Dejours) J. Physiologie 51:163-261, 1959; J. Physiologie 51:929-935, 1959; (Dejours) Lyon Méd. 91:1165-1169, 1959

regulation, during rest at high altitude (Dejours) Rev. Franç. Etud. Clin. Biol. 4:115-127, 1959

regulation, nervous and chemical, muscular work (Torelli and others) Boll. Soc. Ital. Biol. Sper. 39: 1747-1750, 1750-1753, 1963

resistance to air debt, influence of on, and on arterial oxygen saturation during muscular exercise (Namur) Arch. Int. Physiol. 68:608-617, 1960

respiratory minute volume during moderate exercise (Kumar) Indian J. Physiol. Pharmacol. 8:104-111, 1964

respiratory, multiple factor theory (Gray) Science 103:739-744, 1946

stimulus for increased, during muscular exertion (Barman and others) J. Clin. Invest. 22:53-56, 1943

Ventilation (Cont.)

    total, effects of by obstructing blood vessels and muscular effort (Delucchi) J. Aviation. Med. $\underline{14}$:23-27,

        1943

    variations during dynamic muscular exercise (Dejours and Teillac) Rev. Franç. Etud. Clin. Biol. $\underline{8}$:439-444, 1963

    ventilatory response to CO_2 during work, normal and low oxygen tensions (Asmussen and Nielsen) Acta Physiol.

        Scand. $\underline{39}$:27-35, 1957

    ventilatory response to exercise in chronic obstructive lung disease (Gandevia) Amer. Rev. Resp. Dis.

        $\underline{88}$:406-413, 1963

    ventilatory stimuli, autonomy of oxygen CO_2 and nervous (Dejours and others) J. Physologie $\underline{52}$:63-64,

        1960

    <u>see also</u> Alveolar air; Hyperventilation; Lungs; Pulmonary; Respiration

Ventricle

    heart performance, changes in left ventricular end-diastolic pressure and stroke work during infusion and

        following exercise (Gregg and others) Physiol. Rev. $\underline{35}$:130-136, 1955

    left, adaptation mechanism of, to muscular exercise (Mitchell) Pediatrics $\underline{32}$(Suppl.):660-670, 1963

    left, diameter, posture and exercise (Wilson) Circ. Res. $\underline{11}$:90-95, 1962

    left, function at rest and during exercise (Chapman and others) J. Clin. Invest. $\underline{38}$:1202-1213, 1959

    left, function, indirect measurement during exercise (Cumming and Edwards) Canad. Med. Ass. J. $\underline{89}$:

        219-221, 1963

    left heart, blood, quantity expelled (Tigerstedt) Scand. Arch. Physiol. $\underline{22}$:115-190, 1909

    left, hemodynamic determinants of rate of change in pressure during isometric contraction (Reeves and

        others) Amer. Heart J. $\underline{60}$:745-761, 1960

    minute-output time, effect of exercise (Cope) Amer. J. Physiol. $\underline{94}$:140-143, 1930

    responses to exertion, constancy of stroke volume (Rushmer) Amer. J. Physiol. $\underline{196}$:745-750, 1959

Ventricular conduction

    aberrant conduction in supraventricular extrasystoles eliminated by exercise (Boikan and Gunnar) Amer.

        Heart J. $\underline{47}$:626-629, 1954

    auriculoventricular, in the electrocardiogram after exercise (Giusti) Cuore Circ. $\underline{45}$:193-203, 1961

    right, ventricle, influence of muscular exercise on changes (Giusti) Cuore Circ. $\underline{44}$:89-102, 1960

Ventricular function

    contractions, premature, and exercise (Mann and Burchell) Proc. Staff Meet. Mayo Clin. $\underline{27}$:383-389, 1952

    'echoes' (Rosenblueth) Amer. J. Physiol. $\underline{195}$:53-60, 1958

    ejection, left, determinants of duration, in normal young men (Jones) J. Appl. Physiol. $\underline{19}$:279-283, 1964

    ejection rate, left, effect of exercise (Levine and others) J. Clin. Invest. $\underline{41}$:1050-1058, 1962

Ventricular rupture

    rupture by strenuous physical exertion (Guy and Wichowski) Amer. J. Surg. $\underline{85}$: 418-423, 1953

Vision

    expediting adaptation to darkness (Kekcheyev) Nature $\underline{151}$:617-618, 1943

Water

loss, evaporative, measurement by a thermal conductivity cell (Adams and others) J. Appl.
Physiol. 18:1291-1293, 1963

and salts, loss through skin, physiological adjustments (Hancock and others) Proc. Roy. Soc. 105B:
43-59, 1930

vapor loss, respiratory tract, during outdoor exercise (Brebbia and others) J. Appl. Physiol. 11:219-222,
1957; U. S. Army Tech. Rep. EP-57, 1957

work beneath, hygiene (Haldane) Ann. Hyg. Publ. 11:102-127, 1909

Weight, body

central nervous system, influence of exercise on albino rat (Donaldson) J. Comp. Neurol. 21:129-137, 1911

control, and exercise (Mayer) Postgrad. Med. 25:325-332, 1959

diet and activity, women (Taggart) British J. Nutrition 16:223-235, 1962

energy expenditure, influence on (Malhotra and others) J. Appl. Physiol. 17:433-435, 1962

exercise and excess fat (Wells and others) J. Ass. Phys. Ment. Rehab. 16:35-40, 1962

food intake and exercise, normal rats and genetically obese adult mice (Mayer and others) Amer. J. Physiol.
177:544-548, 1954

gain, and body composition, effect on performance in dog (Young) J. Appl. Physiol. 15:493-495, 1960

organ weights, effects of exercise, albino rat (Donaldson) Amer. J. Anat. 56:57-70, 1935

organ weights, effects of increased physical activity, mice (Class) Zeits. Anat. Entwicklungsgesch. 122:
251-265, 1961

reduction, effect on specific gravity and body fat, female adolescents (Goldman and others) Ann. N.Y.
Acad. Sci. 110:913-917, 1963

see also Obesity

Wheat germ oil

octacosanol, and vitamin E, effect on swimming performance, rats (Consolazio and others) J. Appl. Physiol.
19:265-267, 1964

Women

energy intake and expenditure of medical college women (Banerjee and Mahindra) J. Appl. Physiol. 17:
971-973, 1962

physical efficiency, effect of prescribed strenuous exercises (Walters) Res. Quart. 24:102-111, 1953

strenuous exercise, effect of (Ryde) J. Roy. Army Med. Corps 103:40-42, 1957

Work

adjustment of monkeys to five continuous days (Byck and Hearst) Science 138:43-44, 1962

aerobic capacity, special reference to age (Åstrand) Acta Physiol. Scand. 49(Suppl. 169):1-92, 1960

agricultural, and isometric contraction (Monod and Laville) Concours Med. 86:521-522, 1964

anaerobic, relationship between range of tissue temperature and local oxygen uptake in forearm, post-
exercise period (Abramson and others) J. Clin. Invest. 38:1126-1133, 1959

-"blood", autotransfusion, effect on pulmonary ventilation (Asmussen and Nielsen) Acta Physiol. Scand.
20:79-87, 1950

duration, effect on efficiency of muscular work (Crowden) J. Physiol. 80:394-408, 1934

Work (Cont.)

efficiency of underwater swimmers (Goff and others) J. Appl. Physiol. 10:197-202, 1957

equilibrium factor (Korotkoff) Concours Med. 85:5951-5954, 1963

and the heart (Rosenbaum) New York, Paul Hoeber 1959; (Acker) J. Tenn. Med. Ass. 56:46-48, 1963

heavy physical, short-term after-effects (Mark) Arbeitsphysiol. 2:129-147, 1930

heavy, regulation of respiration in (Asmussen and Nielsen) Acta Physiol. Scand. 12:171-188, 1946

load, and environment, physiological responses (Suggs and Splinter) J. Appl. Physiol. 16:413-420, 1961

load and work capacity, relation between (Bink) T: Soc. Geneesk. 41:698-701, 1963

maximal and submaximal, relationships between performance tests and physiological measures (Hodgson) Res. Quart. 17:208-224, 1946

mechanical, interrelation between diet and body condition and the energy production during, dog (Anderson and Lusk) Proc. Nat. Acad. Sci. 3:386-389, 1917

muscular, adaptation, metabolic consequences (Pařízková and Poupa) Brit. J. Nutr. 17:341-345, 1963

muscular, adenopathy (Chevallier) Rev. Med. Moyen Orient 18:7-10, 1961

muscular, aerobic, measurement of human capacity (Billings and others) J. Appl. Physiol. 15:1001-1006, 1960

muscular, ballistocardiogram after, quantitative evaluation of (Busnengo) Riv. Med. Aero. 23:385-396, 1960

muscular, biochemical basis (Konttinen) Duodecim 80:110-114, 1964

muscular, blood coagulation in (Casula and others) Gior. Clin. Med. 42:619-638, 1961

muscular, blood lactic acid during (Bang) Bibliot Laeger 128:106-110, 1936; Levin and Munksgaard, 1935

muscular, blood reaction in (Arborelius and Liljestrand) Skand. Arch. Physiol. 44:215, 1923

muscular, capacity, modification during formation and disorders of motor dynamic stereotype of varied complexity (Chebanova) Gig. Tr. Prof. Zabol.' 7:21-27, 1963

muscular, cardiac output during, and its regulation (Asmussen and Nielsen) Physiol. Rev. 35:778-800, 1955

muscular, casein hydrolyzate, ingested, influence on high energy nucleotide content of working muscle (Afar and Rogozkin) Canad. J. Biochem. Physiol. 41:1531-1536, 1963

muscular, circulatory and respiratory adaptation to severe (Åstrand and others) Acta Physiol. Scand. 50:254-258, 1960

muscular, duration and intensity, and free fatty acids in blood (Cerretelli and others) Boll. Soc. Ital. Biol. Sper. 37:1660-1662, 1961

muscular, economy (Gessler) Deutsch. Arch. klin. Med. 157:36-45, 1927

muscular, efficiency of mechanical power development during muscular shortening and its relation to load (Hill) Proc. Roy. Soc. 159:319-324, 1964

Work (Cont.)

muscular, stroke volume behaviour, and determination of arterial and venous CO_2 (Brandi and Soro)
Arch. Fisiol. 62:1-12, 1963

muscular, voluntary and electrically induced, comparison between (Krogh and Lindhard) J. Physiol. 51:
182-201, 1917

negative, physiological cost (Abbott and others) J. Physiol. 117:380-390, 1952

negative, rate of oxygen consumption, effects of force and speed changes (Abbott and Bigland) J. Physiol. 120:
319-325, 1953

performance, physiological changes during, porcelain factory, women (Okhrimenko) Gig. Tr. Prof. Zabol.
7:9-13, 1963

physical, as cause of lung emphysema (Podkaminsky) Arbeitsphysiol. 1:577-585, 1929

physical, automatic mechanochronometry (Gumener and others) Gig. Sanit. 29:58-62, 1964

physical test, reliability and validity of (Borg and Dahlström) Acta Physiol. Scand. 55:353-361, 1962

physiological and its equivalent (Chauveau) Paris, Quantin, 1888; Rev. Scient. 3rd series, 15:129-139, 1888

production, maximal (Fletcher) J. Appl. Physiol. 15:764-768, 1960

respiratory changes, initial, at transition from rest to work and work to rest (Asmussen and Nielsen) Acta
Physiol. Scand. 16:270-285, 1948

-rest cycle, human performance as a function (Ray and others) National Academy of Sciences - National
Research Council, Publication No. 882, 1961

speed of, influence on mechanical efficiency (Cathcart and others) J. Physiol. 58:355-361, 1924

static, observations (Monod) Paris, Thesis No. 721, Université Faculté de médecine, 1956

static, physiological researches into (Kektscheew) Arbeitsphysiol. 2:526-540, 1930

static, physiology (Dolgin) Arbeitsphysiol. 2:205-214, 1929

static, recovery pause, determination (Rohmert) Int. Zeits. angew. Physiol. 18:123-164; 191-212, 1960

submaximal and maximal, cardiac output during (Åstrand and others) J. Appl. Physiol. 19:268-274, 1964

submaximal, nomogram for calculation of aerobic capacity from pulse rate during (Åstrand and Rhyming)
J. Appl. Physiol. 7:218-221, 1954

time, and rest time (Lammers) T. Soc. Geneesk. 41:631-633; 625-626, 1963

time and rest time, social aspects (Dop) T. Soc. Geneesk. 41:626-628, 1963

work power (Blix) Scand. Arch. Physiol. 15:122-146, 1904

Work performance, see Capacity, physical working

Workers

50-64 years old, physical work capacity (Åstrand) Acta Physiol. Scand. 42:73-87, 1958

manual, 50-64 years old, at rest and work, clinical and physiological studies (Åstrand) Acta Med. Scand. 162:
155-164, 1958

see also Longshoremen; Lumber workers; Miners and other individual headings

Wound healing

    effect of exercise, rats (Newburger) Surgery 13:692-695, 1943

X

X-rays, see Radiation